Toxoplasmosis

A comprehensive clinical guide

This authoritative and comprehensive account looks at the re-emergence of toxoplasmosis as a significant and potentially fatal infection. A team of acknowledged international experts reviews the latest diagnostic techniques, and the management of infection in pregnant women, neonates, the eye, transplant and other immunosuppressed patients and those with acquired immuno-deficiency syndrome (AIDS). The contentious issue of the role of screening during pregnancy and in the newborn is covered in depth. The introductory chapters on biology, immunology and epidemiology of the infection provide an essential background to understanding the clinical disease. The full range of treatment strategies is presented in an easily accessible form.

Although the burden of this disease varies greatly from country to country, it remains a global public health problem which affects about one billion individuals. The natural history and life-cycle of the causative organism, *Toxoplasma gondii*, provide a fascinating insight into one of the most successful parasites on Earth.

This will be an essential source of reference for infectious disease specialists, microbiologists, parasitologists and obstetricians and gynaecologists.

David H. M. Joynson is Consultant in Medical Microbiology and Director of the Toxoplasma Reference Unit, Public Health Laboratory Service at Singleton Hospital, Swansea.

Tim G. Wreghitt is Deputy Director of the Public Health and Clinical Microbiology Laboratory at Addenbrooke's Hospital, Cambridge.

Toxoplasmosis

A comprehensive clinical guide

Edited by

David H. M. Joynson

and

Tim G. Wreghitt

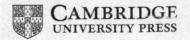

CAMBRIDGE UNIVERSITY PRESS
Cambridge, New York, Melbourne, Madrid, Cape Town, Singapore, São Paulo

Cambridge University Press
The Edinburgh Building, Cambridge CB2 2RU, UK

Published in the United States of America by Cambridge University Press, New York

www.cambridge.org
Information on this title: www.cambridge.org/9780521443289

© Cambridge University Press 2001

First published 2001
This digitally printed first paperback version 2005

A catalogue record for this publication is available from the British Library

Library of Congress Cataloguing in Publication data

Toxoplasmosis : a comprehensive clinical guide / edited by David H. M. Joynson and
Tim G. Wreghitt.
    p. ;   cm.
  Includes bibliographical references and index.
  ISBN 0 521 44328 8 (hb)
    1. Toxoplasmosis. I. Joynson, David H. M. (Huw Malcolm), 1943 – II. Wreghitt, T. G.
    [DNLM: 1. Toxoplasmosis. WC 725 T7551 2001]
  RC186.T75 T686 2001
  616.9´36–dc21   2001025511

ISBN-13 978-0-521-44328-9 hardback
ISBN-10 0-521-44328-8 hardback

ISBN-13 978-0-521-01942-2 paperback
ISBN-10 0-521-01942-7 paperback

Contents

Contributors

D. Buxton
Animal Diseases Research Association,
Moredun Research Institute,
408 Gilmerton Road,
Edinburgh,
Scotland

J. Couvreur
Institute de Puériculture de Paris,
ADHMI,
Laboratoire de Serologie et de Recherche sur
la Toxoplasmose,
26 Boulevard Brune,
Paris,
France

J. P. Dubey
U.S. Department of Agriculture,
Zoonotic Disease Laboratory,
Beltsville MD,
USA

G. N. Dutton
Tennet Institute of Ophthalmology,
Gart Naval General Hospital,
1053 Great Western Road,
Glasgow,
Scotland

R. B. Eaton
Newborn Toxoplasmosis Screening Program,
State Laboratory Institute,
305 South Street,
Jamaica Plain,
MA,
USA

J. L. Fishback
School of Medicine,
Department of Pathology & Oncology,
The University of Kansas Medical Center,
3901 Rainbow,
Boulevard,
Kansas City,
USA

J. K. Frenkel
1252 Vallecita Drive,
Santa Fe,
NM,
USA

R. E. Gilbert
Department of Paediatric Epidemiology,
Institute of Child Health,
University of London,
30 Guildford Street,
London, UK

G. F. Grady
Newborn Toxoplasmosis Screening Program
State Laboratory Institute,
305 South Street,
Jamaica Plain,
MA,
USA

E. C. Guy
Toxoplasma Reference Unit,
Public Health Laboratory,
Singleton Hospital,
Swansea,
Wales

S. Hall
Storrs House Farm,
Storrs Lane,
Sheffield, UK

D. O. Ho-Yen
Toxoplasma Reference Laboratory,
Raigmore Hospital,
Inverness,
Scotland

H.-W. Hsu
Newborn Toxoplasmosis Screening Program,
State Laboratory Institute,
305 South Street,
Jamaica Plain,
MA,
USA

C. A. Hunter
Department of Pathobiology,
University of Pennsylvania,
3800 Spruce St,
Philadelphia,
USA

D. H. M. Joynson
Toxoplasma Reference Unit,
Public Health Laboratory,
Singleton Hospital,
Swansea,
Wales

R. Lynfield
Newborn Toxoplasmosis Screening Program,
State Laboratory Institute,
305 South Street,
Jamaica Plain,
MA,
USA

P. Mariuz
Infectious Disease Unit,
Department of Medicine,
University of Rochester,
School of Medicine and Dentistry,
Rochester NY,
USA

R. E. McCabe
School of Medicine,
Department of Internal Medicine,
University of California,
Davis Veterans Administrative Medical
Centre (612/111),
150 Muir Road,
Martinez,
California,
USA

C. S. Peckham
Department of Paediatric Epidemiology,
Institute of Child Health,
University of London,
30 Guildford Street,
London, UK

E. Petersen
Laboratory of Parasitology,
Division of Biotechnology,
Statens Seruminstitut,
Artillerivej 5,
Copenhagen 5,
Denmark

G. Reichmann
Institute for Medical Microbiology and
Virology,
Heinrich-Heine University,
Dusseldorf,
Germany

M. Ryan
Communicable Disease Surveillance Centre,
61 Colindale Avenue,
London, UK

R. T. Steigbigel
Division of Infectious Diseases,
Health Science Centre,
SUNY Stony Brook,
Stony Brook NY,
USA

P. Thulliez
Institute de Puériculture de Paris,
ADHMI,
Laboratoire de Serologie et de Recherche sur
la Toxoplasmose,
26 Boulevard Brune,
75014 Paris,
France

T. G. Wreghitt
Clinical Microbiology and Public
Health Laboratory,
Addenbrooke's Hospital,
Hills Road,
Cambridge, UK

Preface

Exactly one hundred years ago, the first description of *Toxoplasma gondii* was recorded but a further 60 years were to elapse before the final identification of the cat family as the definitive host was made. The heteroxenous nature of the parasite, its ability to infect any warm-blooded creature, the territorial range of its hosts (especially birds) and the production of tissue cysts that can survive for many years have contributed to the world-wide dissemination of the infection. Indeed, it is reasonable to conclude that perhaps *T.gondii* is one of the most successful parasites on Earth. About one billion people throughout the world are infected though the prevalence of infection shows consideration geographical variation.

Transmission of infection is by ingestion of either oocysts as a result of environmental contamination or tissue cysts in raw or undercooked meat. It is probable that the favoured route of transmission varies in different parts of the world – the epidemiology of the infection is still not completely known. It is also possible that other vectors, for example water and aerosols, may be involved.

Toxoplasma infection can be acute, chronic, latent/quiescent or re-activated, while the clinical presentation, investigation and management can vary according to the specific patient group involved. Infection in the immunocompetent, though very common, is generally regarded as a trivial event though there are suggestions that it may in fact be a more debilitating illness than was previously supposed.

It has been known since the first quarter of the last century that toxoplasma can cause a devastating congenital infection but this was thought to be a relatively infrequent occurrence. However, there is now an increasing awareness that the effects of foetal infection are protean and may first present years or decades after birth. To try to reduce the risk of congenital infection, some countries have introduced prenatal or newborn screening. In other countries, the debate regarding the cost-benefit of screening is often controversial yet inconclusive due to lack of data and the failure to fund appropriate studies to address the issue.

The end of the twentieth century has witnessed a significant increase in the number of immunosuppressed and immunocompromised patients. This has occurred in the main as a corollary to advances in medical treatment and to the advent of HIV infection and AIDS. Consequently, *T.gondii* has re-emerged as a significant cause of morbidity and mortality. This has spurred research and given new insights into the pathogenesis and immunology of the infection. These have revealed subtle inter-reactions with, for example, the host's immune system and HIV. This work may eventually lead to the development of an effective vaccine.

Fifty years ago, the diagnosis of toxoplasma infection took a huge step forward with the introduction of the Sabin and Feldman Dye Test. Remarkably, this has stood the test of time and is still regarded as the 'gold standard". However, it is unwise to rely solely on one laboratory test. It is now usual practice to choose from a range of serological tests and methods of detection of the parasite by culture, nucleic acid detection or specific stains according to the specific patient group being investigated and the clinical questions that need to be addressed. Despite the plethora of tests now available, clinical acumen and awareness are still paramount.

Sadly, the mainstay of treatment is still a combination of ancient antibiotics that are not effective against the tissue cyst and can be both toxic and teratogenic. The apparent lack of interest in the pharmaceutical industry to develop new chemo-therapeutic agents is to be regretted. A safe antibiotic that is effective against all forms of the parasite and crosses the placental and brain barriers is urgently required. The availability of such a drug and the prospect of a genuine cure would undoubtedly transform attitudes towards the infection.

Toxoplasma gondii has developed a complex biological relationship with humans. The manifestations of the infection that it causes are protean, unpredict-able and subtle and can be difficult to diagnose, treat and prevent. The key factor in solving such problems is understanding based on knowledge and evidence. Thus, contributions have been invited from experts from a variety of scientific, epi-demiological and medical fields so that a greater understanding of the disease as a whole is attained. The purpose of this book, therefore, is to be an easily accessible resource of information to clinicians, epidemiologists, microbiologists, midwives and nurses and others involved in caring for patients who are at risk or suffering from toxoplasmosis. It is hoped that this aim has been achieved.

D.H.M.J.

Historical perspective

1900	Laveran – detected the organism in the blood of a bobolink, a common American songbird.
1908	Nicholle & Manceaux – observed the causative agent in an African rodent *Ctenodactylus gondii* and gave it the name *Toxoplasma gondii*. '*Toxon*' the Greek word for bow or arc and '*plasma*' meaning form.
1908	Splendore – found the parasite in a rabbit.
1923	Janku – reported the first case of chorioretinitis in a child, found parasites in the eye and called them 'sporozoa'.
1928	Levaditi – identified these 'sporozoa' as *Toxoplasma gondii*.
1938	Wolf & Cowan – identified toxoplasma as the cause of neonatal encephalitis: the first report of congenital transmission of *T. gondii*.
1940	Pinkerton & Weinman – reported a fatal case of disseminated toxoplasmosis in an adult.
1941	Sabin – described a triad of signs (retinochoroiditis, hydrocephalus and cerebral calcification) in an infant with congenital toxoplasmosis.
1948	Sabin & Feldman – development of the dye test, still the 'gold standard' half a century later.
1952	Slim – description of the 'glandular' form of acquired toxoplasma infection.
1954	Jacobs *et al.* – isolation of *T. gondii* from the eye of a patient with chorioretinitis.
1954	Weinman & Chandler – suggested that transmission of toxoplasma may be related to eating undercooked pork.
1960	Jacobs, Remington *et al.* – demonstration that tissue cysts were resistant to proteolytic enzymes.
1965, 1969	Hutchinson – discovered *T. gondii* in feline faeces and recognized that the cat was the definitive host.

1969   Wallace – an epidemiological study of the population of some
            Pacific islands indicated the importance of the cat in the
            transmission of infection to humans.

1970   Dubey, Millar & Frenkel – the finding of sexual stages and the
            oocyst in the small intestine of the cat clarified the lifecycle of
            toxoplasma and indicated that it was a coccidian parasite.

1970s   Increasing awareness of the risk to the foetus as a consequence of an
            acute toxoplasma infection in a pregnant woman.

1980s   Emergence of *T. gondii* as a life-threatening infection in
            immunocompromised patients especially those with AIDS.

Biology of toxoplasmosis

E. Petersen[1] and J. P. Dubey[2]

[1] Statens Seruminstitut, Copenhagen, Denmark
[2] U.S. Department of Agriculture, Beltsville, USA

History

Toxoplasma gondii is a coccidium, with the domestic cat and other felids as its definitive host and a wide range of birds and mammals as intermediate hosts. It was first detected by Nicolle and Manceaux (1908, 1909) in a rodent *Ctenodactylus gondi*, and by Splendore (1908) in a rabbit. The name *Toxoplasma* is derived from the crescent shape of the tachyzoite (in Greek: toxo = arc, plasma = form). Knowledge of the full lifecycle of *T. gondii* was not completed until 1970, when the sexual phase of the lifecycle was identified in the intestine of the cat, by demonstrating oocysts in cat faeces and characterizing them biologically and morphologically (Dubey et al. 1970*a*, *b*).

Taxonomy

Toxoplasma gondii is placed in the phylum Apicomplexa (Levine 1970), class Sporozoasida (Leukart 1879), subclass Coccidiasina (Leukart 1879). Traditionally, all coccidia until 1970 were classified in the family Eimeriidae. After the discovery of the coccidian cycle of *T. gondii* in 1970, *T. gondii* has been placed by different authorities in the families Eimeriidae, Sarcocystidae or Toxoplasmatidae. Phylogenetic analysis of *T. gondii* and order Apicomplexa is shown in Figure 1.1.

Lifecycle

The definitive host is the domestic cat and other Felidae (Frenkel et al. 1970; Jewell et al. 1972), where the sexual cycle takes place in the intestinal epithelial cells. Infected cats excrete oocysts which are infectious to virtually all warm-blooded animals. There are three infectious stages of the parasite: the tachyzoite (the rapidly dividing form) in tissues, the bradyzoite (the slowly dividing form) inside cysts in tissues and the sporozoites in the oocyst in cat faeces (Figure 1.2).

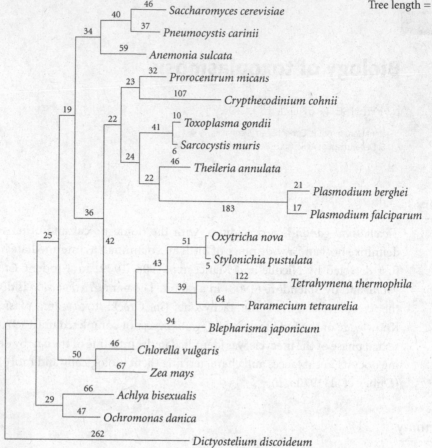

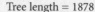

Figure 1.1   Phylogenetic analysis of *Toxoplasma gondii* and other Apicomplexa. Numbers represent character changes between organisms on the branch of the tree. The tree length represents the overall change of characters that result in the most parsimonious tree obtained. (From Gagnon, S., Levesque, R. C., Sogin, M. L., & Gajadhar, A. A. (1993). Molecular cloning, complete sequence of the small subunit ribosomal RNA coding region and phylogeny of *Toxoplasma gondii*. *Molecular and Biochemical Parasitology*, **60**, 145–8. With permission from the authors and the publisher.)

The enteroepithelial cycle in the definitive host – the cat

Five morphologically distinct asexual stages (types A–E) of *T. gondii* develop in enterocytes before gametogony begins (Dubey & Frenkel 1972). The origin of the gametes has not been finally established, but it is believed that merozoites (stages D and E) develop into gametes. Gametes occur throughout the small intestine, but are most prevalent in the ileum, where they are found 3–15 days after infection.

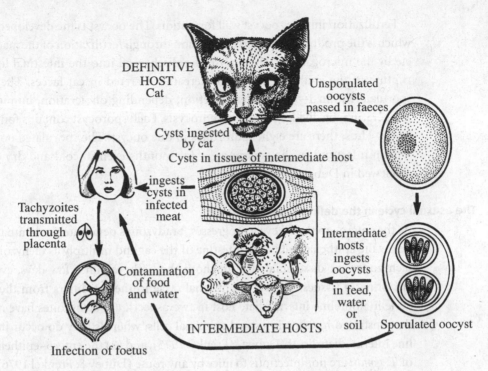

Figure 1.2 Lifecycle of *Toxoplasma gondii*.

The microgamete (the male gamete) is biflagellate and fertilizes the macrogamete (the female gamete) within the enterocyte. Oocysts are formed when a wall is laid around the fertilized gamete (zygote). Oocysts are expelled into the intestinal lumen after the rupture of enterocytes and are unsporulated when excreted in faeces.

The prepatent period (interval between ingestion and shedding of oocysts) after the ingestion of tissue cysts is 3–10 days, with peak oocyst production between 5 and 8 days after a patent period varying from 7 to 20 days (Dubey & Frenkel 1972, 1976). Cats not previously infected with *T. gondii* shed oocysts after ingesting each of the infective stages of the parasite: the tachyzoite, the bradyzoite and the sporozoite (Frenkel et al. 1970; Dubey & Frenkel 1976). The prepatent period varies according to the stage of *T. gondii* with which the cat is infected, with a short (3–10 days) prepatent period when the oral inoculum contains bradyzoites and a long prepatent period (>13 days) when the inoculum contains tachyzoites (Dubey 1998b) or sporozoites (Freyre et al. 1989; Dubey 1996). Cats previously infected with *T. gondii*, and which produced oocysts during the previous infection, are generally immune to renewed oocyst shedding, but immunity is not life long (Dubey & Frenkel 1974; Frenkel & Smith 1982; Dubey 1995).

Fertilization initiates oocyst wall formation. The oocyst is the developed zygote, which is the product of sexual reproduction through fertilization of the macrogamete by the microgamete. The oocysts are discharged into the intestinal lumen by rupture of the epithelial cells, and thereafter excreted in cat faeces. The oocysts sporulate within 1–5 days after excretion, depending on aeration, humidity and temperature, by dividing into two sporocysts. Each sporocyst contains four sporozoites. Thus, there are eight sporozoites in one oocyst. The sporulated oocyst can remain infectious in the environment for months even in cold and dry climates (reviewed in Dubey 1977).

The asexual cycle in the definitive host – the cat

As the entero–epithelial cycle progresses, bradyzoites penetrate the lamina propria below the epithelial cell in the intestine of the cat and multiply as tachyzoites. The tachyzoites are disseminated throughout the body within a few days, eventually encysting in tissues. The extra-intestinal cycle in the cat differs from the similar cycle in nonfeline intermediate host in two aspects: (1) tachyzoites have not been demonstrated in feline intestinal epithelial cells, whereas they do occur in nonfeline intermediate hosts (Dubey & Frenkel 1973), and (2) the entero–epithelial types of *T. gondii* are noninfectious to mice by any route (Dubey & Frenkel 1976), which suggests that the feline entero–epithelial forms do not give rise to tachyzoites.

Intermediate host

Toxoplasma gondii tachyzoites are disseminated throughout the body of the intermediate host in macrophages and lymphocytes as well as free in the plasma. Tachyzoites continue to divide within the host cell by endodyogeny (internal division into two) until the host cell is filled with parasites. At a given time the dividing tachyzoites cannot be contained within the host cell, which bursts. The tachyzoites are released and seek new host cells to repeat the process. Depending on the strain of *T. gondii* and the host resistance, tachyzoites may be found for days or even months after acute infection. For example, tachyzoites persist in foetal membranes for weeks after infection of the mother or the dam, and are nearly always present in placentas of mothers at the time of parturition, if the foetus was infected *in utero*.

At some time after infection the tachyzoites transform to bradyzoites in tissue cysts. The signals responsible for the transformation are not known, and the debate continues as to whether signals from the host immune system are needed. Bradyzoites also divide by endodyogeny. Bradyzoites are enclosed in a thin cyst wall. Tissue cysts may be found as early as 3 days after infection but are usually not numerous until 7 weeks after infection (Dubey & Frenkel 1976; Derouin & Garin 1991; Dubey et al. 1998). Intact tissue cysts probably do not cause any inflammation and may persist for life. It has been suggested that tissue cysts may switch from the bradyzoite stage to the tachyzoite stage during the life of the tissue cysts, producing new tachyzoites which may give rise to new tissue cysts thus ensuring a prolonged infective stage (Hérion & Saavedra 1993). If the intermediate host is eaten by another warm-blooded animal, tissue cysts are able to infect a new host.

Fewer than 50% of cats shed oocysts after ingesting tachyzoites or oocysts, whereas almost all cats shed oocysts after ingesting tissue cysts (Dubey & Frenkel 1976). Cats infected with oocysts and tachyzoites probably give rise to bradyzoites, which after a variable period of time may disseminate to the intestinal mucosa and start the entero–epithelial cycle with the resulting production of oocysts (Freyre et al. 1989). For comparison, the lifecycles of major coccidian genera are shown in a simplified form in Figure 1.3.

Morphology, ultrastucture and antigens

The tachyzoite

The tachyzoite (previously called trophozoite) is crescent shaped and is approximately 2×6 µm in size (Figure 1.4). The tachyzoite has a pellicle, subpellicular microtubules, a polar ring, a conoid, rhoptries, micronemes, mitochondria, endoplasmatic reticulum, Golgi apparatus, ribosomes, rough surface endoplasmatic reticulum, micropores and a well-defined nucleus (Figure 1.5).

The nucleus is situated in the central or posterior part of the cell (Sheffield & Melton 1968). The pellicle consists of three membranes. The inner membrane is discontinuous in three areas: at the polar ring (anterior), at the micropore (lateral) and towards the posterior end. The polar ring is an osmiophilic thickening of the inner membrane at the anterior end of the tachyzoite. The polar ring encircles the conoid, a cylindrical cone which consist of six to eight fibrillar elements arranged like a compressed spring. The 22 subpellicular microtubules originate from the polar ring and run longitudinally for almost the entire length of the cell (Sulzer et al. 1974) and probably provide a frame for the parasite.

The rhoptries are four to ten club-shaped, gland-like structures with an anterior narrow neck and posterior-sac-like end reaching as far as the nucleus. The rhoptries contain a honey-combed structure and are thought to have a secretory function associated with host cell penetration. When the parasite has attached to the host cell, the contents of the rhoptries are discharged through the conoid (Nichols et al. 1983). The micronemes are rice-grain-like structures, usually fewer than 100 in number, situated at the conoidal end of *T. gondii* without any defined function, but they may participate in invasion of the host cell (Joiner & Dubremetz 1993). In addition to the rhoptries and the micronemes, the parasite contains dense granules which also appear to have a secretory function (Charif et al. 1990).

SIMPLIFIED LIFE-CYCLES OF MAJOR COCCIDIAN GENERA

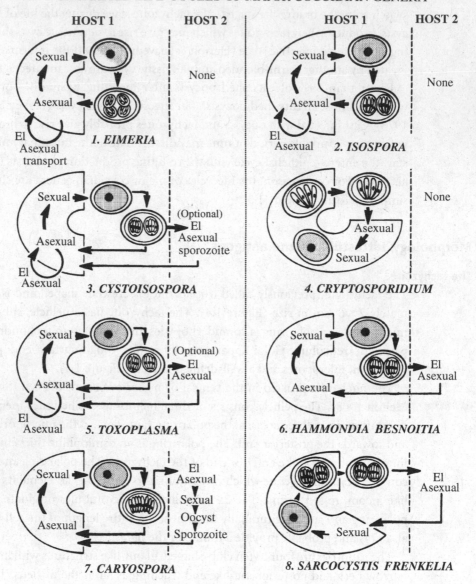

Figure 1.3   Simplified lifecycles of major coccidian genera. For each genus, a diagrammatic
representation of the intestinal tract appears on the left of the dotted line, under 'HOST 1'
(the definitive host), where oocyst morphology is also shown. On the right, under 'HOST
2', the extraintestinal stages that develop in the intermediate host are listed in order of
development. (From Fayer, R. & Dubey, J. P. (1987). *Int J Parasitol*, **17**, 615. With
permission.)

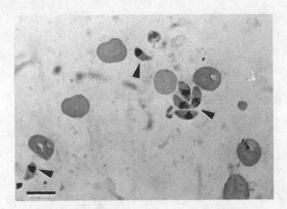

Figure 1.4   *Toxoplasma gondii* tachyzoites (arrowheads) in smear. Mouse peritoneum. Giemsa stain. ×750. Bar = 10 μm.

The functions of the conoid, rhoptries and micronemes are not fully known. The conoid can rotate, extend and retract and is important when the parasite searches for an attachment site at the host cell, as the parasite can rotate, glide and twist. Myosin has been found in the apical end of the parasite (Schwartzman & Pfefferkorn 1983), and actin has been found both at the apical end and distributed throughout the cytoplasm (Endo et al. 1988). The motion observed during parasite entry corresponds to the orientation of the subpellicular microtubules, and it is likely that the microtubules are the basis of the motility system. The microphores are sites specialized for the uptake of nutrients through endocytosis (Nichols et al. 1994).

After entry into the host cell, the parasite is surrounded by a parasitophorous vacuole membrane (PVM). The PVM contains numerous intravacuolar tubules (Sheffield & Melton 1968; Sibley et al. 1985; Sibley & Krahenbuhl 1988; Sibley et al. 1995; Dubey et al. 1998). The intravacuolar tubules appear to be connected to the parasite plasmalemma and consist of host cell vimentin-type intermediate filaments (Halonen & Weidner 1994). *Toxoplasma gondii* enters the host cell by active invasion (Werk 1985).

Endodyogeny is a process in which two progeny form within *T. gondii*, and consume it from within (Sheffield & Melton 1968). The Golgi apparatus divides first, and the anterior cell membranes of the progeny are formed at the anterior end. The nucleus of the parent cell becomes horseshoe-shaped, and part of the nucleus moves towards the anterior end of the developing cells. The nuclear membranes remain intact and the chromosomes do not condense at metaphase. The progeny move towards the cell membrane of the parent parasite as they continue to grow,

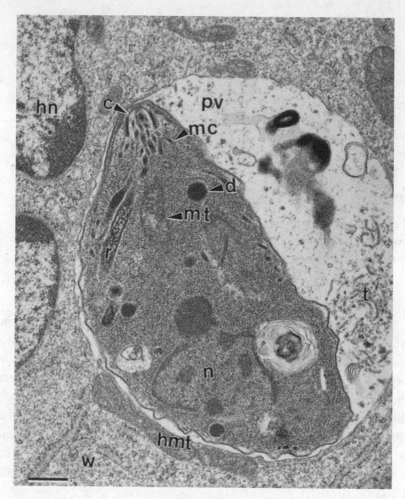

Figure 1.5   Electron micrograph of a *T. gondii* tachyzoite in the parasitophorous vacuole (pv) in the cytoplasm of a human foreskin fibroblast, second day *in vitro* culture after inoculation with GT-1 strain tachyzoites. Note the conoid (c), micronemes (mc), rhoptries (r), dense granules (d), mitochondrion (mt), nucleus (n) in the tachyzoite and numerous intravacuolar tubules (t) inside the parasitophorous vacuole (pv). hmt refers to host cell mitochondrion and hn is host cell nucleus. ×28,300. Bar = 0.35 μm (Courtesy of Dr D. S. Lindsay, Auburn University, Alabama, USA.)

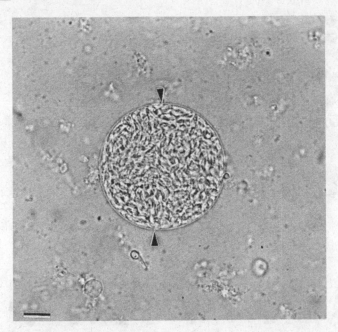

Figure 1.6   *Toxoplasma gondii* tissue cyst in the saline homogenate of
mouse brain. Note the thin cyst wall (arrowheads) enclosing
hundreds of bradyzoites. Unstained ×750. Bar = 10 μm.

and finally the inner membrane of the parent parasite disappears and the outer
membrane fuses with the inner membrane of the progeny, and two new tachyzoites
are formed.

The bradyzoite and tissue cysts

The bradyzoite (brady = slow) is the organism dividing slowly within a tissue cyst
(Frenkel 1973) and is a synonym of cystozoite. A tissue cyst is a collection of bradyzoites surrounded by a well-defined host cell membrane (Figures 1.6, 1.7). The
bradyzoites also multiply by endodyogeny. Tissue cysts are from 5 μm to 60 μm in
size in the brain and 100 μm in other tissues (Dubey 1993) and contain four to
several hundred bradyzoites. Tissue cysts may develop in any tissue but are most
prevalent in neural and muscular organs such as the eye and brain, skeletal and
cardiac muscles (Figure 1.8). The cyst wall is thin (<0.5 μm). The tissue cyst develops in the host cell cytoplasm and its wall is intimately associated with the host cell
endoplasmic reticulum (ER); indeed the cyst wall is partly of host origin (Ferguson
& Hutchison 1987 a,b; Sims et al. 1988). Mature cyst walls are lined with a granular
material which is also found between the bradyzoites (Figure 1.9). In older
cysts, degenerating bradyzoites may occasionally be found (Pavesio et al. 1992). The

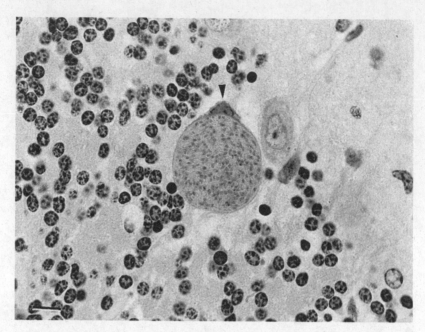

Figure 1.7   Intracellular *T. gondii* tissue cyst in a section of mouse cerebellum. Note the host cell nucleus (arrowhead). Haematoxylin and eosin stain. ×750. Bar= 10 μm.

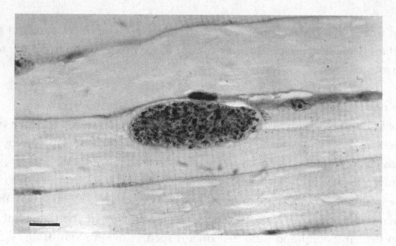

Figure 1.8   *Toxoplasma gondii* tissue cyst in a section of mouse skeletal muscle. Note the cyst is elongated and contains dark-staining polysaccharide granules in bradyzoites. Periodic acid Schiff haematoxylin. ×750. Bar= 10 μm.

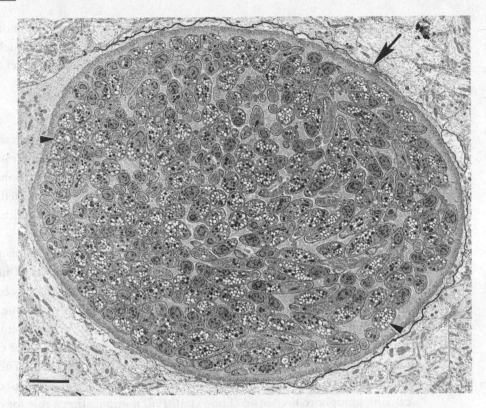

Figure 1.9   Electron micrograph of a well-developed tissue cyst in the brain of a mouse, 1 year after inoculation with *T. gondii*. The cyst is located in a neuron (arrow). The vacuolated areas (arrowheads) in bradyzoites are polysaccharide granules. ×3000. Bar = 3.3 μm. (Courtesy of Dr D. J. P. Ferguson, Oxford University, UK.)

bradyzoites are slender and measure approximately 7 μm × 1.5 μm (Mehlhorn & Frenkel 1980).

Bradyzoites differ only slightly from the tachyzoites. They are more slender than tachyzoites and their nucleus is located more to the posterior end compared to the tachyzoites. The contents of the rhoptries of bradyzoites are electron dense in older cysts (Ferguson and Hutchison 1987a; Dubey & Fenner 1993). Bradyzoites contain several glycogen granules which stain red with the PAS (periodic acid Schiff) reagent, and such granules are few in tachyzoites. Bradyzoites are less susceptible to destruction by proteolytic enzymes than are tachyzoites; tachyzoites are usually killed by acid-pepsin immediately whereas bradyzoites survive for at least two hours (Jacobs et al. 1960; Dubey 1998a). The prepatent period in cats following infection by bradyzoites is shorter (3–10 days) than following infection with tachyzoites (13 days or more) (Dubey & Frenkel 1976; Dubey 1998a). The transition from tachyzoites to bradyzoites can be observed *in vitro* by specific monoclonal antibody surface markers, and occurs through an intermediate stage which usually expresses both exclusive tachyzoite and bradyzoite antigens (Tomavo et al. 1991; Bohne et al. 1992; Soete et al. 1993).

Tissue cyst formation and cyst rupture

The factors that influence tissue cyst formation and all signals for differentiation between different stages are not well known in detail. The transition from tachyzoite to bradyzoite is followed by a shift in stage-specific antigens (Bohne et al. 1993; Gross et al. 1996). Nitric oxide production by *T.-gondii*-infected macrophages seems to be an important mediator in reducing parasite multiplication and the initiation of bradyzoite formation (Bohne et al. 1994).

Tissue cysts are more numerous in animals at the chronic stage of infection with developed immunity, compared to animals in the acute stage of infection, but tissue cysts have been found in mice infected for only 3 days (Dubey & Frenkel 1976), and in tissue cell culture systems not influenced by any immune mechanism (Lindsay et al. 1991, 1993). Therefore, the role of the developing immune response in the formation of tissue cysts remains undecided. The tissue cyst contains both host-derived and *T. gondii* antigens (Sims et al. 1988). The factors determining tissue cyst rupture are unknown. Parasites can be released by the calcium ionophore monensin (Endo et al. 1982), implicating a role for calcium, and permeabilizing the host cell membrane also results in the immediate release of parasites. One theory is that the tissue cysts rupture from time to time and the released bradyzoites are destroyed by the host's immune response or give rise to new cysts or tachyzoites, depending on the immune status of the host. Chronic infection can be reactivated reliably in rodents after exogenous hypercorticism and by stimulating, depleting or interfering with cytokine production (Gazzinelli et al. 1993).

Entero–epithelial stages

The gametes contain the microgamete (the male gamete) and the macrogamete (the female gamete). The oocyst is the developed zygote, which is the product of sexual reproduction through fertilization of the macrogamete by the microgamete. The oocyst is surrounded by a two-layer wall. When excreted in cat faeces, the oocyst contains a sporont, which sporulates within 24–72 hours after excretion by dividing into two round masses called sporoblasts. The sporoblasts elongate and mature into sporocysts, and within each sporocyst four sporozoites develop. Thus, the sporulated oocysts contain eight sporozoites (Dubey et al. 1998).

Five morphologically distinct stages (types) of *T. gondii* develop in intestinal epithelial cells before gametogony begins (Dubey & Frenkel 1972). The types have been called A–E, and each type may exist for several generations before developing into the next stage. When the bradyzoites enter epithelial cells of the proximal part of the small intestine, they lose their PAS-positive granules and divide into two or three organisms: i.e. they become type A parasites. Type A parasites are the smallest of the five asexual intestinal types, and occur as collections of two or three organisms in surface epithelial cells in the jejunum 12–18 hours after infection. Type B organisms are found 12–54 hours after infection and probably divide by endodyogeny and endopolygeny. The type B parasites are characterized by a centrally located nucleus and a prominent nucleolus. Undivided and dividing organisms can occur in the same vacuole, but the undivided organisms stain more darkly than the divided ones. Uncharacteristically, host cells infected with type B parasites are often found in the lamina propria.

Type C merozoites are elongated and have subterminal nuclei and a strongly PAS-positive cytoplasm. They occur 24–54 hours after infection and divide by merogony leaving a residual body. The ultrastructure of types A, B and C parasites has not been described.

Type D merozoites are smaller than type C and contain only a few PAS-positive granules. They are found from 32 hours postinfection and until the cat starts shedding oocysts. It has been proposed that type D parasites divide by merogony (schizogony) (Dubey et al. 1998) and not endopolygeny (Piekarski et al. 1971), but merogony probably also occurs. There is no residual body after division.

Type E parasites resemble type D parasites and probably divide by merogony, but leave a residual body after division. Type E parasites are found 3–15 days after initial infection with tissue cysts. Only late stage parasites (presumably type D) have been studied by electron microscopy. The nucleus divides without any immediate cytoplasmatic division (Sheffield 1970; Ferguson et al. 1974). With repeating nuclear divisions, merozoite formation starts with the development of an anterior membrane complex near the nucleus. Immature merozoites are formed when the new nuclei are included in the newly formed anterior membrane complex. The immature merozoites lie near the outer membrane of the mature meront. The outer membrane invaginates around each merozoite, and the now mature merozoites are released from the meront resulting in host cell death.

Types D or E merozoites released from types D or E parasites undergo gametogony. The gametes are found 3–15 days after infection in the ileum where they are located between the host cell nucleus and the brush border of the host epithelial cell, and are most numerous in cells at the tip of the villi.

The macrogamete (the female gamete) is subspherical and contains a single centrally located nucleus and several PAS-positive granules. Examination of the ultrastructure reveals several micropores, rough and smooth ER, numerous mitochondria, double-membraned vesicles and wall-forming bodies. The double-membraned bodies are located near the nucleus and are probably derived from it (Ferguson et al. 1975).

The microgamete (the male gamete) is ovoid to ellipsoidal in shape. During microgametogenesis, the nucleus of the male gamonts divides to produce 10–21 nuclei (Dubey & Frenkel 1972). The nuclei move towards the periphery of the parasite, entering protuberances in the pellicle of the mother parasite. One or two residual bodies are left in the microgamont after division into microgametes. Each microgamete is biflagellate, appears laterally compressed, and contains mainly nuclear material. At the anterior end is a pointed structure, the perforatorium, which contains the basal bodies from which two long free flagella originate. There is a large mitochodrion anterior to the nucleus. Five microtubules originate near the nucleus and extend posteriorly for a short distance. Microgametes are few in number compared to macrogametes. The microgametes swim to the mature macrogamete, attach by the perforatorium and penetrate the cell membrane, producing the fertilized gamete, the oocyst.

Oocyst wall formation is initiated by fertilization, and five layers are formed around the pellicle of the gamete (Ferguson et al. 1975). The oocyst are now discharged into the intestinal lumen by rupture of the epithelial cells. The mature, unsporulated oocyst, the sporont, is spherical and 10–12 μm in diameter. The wall consists of two colourless layers, and the sporont almost fills the oocyst.

Sporulation

Sporulated oocysts are subspherical to ellipsoidal and are 11 μm × 13 μm in diameter. Each sporulated oocyst contains two ellipsoidal sporocysts, which measure 6 μm × 8 μm. There are four sutures with lip-like thickenings in the sporocyst wall, which open during excystation of the sporozoites (Christie et al. 1978). A sporocyst residuum is present, whereas there is no oocyst residuum. Each sporocyst contains four sporozoites, which are 2 μm × 6–8 μm in size with a subterminal to central nucleus and a few PAS-positive granules in the cytoplasm. Ultrastructurally, the sporozoite is similar to the tachyzoite, except that there is an abundance of micronemes and rhoptries in the former. There is no crystalloid body and nor are there any refractile bodies in the sporozoites found in conventional coccidian sporozoites (Dubey 1993; Dubey et al. 1998).

Genome and antigenic structure

Genome

Toxoplasma gondii is haploid except during sexual division in the intestine of the cat. Sporozoites result from meiosis and seem to follow classic Mendelian laws (Pfefferkorn et al. 1977; Pfefferkorn & Pfefferkorn 1980). The total haploid genome contains approximately 8×10^7 base pairs (bp) (Cornelissen et al. 1984), and a 36-kilobase (kb), circular mitochondrial deoxyribonucleic acid (DNA) (Borst et al. 1984), which has been partly sequenced (Ossorio et al. 1991). Nine chromosomes have been identified by pulsed-field gel electrophoresis (Sibley & Boothroyd 1992*a*), and a molecular karyotype constructed using probes from low-copy number genes (Sibley & Boothroyd 1992*a*). Tubulin genes have been described, and both contain introns (Boothroyd et al. 1987; Nagel & Boothroyd 1988). Only the B1 gene has been found to be tandemly repeated (Burg et al. 1989), but other sequences repeated many times have been identified (McLeod et al. 1991; Blanco et al. 1992). The *T. gondii* DNA has been characterized and a genetic nomenclature for *T. gondii* has been proposed (Johnson et al. 1986; Sibley et al. 1991).

Toxoplasma gondii ribosomal ribonucleic acid (rRNA) has the usual large and small subunit (Gagnon et al. 1993). Sequence analysis of the small subunit RNA suggests that *T. gondii* is phylogenetically related to *Sarcocystis*, but separate from *Plasmodium* (Johnson & Baverstock 1989; Guay et al. 1992, 1993).

Antigens

Two-dimensional gel electrophoresis has identified more then 1000 spots after [^{35}S]methionine labelling of tachyzoites cultured *in vitro* (Handman et al. 1980), which probably reflects at least the number of different proteins present. The different stages of the parasite share common antigens and express stage-specific antigens, both between oocysts and other stages (Kasper et al. 1984; Kasper & Ware 1985), and between bradyzoites and tachyzoites (Kasper & Ware 1989; Woodison & Smith 1990).

The antigens involved in attachment of *T. gondii* to the host cell and the antigens involved in penetration of the host cell and formation of the parasitophorous vacuole have received special attention (Schwartzman 1986; Sadak et al. 1988; Cesbron-Delauw et al. 1989; Schwartzman & Krug 1989; Charif et al. 1990; Achbarou et al. 1991; Leriche & Dubremetz 1991; Saavedra et al. 1991; Ossorio et al. 1992). The major antigens identified so far are summarized in Table 1.1.

Several membrane antigens have been identified (Handman et al. 1980). The most abundant surface antigen is a 30-kDa protein, SAG1 (Kasper et al. 1983; Burg et al. 1988; Santoro et al. 1986; Kasper & Boothroyd 1993). SAG1 appears to be conserved between different *T. gondii* isolates (Bülow & Boothroyd 1991; Sibley & Boothroyd 1992*b*). SAG1 is found only in tachyzoites where it constitutes up to about 5% of the total tachyzoite protein. It is distributed evenly on the surface of the tachyzoite, and in the tubular network of the parasitophorous vacuole, and is shed from the surface of the parasite at the moving junction between the parasite and the host cell during the invasion process (Dubremetz et al. 1985). A *T. gondii* mutant of the RH strain lacking the SAG1 surface antigen has been described

Table 1.1. Major *Toxoplasma gondii* antigens

Localization	Denomination	Mol. Wt. (kDa)	Function	Remarks	Reference
Tachyzoite surface	SAG1 (Surface Antigen 1)	30	Adhesion/penetration	At least two alleles known, GPI anchor	Burg et al. 1988
	SAG2	22	?	GPI-anchor	Prince et al. 1990
	SAG3	43	?		Cesbron-Delauw et al. 1994
Rhoptries	ROP1 (Rhoptry Protein1)	61	Penetration enhancing factor		Schwartzman 1986
	ROP2		Associated with PVM		Saavedra et al. 1991
	ROP3, 4, 5		?		Leriche & Dubremetz 1991
	ROP6		?		Dubremetz et al. 1987
	ROP7	54	?		Saavedra et al. 1991
Dense granules	GRA1 (Granule protein 1)	23	Function in the parasitophorous vacuole, PV	Excreted/secreted antigen, ESA Calcium binding	Cesbron-Delauw et al. 1989 Leriche & Dubremetz 1991
	GRA2	28.5	Function in the PV	ESA	Mercier et al. 1993
	GRA3	30	Inserted into the PVM	ESA	Ossorio et al. 1994
	GRA4	40		ESA, PV network	Cesbron-Delauw & Capron 1993
	GRA5	21	Associated with the tissue cyst wall	ESA	Lecordier et al. 1993
	GRA6	32		ESA, PV network	Lecordier et al. 1995
	p36/38	36/38	Acid phosphatase		Metsis et al. 1995
Micronemes	MIC1 (Microneme Protein 1)	60	Adhesion	Homology to *P. falciparum* TRAP-gene	Fourmaux et al. 1996a
	MIC2	120		Contains EGF-like domains	Fourmaux et al. 1996b
	MIC3	90	?		Fourmaux et al. 1996b
Bradyzoite specific	BAG1	28–30	Heat Shock Protein	Bradyzoite cytoplasm	Bohne et al. 1995
	MAG1	65	?	Bradyzoite cyst wall	Parmley et al. 1995
	SAG4	18	?	Bradyzoite surface	Ödberg-Ferragut et al. 1996

(Kasper 1987). The mutant can be kept in continuous culture. Surface neoglycoproteins have been identified (Robert et al. 1991), but their role in antigenicity and attachment/invasion remains unclear (Table 1.1).

The major surface proteins are anchored by a glycosylphosphatidyl-inositol anchor (Nagel & Boothroyd 1989; Tomavo et al. 1989). Early work suggested the presence of a 'penetration-enhancing factor' secreted from the rhoptries (Lycke & Norrby 1966) later found to be ROP1, and several rhoptry proteins (ROP) were later identified. Five dense granule proteins have been identified and shown to associate with the intravacuolar network and the PVM.

Excreted-secreted antigens (ESA) (Hughes 1981; Chumpitazi et al. 1987; Decoster et al. 1988; Duquesne et al. 1990; Cazabonne et al. 1994) are secreted from the rhoptries and the dense granules. At least three ESAs are located in the dense granules, GRA1(P23), GRA2(GP28.5) and GRA3(P21), and are released inside the parasitophorous vacuole (Charif et al. 1990; Leriche & Dubremetz 1990) (Table 1.1).

Biochemistry

Early work on the biochemistry of coccidia is reviewed by Wang (1982). None of the coccidia, including *T. gondii*, have been grown in cell-free medium. *Toxoplasma gondii* is incapable of purine synthesis and depends entirely on the host cell for preformed purines (Schwartzman & Pfefferkorn 1982; Pfefferkorn 1990). Several purine and pyrimidine salvage enzymes have been identified (Pfefferkorn & Pfefferkorn 1977; Pfefferkorn 1978; Krug et al. 1989; Iltzsch 1993; Manafi et al. 1993). *Toxoplasma gondii* appears only to be able to salvage uracil, and, although it can convert thymine to thymidine, there is no salvage pathway for thymidine (Pfefferkorn & Pfefferkorn 1977; Iltzsch 1993).

Toxoplasma gondii cannot use preformed folates as mammalian cells can, and the dihydrofolate reductase, DHFR, enzyme is therefore a major target for antibiotic agents against *T. gondii* (Derouin & Chastang 1989; Roos 1993). Little is known about the lipids and carbohydrates of *T. gondii*. The parasite has a low cholesterol/phospholipid ratio, many unsaturated fatty acid chains and large amounts of phosphatidylcholine (Gallois et al. 1988). A 6-kDa carbohydrate antigen seems to be responsible for early, *T. gondii*-specific IgM antibody production, and low numbers of concanavalin-A-binding sites have been located on the surface of tachyzoites (Mauras et al. 1980; Johnson et al. 1981). Glycoproteins that bind specific IgG and IgM have been identified on the surface of *T. gondii* (Naot et al. 1983), and it appears that *T. gondii* is capable of both *N*- and *O*-glycosylation (Schwartz & Tomavo 1993).

Host–parasite relationship

Host cell invasion

Early work on invasion of the host cell is reviewed by Werk (1985), and the invasion process has recently been reviewed by Schwartzman and Saffer (1992), Dubremetz and Schwartzman (1993) and Kasper and Mineo (1994). The invasion of the host cell is an active process involving attachment, host cell membrane penetration, formation of a moving junction with the host cell membrane, formation of the PVM and subsequent closure of the host cell membrane after entry. The invasion process is calcium dependent (Bonhomme et al. 1993). SAG1 has been implicated in attachment and penetration (Grimwood & Smith 1992; Mineo et al. 1993), and host cell laminin is also involved in attachment (Joiner 1991b; Furtado et al. 1992a,b). There are higher concentrations of laminin binding proteins (Joiner et al. 1989) and Fc binding sites at one end of the tachyzoite (Budzko et al. 1989). Considering the wide range of animal hosts, it is likely that *T. gondii* has several molecules that may be important in cell adhesion (Dubremetz & Schwartzman 1993; Mineo et al. 1993), and it has even been suggested that cholesterol might be used as a receptor (Pfefferkorn 1990).

After entering a host cell, *T. gondii* is surrounded by the PVM (Figure 1.5), which consists of both host cell membrane and parasite material. The PVM lacks host cell plasma membrane markers, and freeze-fracture analysis indicates that the PVM may completely lack intramembranous particles and may consist of only a phospholipid bilayer. The dense granules probably contribute to intravacuolar tubules (Dubremetz et al. 1993). The main phospholipid of the rhoptries is phosphatidylcholine (Foussard et al. 1991), which may be identical to the phospholipids found in the PVM (Joiner 1991a). *Toxoplasma gondii* phospholipase has been suggested to play a role in invasion, possibly by softening the host cell membrane after attachment (Saffer et al. 1989; Saffer & Schwartzman 1991). The micropore is formed by an invagination of the outer membrane of the pellicle (Nichols et al. 1983; Nichols & Chiappino 1987).

Host pathogenicity

When dealing with pathogenicity and virulence, we will only consider natural infection by the oral route, where infection is acquired from oocysts or tissue cysts, and not artificial infection routes such as intraperitoneal, subcutaneous or intracerebellar inoculation, unless specifically mentioned. Pathogenicity is determined by the virulence of the strain and the susceptibility of the host species, usually the mouse (Kaufman et al. 1959; De Roever-Bonnet 1966; Reikvam & Lorentzen-Styr 1976; Ferguson & Hutchison 1981; Suzuki et al. 1989).

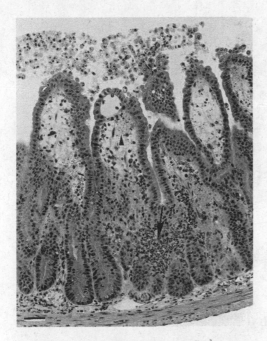

Figure 1.10   Enteritis in a section of mouse small intestine 4
days after feeding *T. gondii* oocysts. Note
desquamation of epithelial cells in the intestinal
lumen, necrosis of the cells in lamina propria
(arrowhead), and inflammation in the glands of
Liberkühn (arrow). Haematoxylin and eosin stain.
×150. Bar=50 μm.

Toxoplasma gondii usually infects the host without producing any clinical signs. After ingestion, bradyzoites or sporozoites penetrate enterocytes, multiplying initially in cells lining the lamina propria and later the epithelium (Figures 1.10, 1.11) (Dubey 1997; Dubey et al. 1997; Speer & Dubey 1998). However, infection may spread to other tissues within a short time after ingestion; *T. gondii* was isolated from mesenteric lymph nodes of cats 4 hours after feeding tissue cysts (Dubey & Frenkel 1972). Infection is disseminated to distant organs through the blood and lymphatics.

An infected host may die from necrosis of the intestine (Figures 1.10, 1.11) and mesenteric lymph nodes (Figure 1.12) before other organs are severely damaged (Dubey & Frenkel 1973), or focal necrosis may develop in many organs. The clinical picture is determined by damage to different organs, especially organs such as the eye, heart and adrenals. Necrosis is caused by the intracellular growth of tachyzoites. *Toxoplasma gondii* does not produce a toxin.

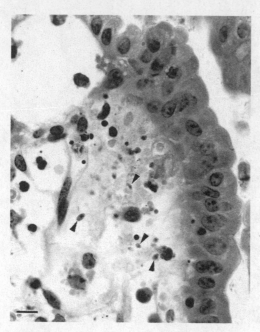

Figure 1.11   Higher magnification of the villus with arrowhead
in Figure 1.10. Note ballooning and necrosis of the
cells of the lamina propria by tachyzoites
(arrowheads). Haematoxylin and eosin stain.
×750. Bar = 10 μm.

Usually by about the third week after infection, the tachyzoites begin to disappear from the visceral tissues (in mice), and tissue cysts are found in increasing
numbers in neural (Figure 1.13) and muscular tissues. Tachyzoites may persist for
longer in the spinal cord and brain because immunity is less effective in neural
organs than in visceral tissues.

The intracellular tachyzoite and later the bradyzoite are found within the parasitophorous vacuole within the host cell's endocytic system. The host cell is unable
to fuse the lysosomes and the parasitophorous vacuole, which explains the parasite's ability to survive intracellularly (Jones & Hirsch 1972; Jones et al. 1972; Joiner
et al. 1990). *Toxoplasma gondii* resists phagosomes by creating a membranous
network between the parasite and the host cell (Sibley & Krahenbuhl 1988).

How *T. gondii* survives intracellularly is not completely known (Frenkel 1967;
Chinchilla & Frenkel 1978). Immunity to *T. gondii* is mainly cell mediated and this
subject was recently reviewed by Gazzinelli et al. (1993). The fate of tissue cysts is
not fully known (Dubey et al. 1998). It has been proposed that tissue cysts may at
times rupture during the life of the host. The released bradyzoites may be destroyed

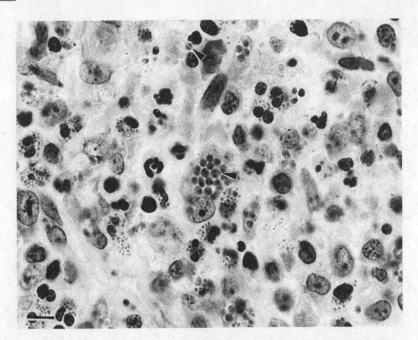

Figure 1.12   Necrosis and inflammation in a mesenteric lymph node of a dog naturally infected with *T. gondii*. Note active division of tachyzoites (arrowheads) in parenchymatous cells. Haematoxylin and eosin stain. ×750. Bar = 10 μm.

by the host's immune response (Frenkel 1953; Frenkel & Escajadillo 1987; Frenkel 1990), which may cause focal necrosis and inflammation, but hypersensitivity may also play a role in such reactions. The rupture of tissue cysts is rarely observed histologically (Ferguson et al. 1989).

Virulence and strain differences

Strain differentiation and population biology

Restriction fragment length polymorphism (RFLP) provides a method for identifying genomic DNA differences between parasites of different isolates or between or among organisms of phylogenic proximity, and has also been applied to *T. gondii* (Cristina et al. 1991a,b; Sibley and Boothroyd 1992b).

Using RFLP on polymerase-chain-reaction-amplified specific single copy genes obtained from different RH lines revealed that there are unique patterns, except from three isolates cloned from the same line (Howe and Sibley 1994).

Strain differences between different isolates of *T. gondii* have been established by isoenzyme electrophoresis (Barnert et al. 1988; Dardé et al. 1988) and by immunological methods (Ware & Kasper 1987), and a relationship between isoenzyme

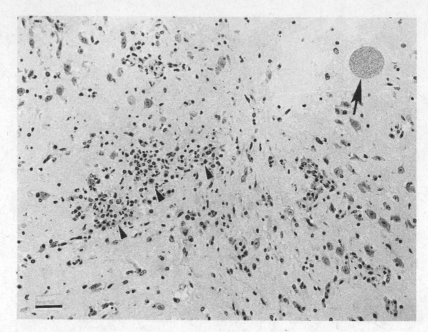

Figure 1.13   Glial nodules (arrowheads) in the cerebrum of a mouse 1 month after inoculation with *T. gondii*. Note a tissue cyst (arrow) away from the area of inflammation. Haematoxylin and eosin stain. ×250. Bar = 30 μm.

pattern (zymodemes) and pathogenicity (virulence) has been described (Dardé et al. 1988, 1992). Furthermore, differences in chromosome size between different isolates have been demonstrated by pulsed-field gel electrophoresis (Candolfi et al. 1989).

Strain-specific differences between different isolates of *T. gondii* have been demonstrated by immunoblot, immune-precipitation with antisera, isoenzyme analysis and DNA typing techniques (Handman et al. 1980; Ware & Kasper 1987; Barnert et al. 1988; Weiss et al. 1988; Bülow & Boothroyd 1991). Polymorphism seems to be limited and, for the few single loci examined in detail, only two alleles have been identified (Boothroyd & Sibley 1993). Virulent strains can now be differentiated from avirulent strains by their reactivity with certain monoclonal antibodies (Gross et al. 1991; Bohne et al. 1993). Virulent strains have conserved restriction fragment patterns, whereas avirulent isolates are polymorphic (Sibley & Boothroyd 1992b). Random amplified polymorphic DNA, RAPD, using arbitrary primers ten nucleotides long has been used to type strains into mouse virulent and nonvirulent isolates (Guo et al. 1997).

Virulence

Most animals can be classified as either resistant or sensitive to *T. gondii* with respect to clinical disease. Generally, humans, cattle, horses, rats and old world monkeys belong to the resistant species, whereas mice, guinea-pigs, hamsters and new world monkeys are sensitive (Darcy and Zenner 1993).

The virulence of *T. gondii* has been traditionally measured in a susceptible host (e.g. mice). Based on studies of mice, some *T. gondii* strains are thought to be more virulent than others, and *in vitro* studies have shown that invasion, multiplication time and cyst production are related to *in vivo* virulence (Appleford & Smith 1997). Virulence is influenced by the stage of the parasite (tachyzoite, bradyzoite and sporozoite), the route of inoculation (oral, intraperitoneal, subcutaneous) and the susceptibility of the host. In mice, oocysts from the M-7741 isolate needed an inoculum size approximately 10–100 times less than that of tissue cysts, producing both earlier symptoms and more deaths than tissue cysts with inocula of the same size (Dubey & Frenkel 1973). However, according to Dubey and Beattie (1988) there are no truly avirulent strains of *T. gondii*; 100,000 oocysts of all strains of *T. gondii* tested were lethal to mice by the oral route.

More severe infections are found in pregnant or lactating mice than in nonlactating mice. Concomitant infection may make the host more susceptible or resistant to *T. gondii* infection (Remington 1970). New-born kittens are more prone to severe toxoplasmosis and death compared to adult, nonimmune cats (Dubey & Frenkel 1972).

The most well-known virulent strain of *T. gondii* (RH strain) was isolated in 1939 from a six-year-old boy (with initials R. H.) in mice (Sabin 1941). Five of the eight mice inoculated with brain tissue from this boy died within 21 days while three mice were not infected. Thus, the RH strain was virulent for mice on its first isolation. Although the RH strain of *T. gondii* can be virulent in many hosts, including humans, it is avirulent in adult rats and adult dogs (Remington et al. 1958; Dubey & Beattie 1988).

Several different mechanisms have been related to virulence in mice. For example, virulence in mice has been related to the expression of heat shock proteins, HSP, in that *T. gondii* isolates capable of expressing high levels of HSP are more virulent (Lyons & Johnson 1995). Increased DNA polymerase activity has been found in the mouse, virulent RH isolate, and it has been hypothesized that the faster, *in vitro* multiplication rate of the RH isolate is reflected in the increased DNA polymerase activity (Makioka & Ohtomo 1995). Increased numbers of a repeat sequence in the promoter region of the *SAG1* gene with fourfold increased expression of SAG1 have been found in virulent isolates (Windeck & Gross 1996).

The virulence of the RH strain has been modified by repeated passage in mice (Yano & Nakabayashi 1986), and it has been suggested that change in virulence is a natural, host-dependent phenomenon (Lecomte et al. 1992). Therefore, intermediate hosts could be important for downregulating the pathogenicity of certain *T. gondii* strains, thus maintaining parasite survival (Lecomte et al. 1992). Mice with severe combined immunodeficiency (SCID) or nude mice die from acute infection with *T. gondii*, but survive if given spleen cells from immune mice (Johnson 1992).

Natural resistance and host specificity

Toxoplasma gondii strains may vary in their pathogenicity in a given host. Certain strains of mice are more susceptible than others (Araujo et al. 1976; Williams et al. 1978; Fujii et al. 1983; McLeod et al. 1984; Suzuki et al. 1993), and appear to be regulated at least in part by H-2- and H-13-linked genes (Williams et al. 1978; Jones & Erb 1985). However, more recently genes of the H-2 and D/L locus have been implicated in the regulation of brain cyst development and *T. gondii* encephalitis (Brown & McLeod 1990; Suzuki and Remington 1994). At least five genes are involved in the regulation of *T. gondii* infection in mice (McLeod et al. 1989; Blackwell et al. 1993). Resistance to *T. gondii* may decrease with the host's age (Gardner & Remington 1977). In mice *T. gondii* can be transferred for several generations during pregnancy from the mother to the litter (Beverley 1959), and *T. gondii* infection in rhesus monkeys has been described as a model for congenital toxoplasmosis (Schoondermark et al. 1993).

Most mammals and birds can be infected with *T. gondii*. The natural resistance to infection varies between species. In general, mice are more susceptible than rats (Lainson 1955; Jacobs 1956). The severity of infection in individual mice within the same strain may also vary (Araujo et al. 1976; Johnson 1984; Suzuki et al. 1989), while certain host species are genetically resistant to symptomatic toxoplasmosis. For example, adult rats do not become ill while young rats can die from toxoplasmosis while mice of any age develop clinical disease. Adult dogs do not experience symtomatic infection, unlike puppies. Cattle and horses are amongst the most resistant intermediate hosts for clinical toxoplasmosis, in contrast to certain marsupials and New World monkeys, which are the most susceptible to overt disease (Dubey & Beattie 1988).

In vivo and *in vitro* cultivation

Animal models

Toxoplasma gondii can be cultured in several laboratory animals, chick embryos and several cell lines (Hughes et al. 1986). Mice, hamsters, guinea-pigs and rabbits are all susceptible, but mice are generally used as hosts because they are more susceptible than others (Abbas 1967), and are not naturally infected when raised in the laboratory on dry food free of cat faeces.

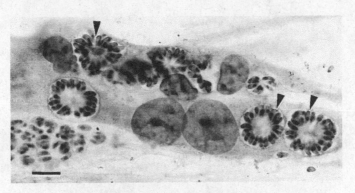

Figure 1.14   *Toxoplasma gondii* tachyzoites in cultured cells. Note rosettes (arrowheads). ×750. Bar = 10 μm.

Tachyzoites grow in the peritoneal cavity of mice and may sometimes produce ascites. They can also grow as free tachyzoites in most other tissues after inoculation with any of the three infectious stages of *T. gondii*. Virulent strains usually produce illness in mice and sometimes kill them within 1–2 weeks. Tachyzoites of a virulent strain can be aspirated from the peritoneal cavity, but avirulent strains grow slowly in mice and free tachyzoites of these strains are often difficult to obtain. Tachyzoites of avirulent strains can be obtained by inducing immunosuppression in the mice with corticosteroids.

Frequent rapid passage of tachyzoites of low virulence may increase their virulence. Most *T. gondii* isolates become virulent in mice after rapid intraperitoneal passage, and repeated frequent passage appears to modify some other biological characteristics as well; for example, the inability of the RH strain and some lines derived from the Beverley and M-7741 isolates to produce oocysts after infecting cats with tissue cysts from these particular strains (Frenkel et al. 1976).

In vitro culture

It is not possible to culture *T. gondii* axenically, i. e. outside host cells, although *T. gondii* contains cytochromes, glycolytic and respiratory systems and can utilize preformed nucleic acids. Several tissue cell culture systems for *in vitro* cultivation of *T. gondii* have been described (Hogan et al. 1960; Matsubayashi & Akao 1963; Buckley 1973; Shimada et al. 1974; Jones et al. 1986; Lindsay et al. 1991; Dimier & Bout 1993). Tachyzoites can be grown in many cell lines in continuous culture (Figure 1.14) (McHugh et al. 1994), and tissue cyst formation can be obtained in cell culture for the RH strain as well (Soete et al. 1994), but the yield is lower compared to mouse infections (Hoff et al. 1977; Jones et al. 1986; Dardé et al. 1989, Lindsay et al. 1991). Tissue cysts formed within 3 days of infecting cell cultures with tachyzoites, and each tissue cyst (Figure 1.15) contained up to 50 bradyzoites (Lindsay

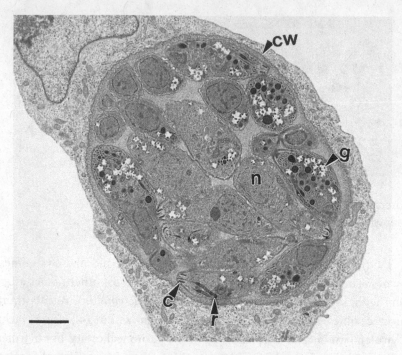

Figure 1.15   Electron micrograph of a tissue cyst of *T. gondii*, 10 days after inoculation of
GT-1 strain sporozoites in M617 cells in culture. Note folding of the cyst wall
(CW), and the granular substance lining the cyst in between bradyzoites.
Bradyzoites have organelles seen in tachyzoites but have more
polysaccharide granules (g) than in tachyzoites. Note the presence of conoid
(c), rhoptries (r) and the nucleus (n) in bradyzoites. The host cell nucleus is
at the upper right. ×6782. Bar = 1.4 µm. (Courtesy of Dr D. S. Lindsay, Auburn
University, Alabama.)

et al. 1993). Many mammalian cells including red blood cells can be infected by *T.
gondii* (Michel et al. 1980). Virulent mouse strains rapidly destroy the cell while
avirulent strains grow slowly causing minimal cell damage.

The mean generation time of RH strain *T. gondii* tachyzoites in cell culture is five
hours, and, unlike the situation in mice, passage of tachyzoites in cell culture is not
known to alter the virulence. Tissue cysts are prominent in mouse brains 8 weeks
after infection. Feline entero–epithelial stages of *T. gondii* have not yet been culti-
vated *in vitro*.

Oocysts (Figure 1.16) can be obtained by feeding tissue cysts from infected mice
to cats that are not immune to *T. gondii*. Normally oocysts will appear in cat faeces
3–10 days after the cat ingests the tissue cysts (Figure 1.17).

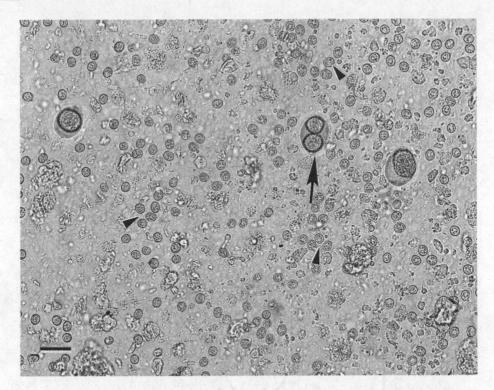

Figure 1.16 *Toxoplasma gondii* unsporulated oocysts (arrowheads) and *Isospora felis* (arrows) in a faecal-float of cat. *Isospora felis* is the commonest coccidium in cat faeces. Its oocysts are about four times the size of *T. gondii* oocysts. It sporulates faster than *T. gondii*; while all *T. gondii* oocysts are unsporulated, *I. felis* has already started to divide (arrow). ×300. Bar = 6 μm.

Summary

Toxoplasma gondii is a coccidian parasite, with the cat as its definitive host and a very wide range of warm-blooded intermediate hosts. The infectious stages are the oocysts shed by the cat and the tissue cysts found in tissues of the intermediate host. There are shared as well as stage-specific antigens. Several coding genes have been described including major surface antigens, and antigens located in the rhoptries and dense granules. Host cell invasion is an active process mediated at least partly by host cell laminin as a receptor, and it appears that *T. gondii* proteins are incorporated in the PVM. Warm-blooded animals differ in their susceptibility to infection and virulence in mice is genetically regulated. Adult cattle, horses, rats and mice and Old World monkeys are resistant, whereas mice, Australian marsupials and New World monkeys are highly susceptible to clinical toxoplasmosis.

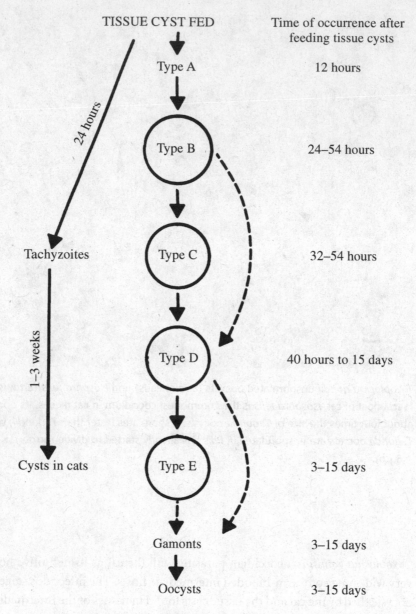

Figure 1.17   Lifecycle of *Toxoplasma gondii* in the tissues of cats fed tissue cysts. Areas of uncertainty are indicated by broken lines. Multiplication within *Toxoplasma* of various types are indicated by straight arrows with solid lines. (Modified with permission from Dubey & Frenkel 1972).

REFERENCES

Abbas, A. M. A. (1967). Comparative study of methods used for the isolation of *Toxoplasma gondii*. *Bulletin of the World Health Organization*, **36**, 344–6.

Achbarou, A., Mercereau-Puijalon, O., Sadak, A., Fortier, B., Leriche, M. A., Camus, D. & Dubremetz, J. F. (1991). Differential targetting of dense granule proteins in the parasitophorous vacuole of *Toxoplasma gondii*. *Parasitology*, **103**, 321–9.

Appleford, P. J. & Smith, J. E. (1997). *Toxoplasma gondii*: the growth characteristics of three virulent strains. *Acta Tropica*, **65**, 97–104.

Araujo, F. G., Williams, D. M., Grumet, F. C. & Remington, J. S. (1976). Strain-dependent differences in murine susceptibility to *Toxoplasma*. *Infection and Immunity*, **13**, 1528–30.

Barnert, G., Hassl, A. & Aspöck, H. (1988). Isoenzyme studies on *Toxoplasma gondii* isolates using isoelectric focusing. *Zentralblat für Bakteriologie und Hygiene A*, **268**, 476–81.

Beverley, J. K. A. (1959). Congenital transmission of toxoplasmosis through successive generations of mice. *Nature*, **183**, 1348–9.

Blackwell, J. M., Roberts, C. W. & Alexander J. (1993). Influence of genes within the MHC on mortality and brain cyst development in mice infected with *Toxoplasma gondii*: kinetics of immune regulation in BALB H-2 congenic mice. *Parasite Immunology*, **15**, 317–24.

Blanco, J. C., Angel, S. O., Maero, E., Pszenny, V., Serpente, P. & Garberi, J. C. (1992). Cloning of repetitive DNA sequences from *Toxoplasma gondii* and their usefulness for parasite detection. *American Journal of Tropical Medicine and Hygiene*, **46**, 350–7.

Bohne, W., Heesemann, J. & Gross, U. (1992). Coexistence of heterogeneous populations of *Toxoplasma gondii* parasites within parasitophorous vacuoles of murine macrophages as revealed by a bradyzoite-specific monoclonal antibody. *Parasitology Research*, **79**, 485–7.

Bohne, W., Gross, U. & Heesemann, J. (1993). Differentiation between mouse-virulent and -avirulent strains of *Toxoplasma gondii* by a monoclonal antibody recognizing a 27-kilodalton antigen. *Journal of Clinical Microbiology*, **31**, 1641–3.

Bohne, W., Heesemann, J. & Gross, U. (1994). Reduced replication of *Toxoplasma gondii* is necessary for induction of bradyzoite-specific antigens: a possible role for nitric oxide in triggering stage conversion. *Infection and Immunity*, **62**, 1761–7.

Bohne, W., Gross, U., Ferguson, D. J. P. & Heesemann, J. (1995). Cloning and characterization of a bradyzoite-specifically expressed gene (*hsp30/bag1*) of *Toxoplasma gondii*, related to genes encoding small heat-shock proteins of plants. *Molecular Microbiology*, **16**, 1221–30.

Bonhomme, A., Pingret, L., Bonhomme, P., Michel, J., Balossier, G., Lhotel, M., Pluot, M. & Pinon, J. M. (1993). Subcellular calcium localization in *Toxoplasma gondii* by electron microscopy and by X-ray and electron energy loss spectroscopies. *Microscopic Research Techniques*, **25**, 276–85.

Boothroyd, J. C. & Sibley, L. D. (1993). Population biology of *Toxoplasma gondii*. *Research in Immunology*, **144**, 14–16.

Boothroyd, J. C., Burg, J. L., Nagel, S. D., Perelman, D., Kasper, L. H., Ware, P. L., Prince, J. B., Sharma, S. D. & Remington, J. S. (1987). Antigen and tubulin genes of *Toxoplasma gondii*. In

Molecular Strategies of Parasitic Invasion, ed. N. Agabian, H. Goodman & N. Nogueira, pp. 237–250. New York: A. R. Liss.

Borst, P., Overdulve, J. P., Weijers, P. J., Fase-Fowler, F. & Van Den Burg, M. (1984). DNA circles with cruciforms from *Isospora* (*Toxoplasma*) *gondii. Biochemical and Biophysical Acta*, **781**, 100–11.

Brown, C. R. & McLeod, R. (1990). Class I MHC genes and CD8+ T cells determine cyst number in *Toxoplasma gondii* infection. *Journal of Immunology*, **145**, 3438–41.

Budzko, D. B., Tyler, L. & Armstrong, D. (1989). Fc receptors on the surface of *Toxoplasma gondii* trophozoites: a confounding factor in testing for anti-*Toxoplasma* antibodies by indirect immunofluorescence. *Journal of Clinical Microbiology*, **27**, 959–61.

Buckley, S. M. (1973). Survival of *Toxoplasma gondii* in mosquito cell lines and establishment of continuous infection in Vero cell cultures. *Experimental Parasitology*, **33**, 23–6.

Bülow, R. & Boothroyd, J. C. (1991). Protection of mice from fatal *Toxoplasma gondii* infection by immunization with p30 antigen in liposomes. *Journal of Immunology*, **147**, 3496–500.

Burg, J. L., Perelman, D., Kasper, L. H., Ware, P. L. & Boothroyd, J. C. (1988). Molecular analysis of the gene encoding the major surface antigen of *Toxoplasma gondii. Journal of Immunology*, **141**, 3584–91.

Burg, J. L., Grover, C. M., Pouletty, P. & Boothroyd, J. C. (1989). Direct and sensitive detection of a pathogenic protozoan, *Toxoplasma gondii*, by polymerase chain reaction. *Journal of Clinical Microbiology*, **27**, 1787–92.

Candolfi, E., Arveiler, B., Mandel, J. L. & Kien, T. (1989). Structure du genome de *Toxoplasma gondii*. Premiers résultats. *Bulletin de la Société Française de Parasitologie*, **7**, 27–32.

Cazabonne, P., Bessieres, M. H. & Seguela, J. P. (1994). Kinetics study and characterisation of target excreted/secreted antigens of immunoglobulin G, M, A and E antibodies from mice infected with different strains of *Toxoplasma gondii. Parasitology Research*, **80**, 58–63.

Cesbron-Delauw, M.-F. & Capron, A. (1993). Excreted/secreted antigens of *Toxoplasma gondii* – their origin and role in the host–parasite interaction. *Research in Immunology*, **144**, 41–4.

Cesbron-Delauw, M.-F., Guy, B., Torpier, G., Pierce, R. J., Lenzen, G., Cesbron, J. Y., Charif, H., Lepage, P., Darcy, F., Lecocq, J. P. & Capron, A. (1989). Molecular characterisation of a 23-kilodalton major antigen secreted by *Toxoplasma gondii. Proceedings of the National Academy of Sciences USA*, **86**, 7537–41.

Cesbron-Delauw, M.-F., Tomavo, S., Beauchamps, P., Fourmaux, M.-P., Camus, D., Capron, A. & Dubremetz, J.-F. (1994). Similarities between the primary structures of two distinct major surface proteins of *Toxoplasma gondii. Journal of Biological Chemistry*, **269**, 16217–22.

Charif, H., Darcy, F., Torpier, G., Cesbron-Delauw, M. F. & Capron, A. (1990). *Toxoplasma gondii*: characterization and localization of antigens secreted from tachyzoites. *Experimental Parasitology*, **71**, 114–24.

Chinchilla, M. & Frenkel, J. K. (1978). Mediation of immunity to intracellular infection (*Toxoplasma* and *Besnoitia*) within somatic cells. *Infection and Immunity*, **19**, 999–1012.

Christie, E., Pappas, P. W. & Dubey, J. P. (1978). Ultrastructure of excystment of *Toxoplasma gondii* oocysts. *Journal of Protozoology*, **25**, 438–43.

Chumpitazi, B., Ambroise-Thomas, P. & Cagnard, M. (1987). Isolation and characterization of

Toxoplasma exo-antigens from *in vitro* culture in MRC5 and Vero cells. *International Journal of Parasitology,* **17**, 829–34.

Cornelissen, A. W. C. A., Overdulve, J. P. & Ploeg, M. van den. (1984). Determination of nuclear DNA of five Eucoccidian parasites, *Isospora* (*Toxoplasma*) *gondii*, *Sarcocystis cruzi*, *Eimeria tenella, E. acervulina* and *Plasmodium berghei* with special reference to gametogenesis and meiosis in *I.* (*T.*) *gondii. Parasitology,* **88**, 531–53.

Cristina, N., Oury, B., Ambroise-Thomas, P. & Santoro, F. (1991a). Restriction-fragment-length polymorphisms among *Toxoplasma gondii* strains. *Parasitology Research,* **77**, 266–8.

Cristina, N., Liaud, M.-F., Santoro, F., Oury, B. & Ambroise-Thomas, P. (1991b). A family of repeated DNA sequences in *Toxoplasma gondii*: cloning, sequence analysis, and use in strain characterization. *Experimental Parasitology,* **73**, 73–81.

Darcy, F. & Zenner, L. (1993). Experimental models of toxoplasmosis. *Research in Immunology,* **144**, 16–23.

Dardé, M. L., Bouteille, B. & Pestre-Alexandre, M. (1988). Isoenzymic characterization of seven strains of *Toxoplasma gondii* by isoelectrofocusing in polyacrylamide gels. *American Journal of Tropical Medicine and Hygiene,* **39**, 551–8.

Dardé, M. L., Bouteille, B., Leboutet, M. J., Loubet, A. & Pestre-Alexandre, M. (1989). *Toxoplasma gondii*: étude ultrastructurale des formations kystiques observées en culture de fibroblastes humains. *Annales de la Parasitologie Humaine et Comparee,* **64**, 403–11.

Dardé, M. L., Bouteille, B. & Pestre-Alexandre, M. (1992). Isoenzyme analysis of 35 *Toxoplasma gondii* isolates and the biological epidemiological implications. *Journal of Parasitology,* **78**, 786–94.

De Roever-Bonnet, H. (1966). Virulence of *Toxoplasma. Tropical and Geographical Medicine,* **18**, 143–6.

Decoster, A., Darcy, F. & Capron, A. (1988). Recognition of *Toxoplasma gondii* excreted and secreted antigens by human sera from acquired and congenital toxoplasmosis: identification of markers of acute and chronic infection. *Clinical and Experimental Immunology,* **73**, 376–82.

Derouin, F. & Chastang, C. (1989). *In vitro* effects of folate inhibitors on *Toxoplasma gondii. Antimicrobial Agents and Chemotherapy,* **33**, 1753–9.

Derouin, F. & Garin, Y. J. F. (1991). *Toxoplasma gondii*: blood and tissue kinetics during acute and chronic infections in mice. *Experimental Parasitology,* **73**, 460–8.

Dimier, I. H. & Bout, D. T. (1993). Rat intestinal epithelial cell line IEC-6 is activated by recombinant interferon-γ to inhibit replication of the coccidian *Toxoplasma gondii. European Journal of Immunology,* **23**, 981–3.

Dubey, J. P. (1977). *Toxoplasma, Hammondia, Besnoitia, Sarcocystis,* and other tissue cyst-forming coccidia of man and animals. In *Parasitic Protozoa,* vol. 3, ed. J. P. Kreier, pp. 101–237, New York: Academic Press.

Dubey, J. P. (1993). *Toxoplasma, Neospora, Sarcocystis,* and other tissue cyst-forming coccidia of humans and animals. In *Parasitic Protozoa,* vol. 6, ed. J. P. Kreier, pp. 1–158, New York: Academic Press.

Dubey, J. P. (1995). Duration of immunity to shedding of *Toxoplasma gondii* oocysts by cats. *Journal of Parasitology,* **81**, 410–15.

Dubey, J. P. (1996). Infectivity and pathogenicity of *Toxoplasma gondii* oocysts for cats. *Journal of Parasitology*, 82, 957–60.

Dubey, J. P. (1997). Brydyzoite-induced murine toxopalsmosis: stage conversion, pathogenesis, and tissue cyst formation in mice fed bradyzoites of different strains of *Toxoplasma gondii*. *Journal of Eukaryotic Microbiology*, 44, 592–602.

Dubey, J. P. (1998a). Re-examination of resistance of *Toxoplasma gondii* tachyzoites and bradyzoites to pepsin and trypsin digestion. *Parasitology*, 116, 43–50.

Dubey, J. P. (1998b). Advances in the life cycle of *Toxoplasma gondii*. *International Journal of Parasitology*, 28, 1019–24.

Dubey, J. P. & Beattie, C. P. (1988). *Toxoplasmosis of Animals and Man*, pp. 1–220. Boca Raton, FL: CRC Press.

Dubey, J. P. & Fenner, W. R. (1993). Clinical segmental myelitis associated with an unidentified *Toxoplasma*-like parasite in a cat. *Journal of Veterinary Diagnostic Investigation*, 5, 472–80.

Dubey, J. P. & Frenkel, J. K. (1972). Cyst-induced toxoplasmosis in cats. *Journal of Protozoology*, 19, 155–77.

Dubey, J. P. & Frenkel, J. K. (1973). Experimental *Toxoplasma* infection in mice with strains producing oocysts. *Journal of Parasitology*, 59, 505–12.

Dubey, J. P. & Frenkel, J. K. (1974). Immunity to feline toxoplasmosis: modification by adminsitration of corticosteroids. *Veterinary Pathology*, 11, 350–79.

Dubey, J. P. & Frenkel, J. K. (1976). Feline toxoplasmosis from acutely infected mice and the development of *Toxoplasma* cysts. *Journal of Protozoology*, 23, 537–46.

Dubey, J. P., Miller, N. L. & Frenkel, J. K. (1970a). The *Toxoplasma gondii* oocyst from cat feces. *Journal of Experimental Medicine*, 132, 636–62.

Dubey, J. P., Miller, N. L. & Frenkel, J. K. (1970b). Characterization of the new fecal form of *Toxoplasma gondii*. *Journal of Parasitology*, 56, 47–56.

Dubey, J. P., Speer, C. A., Shen, S. K., Kwok, O. C. H. & Blixt, J. A. (1997). Oocyst-induced murine toxoplasmosis: life cycle, pathogenicity, and stage conversion in mice fed *Toxoplasma gondii* oocysts. *Journal of Parasitology*, 83, 870–82.

Dubey, J. P., Lindsay, D. S. & Speer, C. A. (1998). Structure of *Toxoplasma gondii* tachyzoites, bradyzoites and sporozoites, and biology and development of tissue cysts. *Clinical Microbiology Reviews*, 11, 267–99.

Dubremetz, J. F. & Schwartzman, J. D. (1993). Subcellular organelles of *Toxoplasma gondii* and host cell invasion. *Research in Immunology*, 144, 31–3.

Dubremetz, J. F., Rodriguez, C. & Ferreira, E. (1985). *Toxoplasma gondii*: redistribution of monoclonal antibodies on tachyzoites during host cell invasion. *Experimental Parasitology*, 59, 24–32.

Dubremetz, J. F., Sadak, A., Taghy, Z. & Fortier, B. (1987). Characterisation of a 43-kDa rhoptry antigen of *Toxoplasma gondii*. In *Host–Parasite Cellular and Molecular Interactions in Protozoal Infection.*, ed. K. P. Chang & D. Snary, pp. 365–9. Berlin: Springer Verlag.

Dubremetz, J. F., Achbarou, A., Bermudes, D. & Joiner, K. A. (1993). Kinetics and pattern of organelle exocytosis during *Toxoplasma gondii* host–cell interaction. *Parasitology Research*, 79, 402–8.

Duquesne, V., Auriault, C., Darcy, F., Declavel, J. P. & Capron, A. (1990). Protection of nude rats against *Toxoplasma* infection by excreted-secreted antigen-specific helper T cells. *Infection and Immunity*, **58**, 2120–6.

Endo, T., Sethi, K. K. & Piekarski, G. (1982). *Toxoplasma gondii*: calcium ionophore A23187-mediated exit of trophozoites from infected murine macrophages. *Experimental Parasitology*, **53**, 179–88.

Endo, T., Yagita, K., Yasuda, T. & Nakamura, T. (1988). Detection and localization of actin in *Toxoplasma gondii*. *Parasitology Research*, **75**, 102–6.

Ferguson, D. J. P. & Hutchison, W. M. (1981). Comparison of the development of avirulent and virulent strains of *Toxoplasma gondii* in the peritoneal exudate of mice. *Annals of Tropical Medicine and Parasitology*, **75**, 539–46.

Ferguson, D. J. P. & Hutchison, W. M. (1987a). An ultrastructural study of the early development and tissue cyst formation of *Toxoplasma gondii* in the brains of mice. *Parasitology Research*, **73**, 483–91.

Ferguson, D. J. P. & Hutchison, W. M. (1987b). The host–parasite relationship of *Toxoplasma gondii* in the brains of chronically infected mice. *Virchows Archives*, **411**, 39–43.

Ferguson, D. J. P., Hutchison, W. M., Dunachie, J. F. & Siim, J. C. (1974). Ultrastructural study of early stages of asexual multiplication and micro-gametogony of *Toxoplasma gondii* in the small intestine of the cat. *Acta Pathologica et Microbiologica Scandinavica Section B*, **82**, 167–81.

Ferguson, D. J. P., Hutchison, W. M. & Siim, J. C. (1975). The ultrastructural development of the microgamete and formation of the oocyst wall of *Toxoplasma gondii*. *Acta Pathologica et Microbiologica Scandinavica Section B*, **83**, 491–505.

Ferguson, D. J. P., Hutchison, W. M. & Pettersen, E. (1989). Tissue cyst rupture in mice chronically infected with *Toxoplasma gondii*: an immunocytochemical and ultrastructural study. *Parasitology Research*, **75**, 599–603.

Fourmaux, M. N., Achbarou, A., Mercereau-Puijalon, O., Biderre, C., Briche, I., Loyens, A., Odberg-Ferragut, C., Camus, D. & Dubremetz, J. F. (1996a). The MIC1 microneme protein of *Toxopalsma gondii* contains a duplicated receptor-like domain and binds to host cell surface. *Molecular and Biochemical Parasitology*, **83**, 201–10.

Fourmaux, M. N., Garcia-Reguet, N., Mercereau-Puijalon, O. & Dubremetz, J. F. (1996b). *Toxoplasma gondii* microneme proteins: gene cloning and possible function. *Current Topics in Microbiology and Immunology*, **219**, 55–8.

Foussard, F., Leriche, M. A. & Dubremetz, J. F. (1991). Characterization of the lipid content of *Toxoplasma gondii* rhoptries. *Parasitology*, **102**, 367–70.

Frenkel, J. K. (1953). Host, strain and treatment variation as factors in the pathogenesis of toxoplasmosis. *American Journal of Tropical Medicine and Hygiene*, **2**, 390–415.

Frenkel, J. K. (1967). Adoptive immunity to intracellular infection. *Journal of Immunology*, **98**, 1309–19.

Frenkel, J. K. (1973). Toxoplasmosis: parasite life cycle, pathology and immunology. In *The Coccidia*, ed. D. M. Hammond & P. L. Long, pp. 344–410. Baltimore, MD: University Park Press.

Frenkel, J. K. (1990). Transmission of toxoplasmosis and the role of immunity in limiting transmission and illness. *Journal of the American Veterinary Medical Association*, **196**, 233–9.

Frenkel, J. K. & Escajadillo, A. (1987). Cyst rupture as a pathogenic mechanism of toxoplasmic encephalitis. *American Journal of Tropical Medicine and Hygiene*, 36, 517–22.

Frenkel, J. K. & Smith, D. D. (1982). Immunization of cats against shedding of *Toxoplasma* oocysts. *Journal of Parasitology*, 68, 744–8.

Frenkel, J. K., Dubey, J. P. & Miller, N. L. (1970). *Toxoplasma gondii*: Fecal stages identified as coccidian oocysts. *Science*, 167, 893–6.

Frenkel, J. K., Dubey, J. P. & Hoff, R. L. (1976). Loss of stages after continuous passage of *Toxoplasma gondii* and *Besoitia jellisoni*. *Journal of Protozoology*, 23, 421–4.

Freyre, A., Dubey, J. P., Smith, D. D. & Frenkel, J. K. (1989). Oocyst-induced *Toxoplasma gondii* infection in cats. *Journal of Parasitology*, 75, 750–5.

Fujii, H., Kamiyama, T. & Hagiwara, T. (1983). Species and strain differences in sensitivity to *Toxoplasma* infection among laboratory rodents. *Japanese Journal of Medical Science and Biology*, 36, 343–6.

Furtado, G. C., Slowik, M., Kleinman, H. K. & Joiner, K. A. (1992a). Laminin enhances binding of *Toxoplasma gondii* tachyzoites to J774 murine macrophage cells. *Infection and Immunity*, 60, 2337–42.

Furtado, G. C., Cao, T. & Joiner, K. A. (1992b). Laminin on tachyzoites of *Toxoplasma gondii* mediates parasite binding to the b1 integrin receptor ab6b1 on human foreskin fibroblasts and Chinese hamster ovary cells. *Infection and Immunity*, 60, 4925–31.

Gagnon, S., Sogin, M. L., Levesque, R. C. & Gajadhar, A. A. (1993). Molecular cloning, complete sequence of the small subunit ribosomal RNA coding region and phylogeny of *Toxoplasma gondii*. *Molecular and Biochemical Parasitology*, 60, 145–8.

Gallois, Y., Foussard, F., Girault, A., Hodbert, J., Tricaud, A., Mauras, G. & Motta, C. (1988). Membrane fluidity of *Toxoplasma gondii*: a fluorescence polarization study. *Biolology of the Cell*, 62, 11–15.

Gardner, I. D. & Remington, J. S. (1977). Age-related decline in the resistance of mice to infection with intracellular pathogens. *Infection and Immunity*, 16, 593–8.

Gazzinelli, R. T., Denkers, E. Y. & Sher, A. (1993). Host resistance to *Toxoplasma gondii*: model for studying the selective induction of cell-mediated immunity by intracellular parasites. *Infectious Agents and Disease*, 2, 139–49.

Grimwood, J. & Smith, J. E. (1992). *Toxoplasma gondii*: the role of a 30-kDa surface protein in host cell invasion. *Experimental Parasitology*, 74, 106–11.

Gross, U., Müller, W. A., Knapp, S. & Heesemann, J. (1991). Identification of a virulence-associated antigen of *Toxoplasma gondii* by use of a mouse monoclonal antibody. *Infection and Immunity*, 59, 4511–16.

Gross, U., Bohne, W., Soête, M. & Dubremetz, J. F. (1996). Developmental differentiation between tachyzoites and bradyzoites of *Toxoplasma gondii*. *Parasitology Today*, 12, 30–33.

Guay, J.-M., Huot, A., Gagnon, S., Tremblay, A. & Levesque, R. C. (1992). Physical and genetic mapping of cloned rDNA from *Toxoplasma gondii*: primary and secondary structure of the 5S gene. *Gene*, 114, 165–71.

Guay, J.-M., Dubois, D., Morency, M.-J., Gagnon, S., Mercier, J. & Levesque, R. C. (1993). Detection of the pathogenic parasite *Toxoplasma gondii* by specific amplification of ribosomal sequences using comultiplex polymerase chain reaction. *Journal of Clinical Microbiology*, **31**, 203–7.

Guo, Z.-G., Gross, U. & Johnson, A. M. (1997). *Toxoplasma gondii* virulence markers identified by random amplified polymorphic DNA polymerase chain reaction. *Parasitology Research*, **83**, 458–63.

Halonen, S. K. & Weidner, E. (1994). Overcoating of *Toxoplasma* parasitophorous vacuoles with host cell vimentin type intermediate filaments. *Journal of Eukaryote Microbiology*, **41**, 65–71.

Handman, E., Goding, J. W. & Remington, J. S. (1980). Detection and characterization of membrane antigens of *Toxoplasma gondii*. *Journal of Immunology*, **124**, 2578–83.

Hérion, P. & Saavedra, R. (1993). The immunobiology of toxoplasmosis. *Research in Immunology*, **144**, 7–79.

Hoff, R. L., Dubey, J. P., Bahbehani, A. M. & Frenkel, J. K. (1977). *Toxoplasma gondii* cysts in cell culture: new biologic evidence. *Journal of Parasitology*, **63**, 1121–4.

Hogan, M. J., Yoneda, C., Feeney, L., Zweigart, P. & Lewis, A. (1960). Morphology and culture of *Toxoplasma*. *Archives of Ophthalmology*, **64**, 655–67.

Howe, D. K. & Sibley, L. D. (1994). *Toxoplasma gondii*: analysis of different laboratory stocks of the RH strain reveals genetic heterogeneity. *Experimental Parasitology*, **78**, 242–5.

Hughes, H. P. A. (1981). Characterization of the circulating antigen of *Toxoplasma gondii*. *Immunology Letters*, **3**, 99–101.

Hughes, H. P. A., Hudson, L. & Fleck, D. G. (1986). *In vitro* culture of *Toxoplasma gondii* in primary and established cell lines. *International Journal of Parasitology*, **16**, 317–22.

Iltzsch, M. H. (1993). Pyrimidine salvage pathways in *Toxoplasma gondii*. *Journal of Eukaryotic Microbiology*, **40**, 24–8.

Jacobs, L. (1956). Propagation, morphology, and biology of *Toxoplasma*. *Annals of the New York Academy of Sciences*, **64**, 154–79.

Jacobs, L., Remington, J. S. & Melton, M. L. (1960). The resistance of the encysted form of *Toxoplasma gondii*. *Journal of Parasitology*, **46**, 11–21.

Jewell, M. L., Frenkel, J. K., Johnson, K. M., Reed, V. & Ruiz, A. (1972). Development of *Toxoplasma* oocysts in neotropical Felidae. *American Journal of Tropical Medicine and Hygiene*, **21**, 512–17.

Johnson, A. M. (1984). Strain-dependent, route of challenge-dependent, murine susceptibility to toxoplasmosis. *Zeitschift für Parasitenkunde*, **70**, 303–9.

Johnson, A. M. & Baverstock, P. R. (1989). Rapid ribosomal RNA sequencing and the phylogenetic analysis of protists. *Parasitology Today*, **5**, 102–5.

Johnson, A. M., McDonald, P. J. & Neoh, S. H. (1981). Molecular weight analysis of the major polypeptides and glycopeptides of *Toxoplasma gondii*. *Biochemical and Biophysics Research Communications*, **100**, 934–43.

Johnson, A. M., Dubey, J. P. & Dame, J. B. (1986). Purification and characterisation of *Toxoplasma gondii* tachyzoite DNA. *Australian Journal of Experimental Medicine and Science*, **64**, 351–5.

Johnson, L. L. (1992). SCID mouse models of acute and relapsing chronic *Toxoplasma gondii* infections. *Infection and Immunity*, **60**, 3719–24.

Joiner, K. A. (1991a). Rhoptry lipids and parasitophorous vacuole formation: a slippery issue. *Parasitology Today*, 7, 226–7.

Joiner, K. A. (1991b). Cell attachment and entry by *Toxoplasma gondii*. *Behring Institute Mitteilungen*, 88, 20–8.

Joiner, K. A. & Dubremetz, F. (1993). *Toxoplasma gondii*: a protozoan for the nineties. *Infection and Immunity*, 61, 1169–72.

Joiner, K. A., Furtado, G., Mellman, I., Kleinman, H., Mietinnen, H., Kasper, L. H., Hall, L. & Fuhrman, S. A. (1989). Cell attachment and invasion by tachyzoites of *Toxoplasma gondii*. *Journal of Cellullar Biochemistry*, 13E, 64.

Joiner, K. A., Fuhrman, S. A., Mietinnen, H., Kasper, L. L. & Mellman, I. (1990). *Toxoplasma gondii*: fusion competence of parasitophorous vacuoles in Fc receptor transfected fibroblasts. *Science*, 249, 641–6.

Jones, T. C. & Erb, P. (1985). H-2 complex-linked resistance in murine toxoplasmosis. *Journal of Infectious Diseases*, 151, 739–40.

Jones, T. C. & Hirsch, J. G. (1972). The interaction between *Toxoplasma gondii* and mammalian cells. II. The absence of lysosomal fusion with phagocytic vacuoles containing living parasites. *Journal of Experimental Medicine*, 136, 1173–94.

Jones, T. C., Yeh, S. & Hirsch, J. G. (1972). The interaction betwen *Toxoplasma gondii* and mammalian cells. I. Mechanism of entry and intracellular fate of the parasite. *Journal of Experimental Medicine*, 136, 1157–72.

Jones, T. C., Bienz, K. A. & Erb, P. (1986). *In vitro* cultivation of *Toxoplasma gondii* cysts in astrocytes in the presence of gamma interferon. *Infection and Immunity*, 51, 147–56.

Kasper, L. H. (1987). Isolation and characterisation of a monoclonal anti-P30 antibody resistant mutant of *Toxoplasma gondii*. *Parasite Immunology*, 9, 433–45.

Kasper, L. H. & Boothroyd, J. C. (1993). *Toxoplasma gondii*: immunology and molecular biology. In *Immunology of Parasitic Infections*, ed. K. S. Warren, pp. 269–84. Cambridge, MA: Blackwell.

Kasper, L. H. & Mineo, J. R. (1994). Attachment and invasion of host cells by *Toxoplasma gondii*. *Parasitology Today*, 10, 184–8.

Kasper, L. H. & Ware, P. L. (1985). Recognition and characterization of stage specific oocyst sporozoite antigens of *Toxoplasma gondii* by human antisera. *Journal of Clinical Investigation*, 75, 1570–7.

Kasper, L. H. & Ware, P. L. (1989). Identification of stage specific antigens of *Toxoplasma gondii*. *Infection and Immunity*, 57, 668–72.

Kasper, L. H., Crabb, J. H. & Pfefferkorn, E. R. (1983). Purification of a major membrane protein of *Toxoplasma gondii* by immunoabsorption with a monoclonal antibody. *Journal of Immunology*, 130, 2407–12.

Kasper, L. H., Bradley, M. S. & Pfefferkorn, E. R. (1984). Identification of stage-specific sporozoite antigens of *Toxoplasma gondii* by monoclonal antibodies. *Journal of Immunology*, 132, 443–9.

Kaufman, H. E., Melton, M. L., Remington, J. S. & Jacobs, L. (1959). Strain differences of *Toxoplasma gondii*. *Journal of Parasitology*, 45, 189–90.

Krug, E. C., Marr, J. J. & Berens, R. L. (1989). Purine metabolism in *Toxoplasma gondii*. *Journal of Biology and Chemistry*, 264, 10601–7.

Lainson, R. (1955). Toxoplasmosis in England II. Variation factors in the pathogenesis of *Toxoplasma* infections: the sudden increase in virulence of a strain after passage in multi-mammate rats and canaries. *Annals of Tropical Medicine and Parasitology*, 49, 397–416.

Lecomte, V., Chumpitazi, B. F. F., Pasquier, B., Ambroise-Thomas, P. & Santoro, F. (1992). Brain-tissue cysts in rats infected with the RH strain of *Toxoplasma gondii*. *Parasitology Research*, 78, 267–9.

Lecordier, L., Mercier C., Torpier, G., Tourville, B., Darcy, F., Liu, J. L., Maes, P., Tartar, A., Capron, A. & Cesbron-Delauw, M. F. (1993). Molecular structure of a *Toxoplasma gondii* dense granule antigen (GRA5) associated with the parasitophorous vacuole membrane. *Molecular and Biochemical Parasitology*, 59, 143–54.

Lecordier, L., Moleon-Borodowski, I., Dubremetz, J. F., Tourvieille, B., Mercier, C., Deslée, D. & Capron, A. (1995). Characterisation of a dense granule antigen of *Toxoplasma gondii* (GRA6) associated to the network of the parasitophorous vacuole. *Molecular and Biochemical Parasitology*, 70, 85–94.

Leriche, M. A. & Dubremetz, J. F. (1990). Exocytosis of *Toxoplasma gondii* dense granules into the parasitophorous vacuole after host-cell invasion. *Parasitology Research*, 76, 559–62.

Leriche, M. A. & Dubremetz, J. F. (1991). Characterisation of the protein contents of rhoptries and dense granules of *Toxoplasma gondii* tachyzoites by subcellular fractionation and mono-clonal antibodies. *Molecular and Biochemical Parasitology*, 45, 249–60.

Lindsay, D. S., Dubey, J. P., Blagburn, B. L. & Toivio-Kinnucan, M. A. (1991). Examination of tisue cyst formation by *Toxoplasma gondii* in cell cultures using bradyzoites, tachyzoites and sporozoites. *Journal of Parasitology*, 77, 126–32.

Lindsay, D. S., Toivio-Kinnucan, M. A. & Blagburn, B. L. (1993). Ultrastructural determination of cytogenesis by various *Toxoplasma gondii* isolates in cell culture. *Journal of Parasitology*, 79, 289–92.

Lycke, N. & Norrby, R. (1966). Demonstration of a factor of *Toxoplasma gondii* enhancing the penetration of *Toxoplasma* parasites into cultured host cells. *British Journal of Experimental Pathology*, 47, 248–56.

Lyons, R. E. & Johnson, A. M. (1995). Heat shock proteins of *Toxoplasma gondii*. *Parasite Immunology*, 17, 353–9.

Makioka, A. & Ohtomo, H. (1995). An increased DNA polymerase activity associated with viru-lence of *Toxoplasma gondii*. *Journal of Parasitology*, 81, 1021–2.

Manafi, M., Hassl, A., Sommer, R. & Aspöck, H. (1993). Enzymatic profile of *Toxoplasma gondii*. *Letters in Applied Microbiology*, 16, 66–8.

Matsubayashi, H. & Akao, S. (1963). Morphological studies on the development of the *Toxoplasma* cyst. *American Journal of Tropical Medicine and Hygiene*, 12, 321–33.

Mauras, G., Dodeur, M., Laget, P., Senet, J. M. & Bourrillon, R. (1980). Partial resolution of the sugar content of *Toxoplasma gondii* membrane. *Biochemical and Biophysical Research Communications*, 97, 906–12.

McHugh, T. D., Holliman, R. E. & Butcher, P. D. (1994). The *in vitro* model of tissue cyst forma-tion in *Toxoplasma gondii*. *Parasitology Today*, 10, 281–5.

McLeod, R., Estes, R. G., Mack, D. G. & Cohen, H. (1984). Immune response to mice ingested *Toxoplasma gondii*. *Journal of Infectious Diseases*, 149, 234–44.

McLeod, R., Skamene, E., Brown, C. R., Eisenhauer, P. B. & Mack, D. G. (1989). Genetic regulation of early survival and cyst number after peroral *Toxoplasma gondii* infection of AXB/BXA recombinant inbred and B10 congenic mice. *Journal of Immunology*, **143**, 3031–4.

McLeod, R., Mack, D. & Brown, C. (1991). *Toxoplasma gondii* – new advances in cellular and molecular biology. *Experimental Parasitology*, **72**, 109–21.

Mehlhorn, H. & Frenkel, J. K. (1980). Ultrastructural comparison of cysts and zoites of *Toxoplasma gondii*, *Sarcocystis muris* and *Hammondia hammondi* in skeletal muscle of mice. *Journal of Parasitology*, **66**, 59–67.

Mercier, C., Lecordier, L., Darcy, F., Deslée, D., Murray, A., Tourvieille, B., Maes, P., Capron, A. & Cesbron-Delauw, M. F. (1993). Molecular characterization of a dense granule antigen (GRA2) associated with the network of the parasitophorous vacuole in *Toxoplasma gondii*. *Molecular and Biochemical Parasitology*, **58**, 71–82.

Metsis, A., Pettersen, E. & Petersen, E. (1995). *Toxoplasma gondii*: characterization of a monoclonal antibody recognising antigens of 36 and 38 kDa with acid phosphatase activity located in dense granules and rhoptries. *Experimental Parasitology*, **81**, 472–9.

Michel, R., Schupp, K., Raether, W. & Bierther, F. W. (1980). Formation of close junction during invasion of erythrocytes by *Toxoplasma gondii in vitro*. *International Journal of Parasitology*, **10**, 309–13.

Mineo, J. R., McLeod, R., Mack, D., Smith, J., Khan, I. A., Ely, K. H. & Kasper, L. H. (1993). Antibodies to *Toxoplasma gondii* major surface protein (SAG–1, P30) inhibit infection of host cells are produced in murine intestine after peroral infection. *Journal of Immunology*, **150**, 3951–64.

Nagel, S. D. & Boothroyd, J. C. (1988). The α- and β-tubulins of *Toxoplasma gondii* are encoded by single copy genes containing multiple introns. *Molecular and Biochemical Parasitology*, **29**, 261–73.

Nagel, S. D. & Boothroyd, J. C. (1989). The major surface antigen, P30, of *Toxoplasma gondii* is anchored by a glycolipid. *Journal of Biological Chemistry*, **264**, 5569–74.

Naot, Y., Guptill, D., Mullenax, J. & Remington, J. S. (1983). Characterization of *Toxoplasma gondii* antigens which react with IgM and IgG antibodies. *Infection and Immunity*, **41**, 331–8.

Nichols, B. A. & Chiappino, M. L. (1987). Cytoskeleton of *Toxoplasma gondii*. *Journal of Protozoology*, **34**, 217–26.

Nichols, B. A., Chiappino, M. L. & O'Connor, G. R. (1983). Secretion from the rhoptries of *Toxoplasma gondii* during host-cell invasion. *Journal of Ultrastructural Research*, **83**, 85–98.

Nichols, B. A., Chiappino, M. L. & Pavesio, C. E. N. (1994). Endocytosis at the microphore of *Toxoplasma gondii*. *Parasitology Research*, **80**, 91–8.

Nicolle, C. & Manceaux, L. (1908). Sur une infection a corps de *Leishman* (ou organismes voisins) du gondi. *Cahiers Recherche de la Herbdomaire Séances Academie Science*, **147**, 763–6.

Nicolle, C. & Manceaux, L. (1909). Sur un protozonim nouveau du gondi. *Cahiers Recherche de la Herbdomaire Séances Academie Science*, **148**, 369–72.

Ödberg–Ferragut, C., Soête, M., Engels, A., Samyn, B., Loyens, A., Beeumen, J. van, Camus, D. & Dubremetz, J. –F. (1996). Molecular cloning of the *Toxoplasma gondi* sag4 gene encoding an 18 kDa bradyzoite specific surface protein. *Molecular and Biochemical Parasitology*, **82**, 237–244.

Ossorio, P. N., Sibley, L. D. & Boothroyd, J. C. (1991). Mitochondrial-like DNA sequences flanked by direct and inverted repeats in the nuclear genome of *Toxoplasma gondii*. *Journal of Molecular Biology*, **222**, 525–36.

Ossorio, P. N., Schwartzman, J. D. & Boothroyd, J. C. (1992). A *Toxoplasma gondii* rhoptry protein associated with host cell penetration has unusual charge assymetry. *Molecular and Biochemical Parasitolology*, **50**, 1–16.

Ossorio, P. N., Dubremetz, J.-F. & Joiner, K. A. (1994). A soluble secretory protein of the intracellular parasite *Toxoplasma gondii* associates with the parasotophorous vacuole membrane through hydrophobic interactions. *Journal of Biological Chemistry*, **269**, 15350–7.

Parmley, S. F., Weiss, L. M. & Yang, S. (1995). Cloning of a bradyzoite-specific gene of *Toxoplasma gondii* encoding a cytoplasmatic antigen. *Molecular and Biochemical Parasitology*, **73**, 253–7.

Pavesio, C. E. N., Chiappino, M. L., Setzer, P. Y. & Nichols, B. A. (1992). *Toxoplasma gondii*: differentiation and death of bradyzoites. *Parasitology Research*, **78**, 1–9.

Pfefferkorn, E. R. (1978). *Toxoplasma gondii*: the enzymatic defect of a mutant resistant to 5-fluorodeoxyuridine. *Experimental Parasitology*, **44**, 26–35.

Pfefferkorn, E. R. (1990). The cell biology of *Toxoplasma gondii*. In *Modern Parasite Biology: Cellular Immunological and Molecular Aspects*, ed. D. J. Wyler, pp. 26–50. New York: Freeman.

Pfefferkorn, E. R. & Pfefferkorn, L. C. (1977). Specific labeling of intracellular *Toxoplasma gondii* with uracil. *Journal of Protozoology*, **24**, 449–53.

Pfefferkorn, L. C. & Pfefferkorn, E. R. (1980). *Toxoplasma gondii*: genetic recombination between drug resistant mutants. *Experimental Parasitology*, **50**, 305–16.

Pfefferkorn, E. R., Pfefferkorn, L. C. & Colby, E. D. (1977). Development of gametes and oocysts in cats fed cysts derived from cloned trophozoites of *Toxoplasma gondii*. *Journal of Parasitology*, **63**, 158–9.

Piekarski, G., Pelster, B. & Witte, H. M. (1971). Endopolygenie bei *Toxoplasma gondii*. *Zeitschrift für Parasitenkunde*, **36**, 122–30.

Prince, J. B., Auer, K. L., Huskinson, J., Parmley, S. F., Araujo, F. G. & Remington, J. S. (1990). Cloning, expression, and cDNA sequence of surface antigen p22 from *Toxoplasma gondii*. *Molecular and Biochemical Parasitology*, **43**, 97–106.

Reikvam, A. & Lorentzen-Styr, A. M. (1976). Virulence of different strains of *Toxoplasma gondii* and host response in mice. *Nature*, **261**, 508–9.

Remington, J. S. (1970). Toxoplasmosis: recent developments. *Annual Review of Medicine*, **21**, 201–18.

Remington, J. S., Jacobs, L. & Kaufman, H. E. (1958). Studies on chronic toxoplasmosis. *American Journal of Ophthalmology*, **46**, 261–8.

Robert, R., Leynia de la Jarrige, P., Mahaza, C., Cottin, J., Marot-Leblond, A. & Senet, J.-M. (1991). Specific binding of neoglycoproteins to *Toxoplasma gondii* tachyzoites. *Infection and Immunity*, **59**, 4670–3.

Roos, D. S. (1993). Primary structure of the dihydrofolate reductase-thymidylate synthase gene from *Toxoplasma gondii*. *Journal of Biological Chemistry*, **268**, 6269–80.

Saavedra, R., Meuter, F. de, Decourt, J. L. & Hérion, P. (1991). Human T-cell clone identifies a potentially protective 54-kDa protein antigen of *Toxoplasma gondii* cloned and expressed in *Escherichia coli*. *Journal of Immunology*, **147**, 1975–82.

Sabin, A. B. (1941). Toxoplasmic encephalitis in children. *Journal of the American Medical Association*, 116, 801–7.

Sadak, A., Taghy, Z., Fortier, B. & Dubremetz, J. F. (1988). Characterization of a family of rhoptry proteins of *Toxoplasma gondii*. *Molecular and Biochemical Parasitology*, 29, 203–11.

Saffer, L. D. & Schwartzman, J. D. (1991). A soluble phospholipase of *Toxoplasma gondii* associated with host cell penetration. *Journal of Protozoology*, 38, 454–60.

Saffer, L. D., Long Krug, S. A. & Schwartzman, J. D. (1989). The role of phospholipase in host cell penetration by *Toxoplasma gondii*. *American Journal of Tropical Medicine and Hygiene*, 40, 145–9.

Santoro, F., Charif, H. & Capron, A. (1986). The immunodominant epitope of the major membrane tachyzoite protein (p30) of *Toxoplasma gondii*. *Parasite Immunology*, 8, 631–9.

Schoondermark, E. Van de Ven, Melchers, W., Galama, J., Camps, W., Eskes, T. & Meuwissen, J. (1993). Congenital toxoplasmosis: an experimental study in rhesus monkeys for transmission and prenatal diagnosis. *Experimental Parasitology*, 77, 200–11.

Schwartz, R. T. & Tomavo, S. (1993). The current status of the glycobiology of *Toxoplasma gondii*: glycosylphosphatidylinositols, *N*- and *O*-linked glycans. *Research in Immunology*, 144, 24–31.

Schwartzman, J. D. (1986). Inhibition of a penetration-enhancing factor of *Toxoplasma gondii* by monoclonal antibodies specific for rhoptries. *Infection and Immunity*, 51, 760–4.

Schwartzman, J. D. & Krug, E. C. (1989). *Toxoplasma gondii*: characterization of monoclonal antibodies that recognize rhoptries. *Experimental Parasitology*, 68, 74–82.

Schwartzman, J. D. & Pfefferkorn, E. R. (1982). *Toxoplasma gondii*: purine synthesis and salvage in mutant host cells and parasites. *Experimental Parasitology*, 53, 77–86.

Schwartzman, J. D. & Pfefferkorn, E. R. (1983). Immunofluorescent localization of myosin at the anterior pole of the coccidian *Toxoplasma gondii*. *Journal of Protozoology*, 30, 657–61.

Schwartzman, J. D. & Saffer, L. D. (1992). How *Toxoplasma gondii* gets into and out of host cells. In *Subcellular Biochemistry, Intracellular Parasites*, vol. 18, ed. J. L. Avila, J. R. Harris, pp. 333–64. New York: Plenum Press.

Sheffield, H. G. (1970). Schizogony in *Toxoplasma gondii*: an electronmicroscopic study. *Proceedings of the Helminthological Society of Washington*, 37, 237–42.

Sheffield, H. G. & Melton, M. L. (1968). The fine structure and reproduction of *Toxoplasma gondii*. *Journal of Parasitology*, 54, 209–26.

Shimada, K., O'Connor, G. R. & Yoneda, C. (1974). Cyst formation by *Toxoplasma gondii* (RH strain) *in vitro*. *Archives of Ophthalmology*, 92, 496–500.

Sibley, L. D. & Boothroyd, J. C. (1992a). Construction of a molecular karyotype for *Toxoplasma gondii*. *Molecular and Biochemical Parasitology*, 51, 291–300.

Sibley, L. D. & Boothroyd, J. C. (1992b). Virulent strains of *Toxoplasma gondii* comprise a single clonal lineage. *Nature*, 359, 82–5.

Sibley, L. D. & Krahenbuhl, J. L. (1988). Modification of host cell phagosomes by *Toxoplasma gondii* involves redistribution of surface proteins and secretion of a 32 kDa protein. *European Journal of Cell Biology*, 47, 81–7.

Sibley, L. D., Weidner, E. & Krahenbuhl, J. L. (1985). Phagosome acidification blocked by intracellular *Toxoplasma gondii*. *Nature*, 315, 416–19.

Sibley, L. D., Pfefferkorn, E. R. & Boothroyd, J. C. (1991). Proposal for a uniform genetic nomenclature in *Toxoplasma gondii*. *Parasitolology Today*, **7**, 327–8.

Sibley, L. D., Niesman, I. R., Parmley, S. F. & Cesbron-Delauw, M.-F. (1995). Regulated secretion of multi-lamellar vesicles leads to formation of a tubulo–vesicular network in host-cell vacuoles occupied by *Toxoplasma gondii*. *Journal of Cell Sciences*, **108**, 1669–77.

Sims, T. A., Hay, T. & Talbot, I. C. (1988). Host–parasite relationship in the brains of mice with congenital toxoplasmosis. *Journal of Pathology*, **156**, 255–61.

Soete, M., Fortier, D., Camus, D. & Dubremetz, J. F. (1993). *Toxoplasma gondii*: kinetics of bradyzoite tachyzoite interconversion *in vitro*. *Experimental Parasitology*, **76**, 259–64.

Soete, M., Camus, D. & Dubremetz, J.-F. (1994). Experimental induction of bradyzoite-specific antigen expression and cyst formation by the RH strain of *Toxoplasma gondii* in vitro. *Experimental Parasitology*, **78**, 361–70.

Speer, C. A. & Dubey, J. P. (1998). Ultrastructure of early stages of infection in mice fed *Toxoplasma gondii* oocysts. *Parasitology*, **116**, 35–42.

Splendore, A. (1908). Un nuovo protoaoz parassita de' conigli incontrato nelle lesioni anatomiche d'une malattia che ricorda in molti punti il Kala–azar dell'uomo. Nota prelininaire pel. *Revista Sociale Science de Sao Paulo*, **3**, 109–12.

Sulzer, A. J., Strobel, P. L., Springer, E. L., Roth, I. L. & Callaway, C. S. (1974). A comparative electron microscopic study of the morphology of *Toxoplasma gondii* by freeze-etch replication and thin sectioning technique. *Journal of Protozoology*, **21**, 710–14.

Suzuki, Y. & Remington, J. S. (1994). MHC class I gene(s) in the D/L region but not the TNF-alpha gene determines development of toxoplasmic encephalitis in mice. *Journal of Immunology*, **153**, 4649–54.

Suzuki, Y., Conley, F. K. & Remington, J. S. (1989). Differences in virulence and development of encephalitis during chronic infection vary with strain of *Toxoplasma gondii*. *Journal of Infectious Diseases*, **159**, 790–4.

Suzuki, Y., Orellana, M. A., Wong, S.-Y., Conley, F. K. & Remington, J. S. (1993). Susceptibility to chronic infection with *Toxoplasma gondii* does not correlate with susceptibility to acute infection in mice. *Infection and Immunity*, **61**, 2284–8.

Tomavo, S., Schwartz, R. T. & Dubremetz, J. F. (1989). Evidence for glycosyl-phosphatidylinositol anchoring of *Toxoplasma gondii* major surface antigens. *Molecular and Cellular Biology*, **9**, 4576–80.

Tomavo, S., Fortier, B., Soete, M., Ansel, C., Camus, D. & Dubremetz, J. F. (1991). Characterization of bradyzoite-specific antigens of *Toxoplasma gondii*. *Infection and Immunity*, **59**, 3750–3.

Wang, C. C. (1982). Biochemistry and physiology of coccidia. In *Biology of the Coccidia*, ed. P. L. Long, pp. 167–228, Baltimore, MD: University Park Press.

Ware, P. L. & Kasper, L. H. (1987). Strain-specific antigens of *Toxoplasma gondii*. *Infection and Immunity*, **55**, 778–83.

Weiss, L. M., Udem, S. A., Tanowitz, H. & Wittner, M. (1988). Western blot analysis of the antibody response of patients with AIDS and toxoplasma encephalitis: antigenic diversity among *Toxoplasma* strains. *Journal of Infectious Diseases*, **157**, 7–13.

Werk, R. (1985). How does *Toxoplasma gondii* enter host cells? *Review of Infectious Diseases*, 7, 449–57.

Williams, D. M., Grumet, F. C. & Remington, J. S. (1978). Genetic control of murine resistance to *Toxoplasma gondii*. *Infection and Immunity*, 19, 416–20.

Windeck, T. & Gross, U. (1996). *Toxoplasma gondii* strain–specific transcript levels of SAG1 and their association with virulence. *Parasitology Research*, 82, 715–19.

Woodison, G. & Smith, J. E. (1990). Identification of the dominant cyst antigens of *Toxoplasma gondii*. *Parasitology*, 100, 389–92.

Yano, K. & Nakabayashi, T. (1986). Attenuation of the virulent RH strain of *Toxoplasma gondii* by passages in mice immunized with *Toxoplasma* lysate. *Biken Journal*, 29, 31–7.

Immunology of toxoplasma infection

C. A. Hunter[1] and G. Reichmann[2]

[1] Department of Pathobiology, University of Pennsylvania, Philadelphia, USA
[2] Institute for Medical Microbiology and Virology, Heinrich-Heine University, Dusseldorf, Germany

Pathogenesis of toxoplasmosis

The infection of immunocompetent individuals with *Toxoplasma gondii* most often results in an asymptomatic infection or occasionally in an infectious mononucleo-sis-type illness (Luft & Remington 1988). However, clinical toxoplasmosis is frequently associated with immune-deficient individuals and maternal–foetal transmission of this parasite causes congenital disease (Remington et al. 1994). In order to appreciate the disease caused by *T. gondii* it is important to have an understanding of the basic biology of this infection and how protective immunity to this parasite is mediated. The ability of the tachyzoite stage of the parasite to invade any nucleated cell, replicate and then lyse the host cell before invading neighbouring cells is an important element that underlies the pathogenesis of this cytolytic infection. In the absence of a protective immune response, the parasite will replicate in an unrestricted manner and destroy infected tissues. Moreover, since the tachyzoite stage of the parasite is intracellular, it is protected from the effects of the humoral immune response. As a consequence, the protective response needed to control this parasite is dominated by cell-mediated immunity, and in particular the production of the cytokine interferon-γ (IFN-γ). The events that lead to the production of IFN-γ and its protective effects are discussed in greater detail below.

The presence of a 'latent' stage of *T. gondii* in the infected host also represents an important aspect of toxoplasmosis. Tachyzoites can transform into bradyzoites which are found within cysts in many tissues, but in particular the brain and muscle. Unlike tachyzoites, bradyzoites are a slow-growing, inactive developmental stage, which fail to provoke an inflammatory response. The persistent nature of the cyst stage ensures that individuals remain infected for life. The biology of toxoplasmosis is further complicated because bradyzoites can transform back into tachyzoites which, in the absence of an appropriate immune response, will replicate and lyse infected cells resulting in the development of disease. However, in

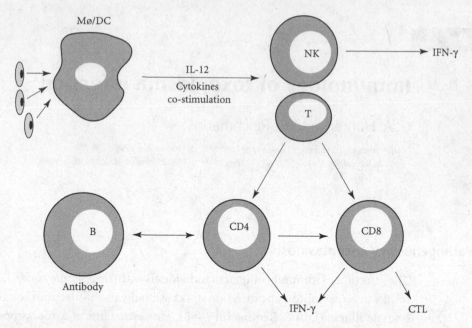

Figure 2.1   Development of the immune response to *Toxoplasma gondii*. Infection with *T. gondii* leads to the production of interleukin-12 (IL-12) by macrophages (Mφ) and/or dendritic cells (DC). These cells also present parasite antigens and provide co-stimulatory signals and other proinflammatory cytokines required for optimal T-cell and natural killer (NK) cell responses. Together, these events lead to the production of interferon-γ (IFN-γ) by NK cells and directs the development of CD4$^+$ and CD8$^+$ T-cells into TH1 cells which produce IFN-γ. CD4$^+$ T-cells provide help for maximal CD8$^+$ T-cells responses as well as for the maturation of B-cell responses. CTL, Cytotoxic lymphocytes.

most individuals there is a protective immune response, which deals with reactivation and this chronic infection normally remains asymptomatic.

Protective immunity to *Toxoplasma gondii*

Development of T-cell responses

As a consequence of the intracellular nature of this parasite, protective immunity to *T. gondii* is characterized by the development of a cell-mediated immune response dominated by the production of IFN-γ by T-cells (a THI-type response). The events that lead to the development of protective T-cell responses are based on the innate ability of accessory cells, such as macrophages and dendritic cells, to present antigen, provide co-stimulation and produce cytokines (see Figure 2.1). Interleukin-12 (IL-12) is produced by accessory cells and is the major factor involved in the differentiation of T-cells into antigen-specific cells which secrete IFN-γ (Hsieh et al. 1993). Following infection with *T. gondii* high levels of IL-12 are produced but the initial cellular source of this cytokine following infection remains unclear. Early reports identified macrophages as the main source of IL-12 (Gazzinelli et al. 1993*c*) and subsequent studies have suggested that dendritic cells (Reis e Sousa et al. 1997) and neutrophils produce IL-12 during toxoplasmosis (Denkers & Marshall 1998). Nevertheless, the production of IL-12 after infection is critical for the development of protective immunity. This is best illustrated by studies which showed that in the absence of IL-12 mice fail to develop protective T-cell responses and die as a consequence of an overwhelming parasitaemia (Khan et al. 1994; Scharton-Kersten et al. 1997). Interestingly, IL-12 is only required at the start of infection for the generation of antigen-specific T-cell responses. However, once antigen-specific T-cells have been generated their production of IFN-γ is independent of IL-12 (Gazzinelli et al. 1994; Khan et al. 1994).

Although IL-12 is a dominant cytokine in the generation of an adaptive immune response, additional factors also have a role in directing the development of T-cell responses. In particular, tumour necrosis factor-α (TNF-α) and IL-1 augment the development of THI-type responses (Shibuya et al. 1998) and these cytokines have been associated with resistance to *T. gondii* (Chang et al. 1990; Johnson 1992*a*; Hunter et al. 1995). However, these cytokines also have a role in the activation of antiparasite effector mechanisms. Other factors that have an important role in T-cell activation are the co-stimulatory CD28 and B7 molecules. The interaction of CD28 on T-cells with B7, present on accessory cells, is one of the most important second signals that regulates T-cell activation. The function of this interaction is to lower the threshold of T-cell activation (Viola & Lanzavecchia 1996) and it is important in enhancing cytokine production, preventing the development of anergy and protecting against apoptosis (Bluestone 1995; Green et al. 1995; Sharpe 1995). The role of the CD28/B7 interaction in the activation of T-cell responses during toxoplasmosis is unclear. One study which has addressed this question demonstrated that, in humans serologically negative for *T. gondii* infection of their monocytes, *T. gondii* resulted in increased expression of B7 and that this was required for the ability of T-cells to proliferate and produce IFN-γ in response to *T. gondii* (Subauste et al. 1998).

The critical role of T-cells in resistance to *T. gondii* is perhaps best illustrated by the patients who are susceptible to toxoplasmosis. However, studies with murine models of toxoplasmosis have also allowed an experimental approach to define the role of T-cells in resistance to *T. gondii*. Both CD4$^+$ and CD8$^+$ T-cell subsets mediate protective immunity (Gazzinelli et al. 1991; Parker et al. 1991; Beaman et al. 1994) and this protective activity depends on the ability of T-cells to produce IFN-γ (Suzuki & Remington 1990). Although both T-cell subsets are important sources of IFN-γ, optimal protective CD8$^+$ T-cell responses depend on the ability of CD4$^+$ T-cells to provide the growth factor IL-2 (Gazzinelli et al. 1992). $\gamma\delta$ T-cells, which are found at mucosal sites, have also been shown to have a role in resistance to *T. gondii* (Johnson et al. 1993; Hisaeda et al. 1995). The ability of naive $\gamma\delta$ T-cells to respond to infected cells and produce IFN-γ may represent a first line of defence against *T. gondii* (Subauste et al. 1995).

Many studies have shown that the protective activity of T-cells is mediated through production of IFN-γ but other T-cell functions could contribute to resistance to *T. gondii*. Since *T. gondii* is intracellular, the ability of T-cells to lyse infected cells may play a role in controlling parasite replication. For example, mouse CD8$^+$ T-cells, human CD4$^+$ T-cell clones and human lymphokine activated killer (LAK) cells are capable of lysing cells infected with *T. gondii* (Khan et al. 1990; Hakim et al. 1991; Subauste et al. 1991, 1992; Curiel et al. 1993). Additional studies with mice that lack perforin-dependent cytolytic activity have shown that they have an increased susceptibility to the chronic stage of infection, supporting a role for cytotoxic activity in the control of *T. gondii* (Denkers et al. 1997).

The same events that lead to the production of IL-12 are also critical for activating natural killer (NK) cells to produce IFN-γ, which represents an innate mechanism of resistance prior to development of adaptive T-cell responses (Figure 2.1) (Gazzinelli et al. 1993c; Hunter et al. 1994). Although IL-12 directly activates NK cells to produce IFN-γ, optimal NK cell responses are only observed in the presence of other cytokines such as TNF-α and IL-1 (Sher et al. 1993; Hunter et al. 1994, 1995). In addition, the CD28/B7 interaction has also been shown to have a role in enhancing NK cell responses during toxoplasmosis (Hunter et al. 1997). Thus, although NK cell responses are traditionally regarded as being a primitive arm of the immune response to infection, it is clear that there are complex regulatory processes that control NK cell activity during infection.

Role of IFN-γ in resistance to *T. gondii*

The protective effects of IFN-γ in resistance to toxoplasmosis appear to be primarily due to its ability to activate macrophages to inhibit the replication of *T. gondii*. Indeed, macrophages from mice infected with *T. gondii* inhibit parasite replication more efficiently than do those from uninfected animals, and this depends on endogenous IFN-γ (Black et al. 1987; Suzuki et al. 1989). TNF-α is a co-factor that is important in IFN-γ's ability to activate macrophages to be microbiostatic. Together, these cytokines upregulate the levels of inducible nitric oxide synthase (iNOS). iNOS is required for macrophage production of reactive nitrogen intermediates (RNI) which inhibit parasite replication (Sibley et al. 1991; Langermans et al. 1992). However, the role of RNI in resistance to *T. gondii* has been questioned by studies in which mice which lack iNOS were shown to be resistant to acute toxoplasmosis (Khan et al. 1996; Scharton-Kersten et al. 1997). Other studies have indicated a role for 5-lipoxygenase arachidonic acid products in human macrophage IFN-γ-induced antitoxoplasma activity (Yong et al. 1994). Moreover, since *T. gondii* can invade nonphagocytic cells, the ability of IFN-γ to activate indolamine dioxygenase and starve parasites of the essential amino acid tryptophan may represent an important mechanism for controlling parasite replication (Pfefferkorn 1984; Nagineni et al. 1996).

Humoral immune response

The induction of a strong cell-mediated immune response is also accompanied by the development of high levels of circulating specific antibody. Early after infection there are high levels of low-affinity circulating IgG. As the B-cell response develops there is affinity maturation, isotype switching occurs and high levels of high avidity IgG can be detected in the serum. The role of antibody in resistance to *T. gondii* is unclear. While the intracellular nature of this infection ensures that the parasite is protected from the effects of antibody, tachyzoites will be exposed to antibody when they lyse their host cell and before they invade a new host cell. At this point antibody may play a role in the killing of parasites, either by activating complement, leading to lysis of the parasite, or opsonizing the parasite for phagocytosis and killing by macrophages (Sibley et al. 1985).

Although levels of antibody fall after the immune response controls the parasite, they remain elevated for the life of the host. The continued presence of cysts and occasional release of tachyzoites may lead to chronic stimulation of the immune response and the maintenance of detectable antibody levels that are characteristic of the latent stage of infection. The antibody responses (rising IgG and the presence of IgM specific for *T. gondii*) allow the identification of individuals who have been exposed to *T. gondii* and can be used to distinguish whether an individual has a recently acquired infection or is latently infected (see Chapter 12).

Toxoplasmosis in the immunocompromised host

Congenital toxoplasmosis

Congenital toxoplasmosis with its associated sequelae continues to be one of the most serious complications associated with this infection (Remington et al. 1994). Congenital disease can occur when a woman becomes infected for the first time during pregnancy. Unlike individuals already infected with *T. gondii* and who have controlled the infection, susceptible women need time to mount a protective primary response. During this period the parasite can disseminate throughout the body, cross the placenta and infect the developing foetus. Since pregnancy is associated with suppression of the immune response, pregnancy may represent an immunocompromised state which allows the parasite more opportunity to disseminate and increase the likelihood of transmission to the foetus.

Congenital disease can be so devastating because of the immunological status of the foetus. If the parasite is transmitted to the foetus during the first trimester, the immune system is poorly developed and the parasite has the opportunity to cause substantial disease. Should the parasite be transmitted during the second or third trimester, the foetal immune system is better developed and can cope more efficiently with this infection and so disease is more likely to be subclinical. Interestingly, transmission is most frequent during the later stages of pregnancy (Remington et al. 1994). This may be a consequence of the time course of placental development and the increased blood supply to the foetus during the later stages of pregnancy, making infection more likely.

The exposure of the foetal immune system to *T. gondii* has long-lasting consequences which have been associated with the occurrence of toxoplasma-induced chorioretinitis in adults who have been affected by congenital toxoplasmosis (Remington et al. 1994). A possible explanation for this observation is that exposure of the developing immune system to *T. gondii* may result in tolerance of T-cells for parasite antigens. This would lead to an inability to deal efficiently with this infection and result in disease later in life. This is supported by studies in which infants with severe congenital disease were shown to have suppressed cellular responses to *T. gondii* (McLeod et al. 1990).

Toxoplasmosis and acquired immunodeficiencies

In recent years the importance of toxoplasmosis in patients with defects in T-cell function has been recognized. Patients with Hodgkin's and nonHodgkin's lymphoma as well as other neoplastic conditions or patients on immunosuppressive therapy (see Chapter 6) are at risk of reactivation of this infection (Britt et al. 1981; Israelski & Remington 1993; Wong & Remington 1993; Slavin et al. 1994). In addition, the incidence of toxoplasmosis in patients has risen dramatically with the increasing population of patients with acquired immunodeficiency syndrome (AIDS) (Israelski & Remington 1992). The close association of T-cell function with resistance to *T. gondii* is perhaps best evidenced by the correlation between the fall in T-cell numbers and the development of toxoplasmic encephalitis in AIDS patients. At the time they present with clinical toxoplasmic encephalitis, such patients almost invariably have CD4$^+$ T-cell counts that have fallen from 800–1200/mm^3 to less than 100/mm^3 with a corresponding reduction in CD8$^+$ T-cell numbers (Israelski & Remington 1992).

Serological evidence indicates that almost all AIDS patients who develop toxoplasmic encephalitis do so as a consequence of reactivation of a latent infection rather than a recently acquired infection (Israelski & Remington 1992). While it has been proposed that disruption of toxoplasma cysts occurs continually in infected individuals, it appears that active toxoplasmosis develops only in immunocompromised individuals (Luft & Remington 1988). This indicates that in immunocompetent individuals there is some form of protective immune response directed against the cyst stage or any bradyzoites/tachyzoites that result from 'leakage' from the cyst or from cyst lysis in the brain. However, in immunocompromised patients these mechanisms are impaired.

Several studies have suggested that there is a synergistic interaction between human immunodeficiency virus (HIV) and *T. gondii* that eventually causes the clinical disease. Infection of macrophages with HIV inhibits the ability of those cells to kill *T. gondii* (Biggs et al. 1995) and monocytes from patients with AIDS are reported to have a reduced ability to kill *T. gondii* (Delemarre et al. 1995). Moreover, peripheral blood mononuclear cells (PBMCs) from patients infected with HIV produce reduced levels of IL-12 and IFN-γ in response to *T. gondii* (Gazzinelli et al. 1995). Thus, infection with HIV compromises the events that lead to resistance to *T. gondii*. In studies directly investigating the interaction between *T. gondii* and HIV, Gazzinelli and colleagues found that *T. gondii* infection of a murine model of HIV gene expression resulted in increased levels of HIV-1 transcripts (Gazzinelli et al. 1996). Thus, the ability of HIV to weaken T-cell-mediated immunity may lead to the reactivation of cysts and the release of tachyzoites. These events would result in further activation of the immune system, a consequence of which is increased viral gene expression. Thus, a vicious cycle would develop in which the immune system is further weakened leading to the development of toxoplasmosis.

Toxoplasmic encephalitis

The brain and toxoplasmosis

In immunocompromised patients, as well as infants suffering from congenital disease, toxoplasmic encephalitis is probably the most common manifestation of disease. The brain is one of the anatomical sites in which cysts persist in greatest numbers and their reactivation and release of tachyzoites can cause severe local disease. This is probably a consequence of the immune-privileged nature of the brain. The lack of immune reactivity at this site is attributed to the presence of the blood–brain barrier which restricts the access of a number of important elements of the immune system (antibodies, cytokines) to the brain (Cserr & Knopf 1993). In addition, the lack of a lymphatic system and low levels of endogenous major histocompatibility complex (MHC) expression and the ability of glial cells to suppress T-cell responses also contribute to the immune-privileged status of the brain (Fontana et al. 1987; Benveniste 1988). Thus, interactions of the systemic immune system with this organ are restricted and it may be easier for the cyst stage of *T. gondii* to persist in this type of environment and, under appropriate conditions, cause disease.

Neuroimmunology of toxoplasmosis

Despite the limited access of the systemic immune system to the brain, there is evidence of active immune surveillance at this site. In murine models, the depletion of T-cell populations results in the reactivation of *T. gondii* infection in the brains of chronically infected mice (Suzuki & Remington 1988; Gazzinelli et al. 1992). The mechanism of T-cell-mediated protection within the central nervous system (CNS) remains to be defined, although there are several possible ways in which this may occur: these cells may lyse parasite-infected cells in the brain; they may be stimulated by glial cells to produce cytokines responsible for mediating resistance (i.e. IFN-γ); or directly stimulate the microbicidal activity of glial cells. Some studies have shown that treatment of chronically infected mice with neutralizing antibodies specific for either TNF-α or IFN-γ resulted in a severe reactivation of toxoplasmic encephalitis (Suzuki et al. 1989; Gazzinelli et al. 1993*a*, *c*). This suggests that the local production of these cytokines is important for continued resistance to *T. gondii*.

Glial cell populations (astrocytes and microglia) have been proposed to be important in mediating immune responses within the brain to *T. gondii* and these cells have been shown to produce proinflammatory cytokines in response to infection with *T. gondii* (Fischer et al. 1997). Murine and human microglia can be activated with IFN-γ to inhibit the replication of *T. gondii* (Peterson et al. 1993; Chao et al. 1994) whereas the stimulation of murine astrocytes with IFN-γ did not affect parasite replication (Peterson et al. 1993). In contrast to these latter results, human astrocytes have been reported to have an RNI-mediated mechanism of killing parasites (Peterson et al. 1995), and Weiss and colleagues have reported that IFN-γ can activate murine astrocytes to inhibit the replication of *T. gondii* (Halonen et al. 1998). In these latter studies the ability of astrocytes to inhibit parasite replication did not involve the production of RNI or tryptophan starvation. These findings imply the presence of an unidentified mechanism for IFN-γ to inhibit the replication of *T. gondii*. Nevertheless, there does appear to be a role for RNI in resistance to *T. gondii* in the brain. This is supported by studies in which treatment with antiTNF-α leads to reactivation of the disease in the brain, associated with decreased levels of iNOS mRNA (Gazzinelli et al. 1993*b*). Further evidence is also provided by studies in which mice deficient in iNOS or treated with inhibitors of iNOS were shown to develop severe toxoplasmic encephalitis, and failed to control parasite replication in the brain (Hayashi et al. 1996; Scharton-Kersten et al. 1997).

Histopathologically, the CNS lesions resulting from toxoplasmic encephalitis in immunocompromised hosts tend to be necrotizing with few infiltrating monocytes (Gray et al. 1989). This is similar to the pathology that occurs in mice with severe combined immunodeficiency (SCID) and which lack functional T-cell responses (Hunter et al. 1992; Johnson 1992b; Schluter et al. 1993). The large areas of necrosis with parasites demonstrable at the periphery of the lesions indicate that parasite growth is unrestricted. In contrast, in most nonAIDS patients with toxoplasmic encephalitis, mononuclear cells tend to predominate with prominent, well-developed cellular infiltrates (Israelski & Remington 1992). The latter pathology is more commonly observed in immunocompetent mice infected with *T. gondii* (Conley & Jenkins 1981; Ferguson et al. 1991).

The pathological differences observed between immunocompetent and immunocompromised hosts may reflect the inability of the compromised host to mount an immune response against the parasites in the lesions which results in uncontrolled proliferation of the parasite and subsequent necrosis. In contrast, despite an antiparasite immune response, susceptibility to progressive toxoplasmic encephalitis in immunocompetent mice is genetically based rather than due to the loss of the ability to mount a protective immune response. The availability of inbred strains of mice, which vary in their resistance or susceptibility to infection with *T. gondii*, has allowed genes that are associated with resistance to this parasite to be identified (Deckert-Schluter et al. 1994). In particular, the *Ld* gene was shown to be associated with resistance to this parasite (Brown et al. 1995). This gene product is a class 1 MHC molecule which is associated with CD8$^+$ T-cell responses and further emphasizes the important role of T-cells in resistance to *T. gondii*. Additional studies with AIDS patients also found an association with HLA-DQ3. Thus, there appears to be a genetic marker of susceptibility to development of toxoplasmic encephalitis in AIDS patients (Suzuki et al. 1996).

Summary

Toxoplasmosis is an important parasitic disease which impacts on individuals with defects in T-cell function. The recent explosion in the availability of reagents to study the immune response in the mouse as well as mice deficient in particular elements of the immune system has allowed a more complete understanding of how immunity to *T. gondii* is regulated. This has led to attempts to modulate and strengthen the protective immune response against *T. gondii*. These studies have shown that treatment with either IL-1 or TNF-α (Chang et al. 1990), IL-2 (Sharma et al. 1985), IL-12 (Gazzinelli et al. 1993c; Khan et al. 1994), or IFN-γ (McCabe et al. 1984), alone or in combination with currently used antitoxoplasma drugs (Araujo & Remington 1992; Araujo et al. 1996), can protect against toxoplasmosis, and that IL-15 can act as a potent adjuvant to direct the development of protective

T-cell responses (Khan & Kasper 1996). An understanding of the immune events that lead to disease may present opportunities to design immune-mediated therapies to manage toxoplasmosis or help in the design of rational vaccination strategies.

Acknowledgements

This work was supported by National Institutes of Health grant numbers AI 42334-01 and AI 41158–01 and CAH is a Burroughs Wellcome New Investigator in Molecular Parasitology.

REFERENCES

Araujo, F. & Remington, J. S. (1992). Recent advances in the search for new drugs for treatment of toxoplasmosis. *International Journal of Antimicrobial Agents*, 1, 153–64.

Araujo, F. G., Hunter, C. A. & Remington, J. S. (1996). Treatment with interleukin-12 in combination with atovaquone or clindamycin significantly increases survival of mice with acute toxoplasmosis. *Antimicrobial Agents and Chemotherapy*, 41, 188–90.

Beaman, M. H., Araujo, F. G. & Remington, J. S. (1994). Protective reconstitution of the SCID mouse against reactivation of Toxoplasmic encephalitis. *Journal of Infectious Diseases*, 169, 375–83.

Benveniste, E. N. (1988). Lymphokine and monokines in the neuroendocrine system. *Progress in Allergy*, 43, 84–120.

Biggs, B. A., Hewish, M., Kent, S., Hayes, K. & Crowe, S. M. (1995). HIV-1 infection of human macrophages impairs phagocytosis and killing of *Toxoplasma gondii. Journal of Immunology*, 154, 6132–9.

Black, C. M., Catterall, J. R. & Remington, J. S. (1987). *In vivo* and *in vitro* activation of alveolar macrophages by recombinant interferon-γ. *Journal of Immunology*, 138, 491–5.

Bluestone, J. A. (1995). New perspectives of CD28-B7-mediated T-cell costimulation. *Immunity*, 2, 555–9.

Britt, R. H., Enzmann, D. R. & Remington, J. S. (1981). Intracranial infection in cardiac transplant recipients. *Annals of Neurology*, 9, 107–19.

Brown, C. R., Hunter, C. A., Estes, R. G., Beckmann, E., Forman, J., David, C., Remington, J. S. & McLeod, R. (1995). Definitive identification of a gene that confers resistance against toxoplasmosis. *Immunology*, 85, 419–28.

Chang, H. R., Grau, G. E. & Pechere, J. C. (1990). Role of TNF and IL-1 in infections with *Toxoplasma gondii. Immunology*, 69, 33–7.

Chao, C. C., Gekker, G., Hu, S. & Peterson, P. K. (1994). Human microglial cell defence against *Toxoplasma gondii*. The role of cytokines. *Journal of Immunology*, 152, 1246–52.

Conley, F. K. & Jenkins, K. A. (1981). Immunohistological study of the anatomic relationship of toxoplasma antigens to the inflammatory response in the brains of mice chronically infected with *Toxoplasma gondii. Infection and Immunity*, 31, 1184–92.

Cserr, H. F. & Knopf, P. M. (1993). Cervical lymphatics, the blood–brain barrier and the immunoreactivity of the brain: a new view. *Immunology Today*, 13, 507–10.

Curiel, T J., Krug, E. C., Purner, M. B., Poignard, P. & Berens, R. L. (1993). Cloned human CD4+ cytotoxic T lymphocytes specific for *Toxoplasma gondii* lyse tachyzoite-infected target cells. *Journal Immunology*, 151, 2024–31.

Deckert-Schluter, M., Schluter, D., Schmidt, D., Schwendmann, G., Wiestler, O. D. & Hof, H. (1994). Toxoplasma encephalitis in congenic B10 and Balb mice: impact of genetic factors on the immune response. *Infection and Immunity*, 62, 221–8.

Delemarre, F. G. A., Stevenhagen, A., Kroon, F. P., Eer, M. Y. van, Meenhorst, P. L. & Furth, R. van (1995). Reduced toxoplasmastatic activity of monocytes and monocyte derived macrophages from AIDS patients is mediated via prostaglandin E_2 *AIDS*, 9, 441–5.

Denkers, E. Y. & Marshall, A J. (1998). Neutrophils as a source of immunoregulatory cytokines during microbial infection. *The Immunologist*, 6, 116–20.

Denkers, E. Y., Yap, G., Scharton-Kersten, T., Charest, H., Butcher, B. A., Caspar, P., Heiny, S. & Sher, A. (1997). Perforin-mediated cytolysis plays a limited role in host resistance to *Toxoplasma gondii*. *Journal of Immunology*, 159, 1903–8.

Ferguson, D. J. P., Graham, D. I. & Hutchison, W. M. (1991). Pathological changes in the brains of mice infected with *Toxoplasma gondii*: a histological, imunocytochemical, and ultrastructural study. *International Journal of Experimental Pathology*, 72, 463–74.

Fischer, K.-G., Nitzgen, B., Reichmann, G. & Hadding, U. (1997). Cytokine responses induced by *Toxoplasma gondii* in astrocytes and microglial cells. *European Journal of Immunology*, 27, 1539–48.

Fontana, A., Frei, K., Bodmer, S. & Hofer, E. (1987). Immune-mediated encephalitis: on the role of antigen- presenting cells in brain tissue. *Immunological Reviews*, 100, 185–201.

Gazzinelli, R. T., Hakim, F. T., Hieny, S., Shearer, G. M. & Sher, A. (1991). Synergistic role of CD4+ and CD8+ T lymphocytes in IFN-γ production and protective immunity induced by an attenuated *Toxoplasma gondii* vaccine. *Journal of Immunology*, 146, 286–92.

Gazzinelli, R., Xu, Y., Hieny, S., Cheever, A. & Sher, A. (1992). Simultaneous depletion of CD4+ and CD8+ T lymphocytes is required to reactivate chronic infections with *Toxoplasma gondii*. *Journal of Immunology*, 149, 175–80.

Gazzinelli, R. T., Denkers, E. Y. & Sher, A. (1993a). Host resistance to *Toxoplasma gondii*: model for studying the selective induction of cell-mediated immunity by intracellular parasites. *Infectious Agents and Disease*, 2, 139–49.

Gazzinelli, R. T., Eltourn, L., Wynn, T. A. & Sher, A. (1993b). Acute cerebral toxoplasmosis is induced by *in vivo* neutralization of TNF-α and correlates with the down-regulated expression of inducible nitric oxide synthase and other markers of macrophage activation. *Journal of Immunology*, 151, 3672–81.

Gazzinelli, R. T., Hieny, S., Wynn, T. A., Wolf, S. & Sher, A. (1993c). Interleukin 12 is required for the T-lymphocyte-independent induction of interferon γ by an intracellular parasite and induces resistance in T-cell deficient hosts. *Proceedings of the National Academy of Science USA*, 90, 6115–19.

Gazzinelli, R. T., Wysocka, M , Hayashi, S., Denkers, E. Y., Hieny, S., Caspar, P., Trinchieri, G. & Sher, A. (1994). Parasite-induced IL-12 stimulates early IFN-γ synthesis and resistance during acute infection with *Toxoplasma gondii*. *Journal of Immunology*, 153, 2533–43.

Gazzinelli, R. T., Bala, S., Stevens, R., Baseler, M., Wahl, L., Kovacs, J. & Sher, A. (1995). HIV infection suppresses type 1 lymphokine and IL-12 responses to *Toxoplasma gondii* but fails to inhibit the synthesis of other parasite-induced monokines. *Journal of Immunology*, **155**, 1565–74.

Gazzinelli, R. T., Sher, A., Cheever, A., Gerstberger, S., Martin, M. & Dickie, P. (1996). Infection of human immunodeficiency virus 1 transgenic mice with *Toxoplasma gondii* stimulates proviral transcription in macrophages *in vivo*. *Journal of Experimental Medicine*, **183**, 1645–55.

Gray, F., Cherardi, R., Wingate, I. L., Wingate, J., Fenlon, G., Gaston, A., Sobel, A. & Porier, J. (1989). Diffuse "encephalitic" cerebral toxoplasmosis in AIDS. *Journal of Neurology*, **236**, 273–7.

Green, J. M., Noel, P. J., Sperling, A. L., Walunas, T. L., Lenschow, D. J., Stack, R., Gray, G. S., Bluestone, J. A. & Thompson, C. B. (1995). T-cell costimulation through the CD28 receptor. *Proceedings of the Association of American Physicians*, **107**, 41–6.

Hakim, F. T., Gazzinelli, R. T., Denkers, E., Hieny, S., Shearer, G. M. & Sher, A. (1991). CD8+ T-cells from mice vaccinated against *Toxoplasma gondii* are cytotoxic for parasite-infected or antigen pulsed host cells. *Journal of Immunology*, **147**, 2310–16.

Halonen, S. K., Chiti, R. C. & Weiss, L. M. (1998). Effect of cytokines on growth of *Toxoplasma gondii* in murine astrocytes. *Infection and Immunity*, **66**, 4989–93.

Hayashi, S., Chan, C. C., Gazzinelli, R. & Roberge, F. C. (1996). Contribution of nitric oxide to the host parasite equilibrium in toxoplasmosis. *Journal of Immunology*, **156**, 1476–81.

Hisaeda, H., Nagasawa, H., Maeda, K., Maekawa, Y., Ishikawa, H., Ito, Y., Good, R. A. & Himeno, K. (1995). γδ T-cells play an important role in hsp65 expression and in acquiring protective immune responses against infection with *Toxoplasma gondii*. *Journal of Immunology*, **154**, 244–51.

Hsieh, C. S., Macatonia, S. E., Tripp, C. S., Wolf, S. F., O'Garra, A. & Murphy, K. M. (1993). Development of Th1 CD4+ T-cells through IL-12 produced by *Listeria* induced macrophages. *Science*, **260**, 547–9.

Hunter, C. A., Roberts, C. W., Murray, M. & Alexander, J. (1992). Detection of cytokine mRNA in the brains of mice with toxoplasmic encephalitis. *Parasite Immunology*, **14**, 405–13.

Hunter, C. A., Subauste, C. S., Van Cleave, V. H. & Remington, J. S. (1994). Production of gamma interferon by natural killer cells from *Toxoplasma gondii*-infected SCID mice: regulation by interleukin-10, interleukin-12, and tumor necrosis factor alpha. *Infection and Immunity*, **62**, 2818–24.

Hunter, C. A., Chizzonite, R. & Remington, J. S. (1995). Interleukin 1β is required for the ability of IL-12 to induce production of IFN-γ by NK cells: a role for IL-1β in the T-cell independent mechanism of resistance against intracellular pathogens. *Journal of Immunology*, **155**, 4347–54.

Hunter, C. A., Ellis-Neyer, L., Gabriel, K., Kennedy, M., Linsley, P. & Remington, J. S. (1997). The role of the CD28/B7 interaction in the regulation of NK cell responses during infection with *Toxoplasma gondii*. *Journal of Immunology*, **158**, 2285–93.

Israelski, D. M. & Remington, J. S. (1992). AIDS associated toxoplasmosis. In *The Medical Management of AIDS*, ed. M. A. Sande & P. A. Volderding, 3rd edn., pp. 319–45. Philadelphia, PA: W. B. Saunders.

Israelski, D. M. & Remington, J. S. (1993). Toxoplasmosis in patients with cancer. *Clinical Infectious Diseases*, 17 [Suppl.], S423–35.

Johnson, L. J., der Vegt, F. P. van & Havell, E. A. (1993). Gamma interferon-dependent temporary resistance to acute *Toxoplasma gondii* infection independent of CD4$^+$ or CD8$^+$ lymphocytes. *Infection and Immunity*, 61, 5174–80.

Johnson, L. L. (1992a). A protective role for endogenous tumor necrosis factor in *Toxoplasma gondii* infection. *Infection and Immunity*, 60, 1979–83.

Johnson, L. L. (1992b). SCID mouse models of acute and relapsing chronic *Toxoplasma gondii* infections. *Infection and Immunity*, 60, 3719–24.

Khan, I. A. & Kasper, L. H. (1996). IL-15 augments CD8$^+$ T-cell-mediated immunity against *Toxoplasma gondii* infection in mice. *Journal of Immunology*, 157, 2103–8.

Khan, I. A., Smith, K. A. & Kasper, L. H. (1990). Induction of antigen-specific human cytotoxic T-cells by *Toxoplasma gondii*. *Journal of Clinical Investigation*, 85, 1879–86.

Khan, I. A., Matsuura, T. & Kasper, L. H. (1994). Interleukin-12 enhances murine survival against acute Toxoplasmosis. *Infection and Immunity*, 62, 1639–42.

Khan, I. A., Matsuura, T., Fonseka, S. & Kasper, L. H. (1996). Production of nitric oxide (NO) is not essential for protection against acute *Toxoplasma gondii* infection in IRF-1-/- mice. *Journal of Immunology*, 156, 636–43.

Langermans, J. A., Van der Hulst, M. E. B., Nibbering, P. H., Hiemstra, P. S., Fransen, L. & Van Furth, R. (1992). IFN-γ induced L-arginine-dependent toxoplasmastatic activity in murine peritoneal macrophages is mediated by endogenous tumor necrosis factor-α. *Journal of Immunology*, 148, 568–74.

Luft, B. J. & Remington, J. S. (1988). Toxoplasmic encephalitis. *Journal of Infectious Diseases*, 157, 1–6.

McCabe, R. E., Luft, B. J. & Remington, J. S. (1984). Effect of murine interferon gamma on murine toxoplasmosis. *Journal of Infectious Diseases*, 150, 961–3.

McLeod, R., Mack, D. G., Boyer, K., Mets, M., Roizen, N., Swisher, C., Patel, D., Beckmann, E., Vitullo, D. & Johnson, D. et al. (1990). Phenotypes and functions of lymphocytes in congenital toxoplasmosis. *Journal of Laboratory and Clinical Medicine*, 116, 623–35.

Nagineni, C. N., Pardhasaraadhi, K., Martins, M. C., Detrick, B. & Hooks, J. J. (1996). Mechanisms of interferon-induced inhibition of *Toxoplasma gondii* replication in human retinal pigment epithelial cells. *Infection and Immunity*, 64, 4188–96.

Parker, S. J., Roberts, C. W & Alexander, J. (1991). CD8$^+$ T-cells are the major lymphocyte subpopulation involved in the protective immune response to *Toxoplasma gondii* in mice. *Clinical and Experimental Immunology*, 84, 207–12.

Peterson, P. K., Gekker, G., Hu, S. & Chao, C. (1993). Intracellular survival and multiplication of *Toxoplasma gondii* in astrocytes. *Journal of Infectious Diseases*, 168, 1472–8.

Peterson, P. K., Gekker, G., Hu, S. & Chao, C. C. (1995). Human astrocytes inhibit intracellular multiplication of *Toxoplasma gondii* by a nitric oxide-mediated mechanism. *Journal of Infectious Diseases*, 171, 516–18.

Pfefferkorn, E. R. (1984). Interferon γ blocks the growth of *Toxoplasma gondii* in human fibroblasts by inducing the host cells to degrade tryptophan. *Proceedings of the National Academy of Science USA*, 81, 908–12.

Reis e Sousa, B. C., Hieny, S., Scharton-Kersten, T., Jankovic, D., Charset, H., Germain, R. N. & Sher, A. (1997). *In vivo* microbial stimulation induces rapid CD40 ligand-independent production of interleukin 12 by dendritic cells and their redistribution to T-cell areas. *Journal of Experimental Medicine*, 186, 1819–29.

Remington, J. S., McLeod, R. & Desmonts, G. (1994) Toxoplasmosis. In *Infectious Diseases of the Foetus and Newborn Infant*, ed. J. S. Remington, J. O. Klein, 4th edn., pp. 140–266. Philadelphia, PA: W. B. Saunders.

Scharton-Kersten, T. M., Yap, G., Magram, J. & Sher, A. (1997). Inducible nitric oxide is essential for host control of persistent but not acute infection with the intracellular pathogen *Toxoplasma gondii. Journal of Experimental Medicine*, 185, 1261–73.

Schluter, D., Deckert-Schluter, M., Schwendemann, G., Brunner, H. & Hof, H. (1993). Expression of major histocompatibility complex class II antigens and levels of interferon-γ, tumor necrosis factor, and interleukin-6 in cerebrospinal fluid and serum in *Toxoplasma gondii*-infected SCID and immunocompetent CB-17 mice. *Immunology*, 78, 430–5.

Sharma, S. D., Hofflin, J. M. & Remington, J. S. (1985). *In vivo* recombinant interleukin 2 administration enhances survival against a lethal challenge with *Toxoplasma gondii. Journal of Immunology*, 135, 4160–3.

Sharpe, A. H. (1995). Analysis of lymphocyte costimulation *in vivo* using transgenic and "knock-out" mice. *Current Opinions in Immunology*, 7, 389–95.

Sher, A., Oswald, I. P., Hieny, S. & Gazzinelli, R. (1993). *Toxoplasma gondii* induces a T-independent IFN-γ response in natural killer cells that requires both adherent accessory cells and tumor necrosis factor-α. *Journal of Immunology*, 150, 3982–9.

Shibuya, K., Robinson, D., Zonin, R., Hartley, S. B., Macatonia, S. E., Somoza, C., Hunter, C. A., Murphy, K. M. & O'Garra, A. (1998). IL-1α and TNF-α are required for IL-12-induced development of Thl cells producing high levels of IFN-γ in BALB/c but not C57BL/6 mice. *Journal of Immunology*, 160, 1708–16

Sibley, L. D., Weidner, E. & Krahenbuhl, J. L. (1985). Phagosome acidification blocked by intracellular *Toxoplasma gondii. Nature*, 315, 416–19.

Sibley, L. D., Adams, L. B., Fukutorni, Y. & Krahenbuhl, J. L. (1991). Tumor necrosis factor-x triggers antitoxoplasmal activity of WN-Y primed macrophages. *Journal of Immunology*, 147, 2340–5.

Slavin, M. A., Meyers, J. D., Remington, J. S. & Hackman, R. C. (1994). *Toxoplasma gondii* infection in marrow transplant recipients: a 20 year experience. *Bone Marrow Transplantation*, 13, 549–57.

Subauste, C. S., Koniaris, A. H. & Remington, J. S. (1991). Murine CD8+ cytotoxic T lymphocytes lyse *Toxoplasma gondii*-infected cells. *Journal of Immunology*, 147, 3955–9.

Subauste, C. S., Dawson, L. & Remington, J. S. (1992). Human lymphokine-activated killer cells are cytotoxic against cells infected with *Toxoplasma gondii. Journal of Experimental Medicine*, 176, 1511–19.

Subauste, C. S., Chung, J. Y., Do, D., Koniaris, A. H., Hunter, C. A., Montoya, J. G., Poreelli, S. & Remington, J. S. (1995). Preferential activation and expansion of human peripheral blood γδ T-cells in response to *Toxoplasma gondii in vitro* and their cytokine production and cytotoxic activity against *T. gondii*-infected cells. *Journal of Clinical Investigation*, 96, 610–19.

Subauste, C. S., de Waal Malefvt, R. & Fuh, F. (1998). Role of CD80 (B7.1) and CD86 (B7.2) in the immune response to an intracellular pathogen. *Journal of Immunology*, **160**, 1831–40.

Suzuki, Y. & Remington, J. S. (1988). Dual regulation of resistance against *Toxoplasma gondii* infection by LyT-2+ and LyT-1+, L3T4 T-cells in mice. *Journal of Immunology*, **140**, 3943–6.

Suzuki, Y. & Remington, J. S. (1990). The effect of anti-IFN-γ antibody on the protective effect of LyT-2+ immune T-cells against toxoplasmosis in mice. *Journal of Immunology*, **144**, 1954–6.

Suzuki, Y., Conley, F. K. & Remington, J. S. (1989). Importance of endogenous IFN-α for prevention of toxoplasmic encephalitis in mice. *Journal of Immunology*, **143**, 2045–50.

Suzuki, Y., Wong., S., Grumet, R., Fessel, J., Montoya, J., Zolopa, A. R., Portmore, A., Schumacher-Perdreau, R., Schrappe, M., Koppen, S., Ruf, B., Brown, B. W. & Remington, J. S. (1996). Evidence for genetic regulation of susceptibility to toxoplasmic encephalitis in AIDS patients. *Journal of Infectious Diseases*, **173**, 265–8.

Viola, A. & Lanzavecchia, A. (1996). T-cell activation determined by T-cell receptor number and tunable thresholds. *Science*, **273**, 104–6.

Wong, S. Y. & Remington, J. S. (1993). Biology of *Toxoplasma gondii*. *AIDS*, **7**, 299–316.

Yong, E. C., Chi, E. Y. & Henderson. W. R. (1994). *Toxoplasma gondii* alters eicosanoid release by human mononuclear phagocytes: role of leukotrienes in interferon-7-induced antitoxoplasma activity. *Journal of Experimental Medicine*, **180**, 1637–48.

The epidemiology of toxoplasma infection

S. Hall[1], M. Ryan[2] and D. Buxton[3]

[1] Storrs House Farm, Storrs Lane, Sheffield, UK
[2] Communicable Disease Surveillance Centre, London, UK
[3] Animal Diseases Research Association, Moredun Research Institute, Edinburgh, Scotland

Introduction

Epidemiology is the study of the distribution and determinants of disease in populations. Its principle purposes are to inform decisions about allocation of healthcare resources, to provide a scientific basis on which prevention strategies can be based and to evaluate the effectiveness of those strategies.

Epidemiology addresses questions about prevalence, incidence and trends in infections and other diseases in different populations. In the case of toxoplasma infection the cause, *Toxoplasma gondii*, is known; nevertheless, epidemiological studies contribute to our understanding of routes of transmission and risk factors for acquiring the organism.

How prevalent is toxoplasma infection and is the incidence changing?

Prevalence

The most widely used method of assessing the frequency with which toxoplasma infection occurs in a given population – be it normal subjects or a particular group of interest such as pregnant women or HIV-positive patients – is to conduct a serological survey. Because, unlike most microbiological agents, the organism persists in its host for life and is capable of reactivating and causing disease, measurement of *T. gondii* IgG antibody provides an estimate of the *prevalence* (as compared to *incidence*, see below) of toxoplasma infection in the population of interest. Such studies using IgG alone cannot tell when their subjects acquired the infection, because IgG probably persists for life, so its presence may (depending on the assay used) indicate infection acquired anything from 2 weeks to decades ago. However, the detection of *T. gondii*-specific IgM is an indicator of relatively recent infection (see below).

Tables 3.1 and 3.2 summarize results from seroprevalence studies conducted throughout the world which show that toxoplasma infection is extremely widespread and often very common. They also illustrate two problems in

Table 3.1. *Toxoplasma gondii* antibody prevalence studies

	Seroprevalence studies in Central/South América and the Caribbean[*]					
Country	Sample	Ages	Test	Titre	% + ve	Reference
Canada						
Ontario (1961–1975)	7,060	All	DT	16	38	Tizard & Caoili 1976
Nova Scotia (1982–1984)	998	<18	IHAT	256	3.3	Pereira et al. 1992
USA						
US military	2,680	–	DT	12	14	Feldman 1968
Portland, Oregon	293	–	DT	16	17	Feldman 1956
California	147	–	IFAT	16	42.9	MacKnight & Robinson 1992
Navajo Indians	236	–	DT	16	4	Feldman 1956
Italy						
Children (1980–1987)	1,494	3–18	ELISA	15 IU	17.9	Moschen et al. 1991
Pregnant women (1991–1994)	3518	–	IC	≥15 IU	40	Buffolano et al. 1996
General population (1987–1991)	19,432	adults	ELISA	–	48.5	Valcavi et al. 1995
Norway						
Military recruits	3,047	18	TST	>2 mm	22.5	Vaage & Midtvedt 1975
Pregnant women (1992)	35,940	–	EIA, DT	–	10.9	Jenum et al. 1998
Sweden						
Pregnant women (1957–1958)	470	–	IHAT	40	47.7	Forsgren et al. 1991
Pregnant women (1987)	1,086	–	IHAT	40	21.1	Forsgren et al. 1991
France						
Pregnant women (1981–1983)	1,074	15–44	IFAT	5 IU	67.4	Jeannel et al. 1988

Table 3.1. (*cont.*)

Country	Sample	Ages	Test	Titre	% + ve	Reference
Seroprevalence studies in North America and Europe[*]						
Spain						
Pregnant women (1993)	191	–	EIA	–	25.7	Guerra & Fernandez 1995
Belgium						
Blood donors (1990)	1,839	–	MEIA	–	67	Luyaso et al. 1997
Pregnant women (1990)	784	–	MEIA	–	50	Luyaso et al. 1997

Country	Sample	Ages	Test	Titre	% + ve	Reference
Seroprevalence studies in Central/South America and the Caribbean						
Mexico						
National	29,279	All	IFAT	16	32	Velasco-Castrejon et al. 1992
Southern (Coastal)	3,229	All	IHAT	25	3.8	Goldsmith et al. 1991
Southern (2 towns)	479	All	IHAT	25	25.5	Goldsmith et al. 1991
Costa Rica						
San Jose + 4 Highland areas	883	15	IFAT	2	64.1	Frenkel & Ruiz 1980
Panama						
Panama City	590	All	DT	2	58.6	Sousa et al. 1988
Chorrera region (1972–1983)	326	All	DT	2	57.5	Sousa et al. 1988
Brazil						
20 States	1,410	All	IFAT	16	61	Ricciardi et al. 1975
Western (Ticuna Indians)	408	All	IHAT	25	20.3	Lovelace et al. 1978
Western (Town dwellers)	61	All	IHAT	25	39.3	Lovelace et al. 1978
Chile						
Regions I, II, III (1982–1983)	19,798	≥4	IHAT	16	32.7	Schenone et al. 1986*a*

Table 3.1. (*cont.*)

Country	Sample	Ages	Test	Titre	% + ve	Reference
				Seroprevalence studies in Central/South America and the Caribbean		
Regions IV, V, VI (1982–1986)	24,164	≥4	IHAT	16	36.1	Schenone et al 1986*b*
Region VII (1985–1986)	1,006	≥9	IHAT	16	42.4	Peña et al. 1986
Santiago (1982–1987)	11,428	5–60	IHAT	16	33.7	Schenone et al. 1987
Countrywide 1982–1994	76,317	All	IHAT	16	36.9	Contreras et al. 1996
French West Indies						
La Guadelope	3,238	0–78	IFAT	50	60	Barbier et al. 1983
Haiti						
Port au Prince	104	All	DT	16	36	Feldman et al. 1956
Rural	719	All	IFAT	20	5.9	Raccurt et al. 1986
				Seroprevalence studies in African countries		
Somalia						
Four districts (1976–1977)	356	18–60	DT	8	53	Zardi et al. 1980
Mogadishu + village	669	All	ELISA	400	48	Ahmed et al. 1988
Kenya						
Four areas	322	>20	HAT	64	54	Griffin & Williams 1983
Nairobi	127	1–10	IHAT	64	42.5	Bowry et al. 1986
Burundi						
Three regions	622	All	IFAT	8 IU	44.1	Excler et al. 1988
Sudan						
Gezira	386	All	LAT	64	41.7	Abdel-Hameed 1991
South Africa						
Four regions	3,379	All	IFAT	16	20	Jacobs & Mason 1978
Nigeria						
Plateau State	210	All	IHAT	256	22.8	Osiyemi et al. 1985
Liberia						
National (1968–1970)	390	All	DT	14	~58	Omland et al. 1977
Mauritania						
17 towns and villages	3,112	6–18	IFAT	150	15.5	Monjour et al (1983)

Table 3.1. (*cont.*)

Country	Sample	Ages	Test	Titre	% + ve	Reference
Seroprevalence studies in African countries						
Ivory Coast						
Four sites	2,000	<30	LAT	–	65.9	Dumas et al (1989)
Niger						
Niger Delta	1,650	All	DT	10	58.9	Arene 1986
Two districts	400	>2	IFAT	40	18.2	Develoux 1988
Niamey 1992	371	All	IFAT	12 IU	18	Julvez et al 1996
Gabon						
Libreville	1,178	All	LAT	8 IU	63	Duong et al. 1992
South West	1,448	All	IFAT	128	52.6	Beauvais et al. 1978
Central African Republic						
North	266	All	LAT	32	40	Dumas et al. 1985
Tanzania						
Pregnant women	849	–	DT	4	35	Doehring et al. 1995
Seroprevalence studies in Middle-East, Southeast Asia and the Pacific						
Papua New Guinea (1972–1973)	315	>9	DT	16	32	Zigas 1976
Laos (Keoudom)	588	>2	CFT	16	15.3	Catar et al. 1992
China						
Guangdong	3,085	–	IHAT	64	0.71	Shen et al. 1990
Chengdu – pregnant women	1,211	–	ELISA		39.1	Sun et al. 1995
Hong Kong (1977–8)	2,499	All	IFAT	16	9.8	Ko et al. 1980
Malaysia	736	All	IFAT	64	20.9	Thomas et al. 1980
West Malaysia	728	All	IHAT	160	13.9	Tan & Zaman 1973
Indonesia						
Central Java (1968)	695	2–75	IHAT	256	2	Cross et al. 1975
Central Sulawesi (1972)	484	All	IHAT	32	27	Clarke et al. 1975
Paniai	188	2–54	IHAT	256	34.6	Gandahusada & Endardjo 1980

Table 3.1. (*cont.*)

Country	Sample	Ages	Test	Titre	% +ve	Reference
		Seroprevalence studies in Middle-East, Southeast Asia and the Pacific				
Borneo (1971–2)	1,050	≥1	IHAT	16	31.4	Durfee et al. 1976
South Sulawesi (1972)	915	All	IHAT	32	28.5	Carney et al. 1978
India						
Kumaon	200	All	IHAT	18	57	Singh & Nautiyal 1991
Women	2,075	Adult	IFAT		7.7	Mittal et al. 1995
New Caledonia	124	All	DT	16	84	Wallace 1976
Tahiti/Society Islands	467	All	DT	16	71	Wallace 1976
Taiwan	231	All	DT	16	4	Wallace 1976
Saudi Arabia	362	4–60	IHAT	64	22.4	Ahmed 1992
Egypt						
Cairo	618	–	DT	16	20.3	Rifaat et al. 1975
Alexandria	161	–	DT	16	29.2	Rifaat et al. 1975
Kena	365	2–72	DT	16	7.7	Rifaat et al. 1975
Al Azhar University	100	–	IHAT	64.	22.4	Rifaat et al. 1975
Kuwait						
Pregnant women	4,000		IHAT	16	58.2	Al-Nakib et al. 1983
Iran: 12 provinces	13,018	All	IFAT	–	51.8	Assmar et al. 1997
Turkey						
Women	996	17–45	EIA	–	39.9	Durmaz et al. 1995
Bangladesh						
Blood donors	49	Adults	LAT	–	12.4	Samad et al. 1997
Pregnant women	617	–	LAT	–	11.2	Samad et al. 1997

Key to Table 3.1. DT, Dye test; CFT, Complement fixation test; IHAT, Indirect haemagglutination test; IFAT, Immunofluorescent antibody test; ELISA, Enzyme linked immunosorbent assay; TST, Toxoplasma skin test; HAT, Haemagglutination test; LAT, Latex agglutination test; EIA, Enzyme immunoassay; MEIA, Microparticle capture enzyme immunoassay; IC, Immunocapture.
*Excluding UK – see Table 3.2.

Table 3.2. *Toxoplasma gondii* antibody prevalence studies carried out in the UK

Area	Source of sample population	n	Ages	Test	Titre	% + ve	References
London	Inpatients + mental handicap	901	All	TST	>1cm	6.7	Fisher 1951
Sheffield (1950s)	General population males	229	>20	DT	4	17.9	Beverley et al. 1954
Sheffield (1950s)	Blood donors + laboratory workers + children for surgery	581	All	DT	4	33.9	Beverley et al. 1954
Sheffield (1989–1992)	Pregnant women	1,621	–	LAT	16	9.9	Zadik et al. 1995
Lincolnshire	Urban and rural adults	1,004	>19	DT	16	31.5	Beattie 1957
Wales	Blood donors + routine child admissions	587	0–60	DT	16	19	Fleck 1963
South Wales	General population	240	0–60	DT	16	25.8	Fleck 1965
London (+ six other cities)	Blood donors	1,440	21–60	DT	16	32.7	Fleck 1969
West of Scotland (1975–1977)	Pregnant women	10,677	–	DT	8	13.4	Williams et al. 1981
Scotland and Midlands	Blood donors , travellers & outpatient attenders	554	All	DT	10	21.5	Jackson et al. 1987
South Yorkshire (1969–1990)	Laboratory samples	1,430	All	LAT	16	22.5	Walker et al. 1992
London (1980–1986)	Pregnant women	6,749	–	ELISA	12	18.8	Gilbert et al. 1993
East Anglia 1992	Pregnant women	13,328	–	MEIA	≥ 6 IU	8.1	Allain et al. 1998
Ireland (1990s)	School children	1,276	4–18	LAT	4	12.8	Taylor et al. 1997

Abbreviations as in Table 3.1.

comparing findings between studies: the range of tests used and also of antibody titres (even using the same test) which are considered 'positive'. Some earlier studies used the toxoplasma skin test which is akin to IgG serology and not suitable for indicating recent infection. Another problem is the different age ranges studied.

Nevertheless there are striking differences in seroprevalence both between countries and within countries. For example that in Costa Rica (Frenkel & Ruiz 1980) was 61.4% compared with 0.71% in China (Shen et al. 1990). A study in Papua New Guinea (Zigas 1976) demonstrated a ninefold difference in seropositivity between regions (7–63%). In the UK 14 studies since 1951 found overall seroprevalence rates ranging from 6.7% to 33.9%. By contrast, 67.4% of pregnant women in a French study conducted in the 1980s were *T. gondii* antibody positive (Jeannel et al. 1988).

Incidence

It is also important to know how many *new* infections are occurring per unit time in a given population (*incidence*). This information might be used, for example, in assessing the need for preventive programmes such as prenatal screening or, if one became available, for vaccination. Incidence data can elucidate target populations (for example, certain age groups) for focused intervention and serve as outcome measures for evaluating the effectiveness of such programmes. They may also be used to predict future patterns in the incidence of toxoplasma infection (Ades & Nokes 1993).

Because most toxoplasma infections are asymptomatic, estimates of incidence, like prevalence, must also be derived from serological studies. There are two options: the first is direct and depends on measuring either specific IgM, or seroconversion, or both. Such studies require large numbers of subjects to maximize precision of the incidence estimate because numbers of new cases occurring in a time period practical to study will be relatively low; those studies measuring seroconversion also require serial specimens from the same identifiable subjects. Thus particular 'at risk' patient groups such as pregnant women or HIV-positive individuals are often used in incidence studies.

Such incidence studies have been criticized for not making best use of their data (Ades 1992). For example, periods at risk have not been taken into account and the implications of IgM persistence (which can be for several years in some subjects, using the most sensitive tests) have been overlooked. Confidence intervals are rarely calculated. Reanalysing the data from six UK studies, Ades derived a range of estimated incidence per 1000 pregnancies of between 1.1 and 14.5. This compared with the figure of 2 per 1000 widely cited for the incidence of toxoplasma infection in pregnancy in the UK. Subsequently, using a more sophisticated technique of mathematical modelling, Ades and Nokes (1993) estimated the incidence of toxo-plasma infection among women of childbearing age in the UK in the 1990s to be 0.7 or less per 1000 susceptibles per year. This is in line with the findings of Zadik et al. 1995, who found an annual incidence per thousand susceptibles of 0.34. This was a study of seroconversion among pregnant women in Sheffield, England, between 1989 and 1992.

The second means of estimating incidence is indirectly, from seroprevalence studies; these have several advantages. They are relatively cheap to undertake on a large scale, 'banked' sera taken for other purposes can be used and the anonymity of study subjects can be preserved. The findings of such studies should, however, be viewed critically because some have used cross-sectional seroprevalence data (the proportions *T. gondii* antibody positive at each year of age in a study sample examined at one point in time) to calculate the 'antibody acquisition rate' or 'annual increase in seroprevalence' (e.g. Broadbent et al. 1981). These are not the same as incidence because they take no account of the declining number of suscep-tible subjects with age.

Recently, however, mathematical modelling techniques – largely made possible by modern computing power – have been developed to derive incidence figures from seroprevalence data (Ades 1992; Ades & Nokes 1993; Marschner 1997). Allain et al. (1998) derived an estimated incidence range of 0.7–3.4 infections per 1000 pregnancies among pregnant women living in East Anglia, UK, in 1992, using a method combining the prevalence of both anti- *T. gondii* IgM and IgG. This is an important new area in the study of the epidemiology of toxoplasma infection. Nevertheless, such studies sometimes make assumptions; for example, that toxo-plasma IgG antibody does not become undetectable over time in most people, that the probability of being selected in a cross-sectional sample is the same for both infected and uninfected individuals and that transmission modes are the same at all ages. The most recent models allow for the latter two assumptions, but authors nevertheless draw attention to these important caveats to the use of serial preva-lence data for assessing incidence (Marschner 1997).

As a measure of the size of the problem of toxoplasma infection, sero-epidemiology can only provide information about numbers of persons infected. The other half of the equation, essential for assessing the need for prevention pro-grammes, is the associated morbidity and mortality burden. On a population basis, this can be estimated by extrapolating from *ad hoc* studies and case series. For example, the annual number of neonates and infants in England and Wales who are born with clinically obvious severe manifestations of congenital toxoplasma infec-tion (central nervous system (CNS) involvement, retinochoroiditis, systemic disease) has been estimated at about 30–40 (Joynson 1992). This figure was derived from annual total births applying the following assumptions: an estimated incidence of maternal toxoplasma infection of 2 per 1000 pregnancies; a transplacental transmission rate of about 40% and a proportion of infected neonates manifesting severe disease of about 8% (Remington & Desmonts 1990).

Similar estimates based on the same assumptions have also been made for other countries, including Scotland (Joss et al. 1990) and Holland (Conyn van Spaendonck 1991). In the latter country it was estimated by this means that 800 babies infected both clinically and subclinically were born annually (0.5% live births). A prospective survey to determine the 'true' incidence of toxoplasma infection in pregnancy and the birth prevalence of congenital toxoplasma infection produced findings which were discrepant from these estimates (Conyn van Spaendonck 1991). The observed birth prevalence was one and a half times less than that expected, and the number of maternal infections was one-fifth of that predicted. It was suggested that a primary and secondary prevention programme instituted concurrently with the survey explained part of the discrepancy. However, the problems associated with deriving incidence from seroprevalence data, already described, as well as a probable 'cohort effect' (see below) were also thought to have biased the original estimate. It was calculated that, had the intervention programme not been in place, the 'true' numbers of infected newborns would have been 160 – still highly discrepant from the 800 estimated.

Some studies, using methods to estimate the frequency of congenital toxoplasma infection like those above, have attempted to calculate the cost of the mental and physical handicap caused by the infection, in order to determine the cost–benefit ratio of introducing prevention by prenatal screening or health education (Henderson et al. 1984; Joss et al. 1990). Such studies depend on a number of assumptions and their conclusions should therefore be viewed with caution.

Another method of estimating the size of the clinical burden is to use data on toxoplasma seroprevalence among HIV-positive individuals, in conjunction with information on the proportion of those with both antibodies who go on to develop severe systemic toxoplasma infection, to predict the number of individuals in a population who may need the health-care resources associated with toxoplasma encephalitis. In the UK, a study of HIV-positive individuals demonstrated a seroprevalence of 27% for toxoplasma antibodies and suggested that a further 0.5–1% per year may suffer primary toxoplasma infection (Holliman 1990). Using the data of Grant et al. (1990), it could be predicted that 3.5% to 10.3% of AIDS patients in the UK would develop cerebral toxoplasma infection at some time. The advent of highly active antiretroviral therapy (HAART) has now of course had a significant effect on such predictions in those populations where it is available.

Such extrapolated estimates of the burden of toxoplasma infection make good use of available data. However, they have two main disadvantages. First, they often depend on data collected in a range of countries at different times, which may not apply to the population in question because of geographical and temporal differences in the epidemiology of toxoplasma infection (see below), and, second, they cannot be used to monitor the effectiveness of intervention programmes.

An alternative method of assessing the clinical burden of toxoplasma infection is by laboratory-based surveillance, enhanced by clinical information on reported cases. The Communicable Diseases (Scotland) Unit and the Communicable Disease Surveillance Centre (CDSC) of the Public Health Laboratory Service run such schemes covering Scotland and England and Wales respectively. Patients with toxoplasma infection are reported to these national surveillance centres mainly by reference laboratories (thus ensuring optimal microbiological confirmation of the diagnosis). Each reported case is accompanied by a limited amount of epidemi-ological and clinical information. These data provide national trends in the different clinical manifestations of toxoplasma infection which are valuable for health-care and intervention planning and evaluation purposes. However, they have some disadvantages; for example, they under-ascertain to an unknown extent not only subclinical, but also symptomatic cases, because of incomplete reporting and because the diagnosis of toxoplasma infection in patients with nonspecific symptoms and signs may not be considered. Furthermore some cases, particularly of retinochoroiditis, may be diagnosed clinically without recourse to microbiolog-ical investigation.

Another problem, relevant to toxoplasma infection epidemiology generally, is the lack of internationally accepted case definitions for its various manifestations. This is particularly problematic for congenital toxoplasma infection (Hall 1983) and toxoplasmic retinochoroiditis (Holliman et al. 1991). The issue of case definitions for congenital toxoplasmosis has, however, recently been addressed (Lebech et al. 1996) and is discussed further below.

In conclusion, there are no simple, reliable methods of measuring the 'size of the problem' of toxoplasma infection and published estimates must therefore always be viewed critically. Nevertheless, both serological studies and laboratory-based national surveillance have yielded some interesting trends which show a degree of consistency and which will now be described.

Time trends in toxoplasma infection – is the incidence changing ?

There is evidence from a number of *T. gondii* antibody surveys that the incidence of toxoplasma infection has been falling in parts of Europe, Scandinavia, the UK and the United States. Using the new mathematical modelling techniques referred to above, both Ades and Nokes (1993) and Marschner (1997) showed that the inci-dence in a region of England fell sixfold between 1915 and 1970, but then remained stable for the next 20 years. Ades and Nokes also predicted little change in the first half of the 1990s. Their central estimates of incidence in 25 year olds ranged between 0.07 and 0.1 per 100 susceptibles per year for 1995; this compared with 0.5 to 0.8 for the same age group in the 1980s. This finding emphasizes the danger of neglecting a possible 'cohort effect' when making inferences about *incidence* from cross-sectional sero-*prevalence* studies (Ljungstrom et al. 1995). A 'cohort effect' is the variation in health status that arises from the different causal factors to which each birth cohort in the population is exposed as the environment and society change over time.

Sousa et al. (1988) also demonstrated a cohort effect in toxoplasma infection among inhabitants of a recently founded village in Panama. The younger population had been born there, whereas the older people had moved in from elsewhere. The seroprevalence data showed two distinct curves for each cohort. In a detailed study in The Netherlands, in which incidence data derived from a prospective antenatal survey were compared with incidence estimates derived from a number of seroprevalence surveys, Conyn van Spaendonck (1991) found discrepancies which were, at least in part, due to cohort effects. She found a much higher seroprevalence among women born in 1948–1952 than in subsequent birth cohorts.

In line with the data of Ades and Nokes (1993), Forsgren et al. (1991) showed that the prevalence of toxoplasma antibody among nonimmigrant pregnant women in Southern Sweden fell from 47% in 1957–1958 to 18% in 1987 (it was higher and changed little among immigrants). The decline occurred in all age groups, although it may have reversed in recent years (Ljungstrom et al. 1995). Antenatal serological studies in Paris also suggest that the incidence of toxoplasma infection has been falling there, with 70% positive in 1985 compared to 87% 1960–1970 (Remington & Desmonts 1990). Comparable data for Liege, Belgium were 47% and 70% respectively (European Network on Congenital Toxoplasma Infection 1993). In Palo Alto, California, only 10% of pregnant women were *T. gondii* antibody positive in 1987 compared to 24% in 1974 (Remington & Desmonts 1990). By contrast, a number of antenatal serological studies in inner London do not reveal striking trends: 22% *T. gondii* antibody positive in the 1960s (Ruoss & Bourne 1972) compared to 19.5% in 1991 (Ades et al. 1993). However, trends among populations of large conurbations are difficult to interpret because of likely multiple cohort effects associated with mobility and changing ethnic mix (see below).

A review of laboratory reports of toxoplasma infection in England and Wales showed no remarkable changes in annual totals over the 17-year period 1976–1992 (Ryan et al. 1995). However, when the data were analysed by clinical subgroup some interesting trends emerged which tended to counterbalance each other, thus causing the unchanging overall totals. This observation emphasizes the heterogeneous nature of toxoplasma infection – each clinical manifestation having its own descriptive epidemiological features and risk factors.

Ryan et al. (1995) observed a marked fall in reports of toxoplasmic lymphade-nopathy in children and teenagers during the 1980s. This also occurred, but to a lesser extent, among young adults, although there was no change among the older age group. By contrast, reports of acute toxoplasma infection in pregnant women changed little between 1981 and 1988, then increased eightfold in 1989 (probably as a result of heightened public awareness – see below) and then declined slightly but remained at a higher level from 1990 to 1992.

Reports of severe toxoplasma infection in immunocompromised persons and of toxoplasmic retinochoroiditis both represent, by and large, reactivation of latent infection – whether acquired or congenital. The numbers of reports of immuno-suppressed patients with severe systemic toxoplasma infection increased tenfold in England and Wales over the 1980s – transplant surgery and human immunodeficiency virus (HIV) infection being the main underlying risk factors. By contrast, reports of toxoplasma eye disease fell by two-thirds in 1981–1992.

National trends in congenital toxoplasma infection manifesting in infancy and childhood were more difficult to assess through this laboratory-based surveillance scheme, mainly because of difficulties in using the limited information available with each report, and in confirming the diagnosis in babies and children with com-patible, but nonspecific, clinical signs. A review of these data for the years 1975–1980 had yielded a total of 34 possible cases conforming to a preset clinical and serological case definition, including four with the classic triad (Hall 1983). There were, however, no reports of infants with the classic triad in 1989–1992. These data on congenital infection were clearly discrepant from the predicted 30–40 cases per annum manifesting in the first year of life with severe congenital toxoplasma infection cited in the previous section. In order to determine whether this was an artefact of the laboratory reporting system, congenital toxoplasma infection was made a reportable condition for 12 months, 1989–1990, via an active clinical reporting scheme (The British Paediatric Surveillance Unit). This yielded a total of 14 cases for that birth cohort, only seven of whom had CNS involvement (Hall 1992).

A similar discrepancy between observed and expected numbers has also been described in Scotland (Joss et al. 1990). These observations reflect major difficulties in defining the size of the problem of congenital toxoplasma infection in any country and in monitoring trends if a preventive programme is instituted. France and Austria, which have national prenatal screening programmes for toxoplasma infection, have no national surveillance for congenital toxoplasma infection to eval-uate their effectiveness (Remington & Desmonts 1990). Before such surveillance can be instituted and provide valid data, there is a need for case definitions of con-genital toxoplasma infection to be agreed and laboratory investigations of all sus-pected cases to be standardized.

A classification system and case definitions of toxoplasma infection in immuno-competent pregnant women and their congenitally infected offspring was devised by the European Research Network on Congenital Toxoplasmosis (Lebech et al. 1996). In this, four separate groups – pregnant women, foetuses, infants and individuals over one year of age – are identified. For each, the likelihood of infection is separated into five mutually exclusive categories: 'definitely', 'probably', 'possibly', 'unlikely to be' and 'not' infected. Inclusion of a case in any one category depends on the available serological, parasitological and clinical information, which the authors define for each possible scenario. The system is designed to be usable in different countries and to aid large epidemiological studies, as well as the diagnosis and management of individual cases.

Monitoring changing patterns in the occurrence of toxoplasma infection as described above is of little value for its own sake. Increases or declines in incidence require explanation and appropriate public health intervention. The upsurge in severe toxoplasma infection in England and Wales in the 1980s was clearly associated with the underlying increase in immunocompromised subjects. Toxoplasma infection has been associated with immunosuppression, mainly due to malignancy, since the 1960s and published case reports of what used to be extremely rare manifestations of the infection support the trends obtained from routine surveillance. For example, of 46 case reports of pulmonary toxoplasma infection in the world literature, 1940–1991, 35 were after 1980 (Pomeroy & Filice 1992). Thirty one patients were immunocompromised among whom there were six patients with recent transplant surgery and 19 with HIV infection – all of these 25 were reported after 1980. Sixteen of 21 reports in the world literature of toxoplasmic encephalitis in immunocompromised children (excluding HIV infection) between 1954 and 1994 were after 1980 (Khan & Correa 1997). Reviews of adult cerebral toxoplasma infection show an identical pattern (Luft & Remington 1985).

It is, however, also clear that in the era before HAART the rates of severe toxoplasma infection complicating AIDS varied from country to country; for example, the proportion of AIDS patients presenting with toxoplasmic encephalitis in France and Belgium was found to be 12–16% compared to 2.5% in the USA (Clumeck 1991). Within the USA, the rates were found to vary according to the individual's country of birth (Luft & Castro 1991). Cerebral toxoplasma infection was diagnosed in the UK in 3.3% of AIDS patients either as an AIDS-defining illness or within one month of AIDS diagnosis. A study analysing risk factors showed that the only independent variable significantly associated with cerebral toxoplasma infection was 'ever lived abroad'. Such subjects were twice as likely to have a diagnosis of cerebral toxoplasma infection (personal communication, M. Ryan 1993). This suggests that those who lived in countries where the incidence of toxoplasma infection was high were more likely to be *T. gondii* antibody positive and hence more likely to develop recrudescence of latent infection. The effect of HAART on the natural history of toxoplasma infection in HIV-positive patients is addressed in Chapter 5. Trends in laboratory reports to CDSC of toxoplasmic encephalitis as an AIDS-defining illness in the UK suggest that it has had a significant impact: there was a steep decline from a peak of 67 such reports in 1994 to 19 in 1999 (M. Wright, 2000 personal communication), even though the reported annual incidence of new cases of HIV infection was relatively unchanged in the 1990s.

The reason for the decline in reports of toxoplasma eye disease in England and Wales in recent years is unknown. No other countries, apart from Scotland, have comparable data available, so it is not known whether this reflects an artefact of ascertainment (for example, a relative increase in numbers of cases diagnosed clinically without serological investigation), or a real change in the epidemiology. Ryan et al. (1995) observed that the mean age of retinochoroiditis cases reported had remained unchanged and that the decline showed substantial geographical variability, thus lending weight to the first explanation. Nevertheless, if the general incidence of toxoplasma infection has been falling, as suggested above, then the incidence of toxoplasma eye disease (believed to result mainly from reactivation of infection acquired *in utero*) might also gradually decline in future generations. However, this trend could be counterbalanced by an increase in ocular toxoplasma infection among HIV-infected individuals – thought to result both from reactivation and from new infections and affecting 3% of such patients in one Paris series (Cocherau-Massin et al. 1992). Again, this trend would be modulated by antiretroviral treatment.

The relative likelihood of these conflicting trends poses difficulties for assessing the size of the problem of toxoplasma eye disease and predicting future trends. They are, like congenital infection, compounded by the lack of case definitions and difficulties in diagnosis (Dutton 1989; Holliman et al. 1991). There may also be 'real' geographical variation; for example, in community surveys in the United States, 0.5% of people examined ophthalmoscopically had fundal lesions characteristic of toxoplasmic retinochoroiditis. In contrast, a similar survey in Brazil found such lesions in 17.7% of the community (Glasner et al. 1992). It was suggested that this very high prevalence of eye disease (long recognized in Brazil) could be associated with particular strains of *T. gondii*, with postnatally acquired as well as congenital infection and with genetic determinants of host susceptibility. Gilbert et al. (1999) studied the incidence of symptomatic toxoplasma eye disease in a UK population using an active clinical reporting scheme involving ophthalmologists. They found a low lifetime risk in white British-born subjects (18 per 100,000) and symptoms were mild and transient in most cases. However, black people born in West Africa had a 100-fold higher incidence of symptomatic toxoplasma eye disease.

The dramatic increase in reported maternal acute toxoplasma infection in England and Wales in the late 1980s illustrates the ascertainment bias to which a voluntary routine epidemiological surveillance system is susceptible. The number of cases in 1989 was still a fraction of that expected on the basis of the findings of *ad hoc* prenatal surveys (Joynson 1992); the upsurge almost certainly represented better ascertainment of the 'true' incidence caused by an increase in public and professional media attention to materno–foetal toxoplasma infection in the UK from the end of 1988 onwards (Hall 1992). By contrast, the decline in toxoplasmic lymphadenopathy in England and Wales in the 1980s may have been 'real', because it paralleled the findings of the *T. gondii* antibody surveys outlined above. The cause of the decline may be changing risk factors for acquiring *T. gondii* (described further below).

This section on time trends in toxoplasma infection would not be complete without reference to time–place clusters or outbreaks of the infection. There are a number of these in the literature which are important because they have increased our understanding of risk factors for acquiring *T. gondii*, as well as routes of transmission. They are described in more detail in the next section. Outbreaks of toxoplasma infection are almost certainly underrecognized because of the relatively long incubation period (about 2–3 weeks) and the absent or nonspecific symptoms. In one outbreak it was estimated that only 3% of infections were diagnosed in spite of intensive media and education campaigns (Bowie et al. 1997). No outbreaks have been detected in England and Wales by the routine laboratory surveillance system. However, serological studies of family members where an index case of toxoplasma infection has been recognized show that common source outbreaks occur relatively frequently (Luft & Remington 1984).

This section has attempted to describe 'the size of the problem' of toxoplasma infection and to assess whether this is changing. It has reviewed various methods of doing this – ranging from serological surveys to laboratory- and clinician-based national surveillance schemes and case series published in the world literature. It has highlighted innovative, recently developed, mathematical modelling techniques which facilitate the estimation of incidence from seroprevalence surveys.

While it is clear that toxoplasma infection is common throughout the world, measuring the clinical burden is more difficult, as is monitoring trends, although both are essential for planning and evaluating the effectiveness of intervention programmes. A major difficulty is the heterogeneous nature of the infection (asymptomatic infection, eye disease, lymphadenopathic illness, congenital infection, severe systemic disease), with each manifestation having its own epidemiological trends and risk factors. Thus, for example, the incidence of severe disease is affected by trends in the numbers of immunocompromised individuals as well as the availability of antiretroviral therapy, while acute lymphadenopathy appears to be on the decline particularly in young people. Another difficulty is the lack of internationally accepted clinical-serological case definitions of all the manifestations of toxoplasma infection.

Thus, 'the size of the problem' remains poorly defined in all countries. Even if numbers of infected persons could be derived more accurately, it is yet a further step to determine the impact of the infection in terms of disability and handicap and cost – both to the individual and to the health-care service.

How is toxoplasma infection acquired?

It was stated at the beginning of this chapter that epidemiology can provide a scientific basis on which disease preventive strategies can be based. For example, increasing our understanding of the sources and routes of transmission of T. gondii can inform strategies for primary prevention of toxoplasma infection (preventing acquisition of the parasite).

Hypotheses on how T. gondii is acquired by human subjects are based on knowledge of the lifecycle of the organism as well as on its biological characteristics; for example, the ability of the oocyst to survive in the environment for long periods given the right conditions of temperature and humidity (see below and Chapter 1). The probable and possible routes of transmission which have been suggested are summarized in Table 3.3. This section of the chapter reviews the epidemiological evidence supporting these hypotheses, of which the two most important are ingestion of environmental oocysts and ingestion of tissue cysts from raw or lightly cooked meat. Although the various routes will be considered separately, this is an artificial distinction because they can interact in complex ways in the same areas at the same time. For example, in a locale highly contaminated with oocysts, where the human population eats meat from locally fed animals, it may be impossible to disentangle the relative risks from oocyst versus tissue cyst ingestion.

Toxoplasma transmission via ingestion of oocysts

Evidence from the lifecycle of T. gondii

The sexual lifecycle of T. gondii is initiated when a cat ingests tissue cysts for the first time. The most important sources of feline toxoplasma infection are persistently infected birds and rodents (Jackson & Hutchison 1989; Peach et al. 1989; Literak et al. 1997). Mice are particularly important because they can pass toxoplasma infection congenitally without causing overt clinical disease (Eichenwald 1948; Beverley 1959; De Roever-Bonnet 1969; Owen & Trees 1998). In this way an occult reservoir of T. gondii tissue cyst infection can be retained in a particular location, with the potential for infecting cats. Rats may also be a significant source of infection but

Table 3.3. Probable and possible routes of transmission of *T. gondii*

1. Oral
   - Ingestion of oocysts
     - *environment*
     - garden soil
     - litter trays
     - floors
     - water
     - *cats* direct contact
   - Ingestion of tissue cysts
     - *meat*
     - eating
     - handling
     - *products of conception*
     - handling farm animals – especially sheep
   - Ingestion of tachyzoites
     - milk (especially goats')
     - blood
     - other body fluids
2. Nonoral
   - Human to human tissue transfer
     - transplanted tissue (tissue cysts, tachyzoites)
     - transplacental transfer (tachyzoites)
     - blood transfusion (tachyzoites)
   - Inoculation
     - laboratory accidents (tachyzoites)
     - handling meat, products of conception, garden soil with non-intact skin (tachyzoites, tissue cysts, oocysts)

unlike mice congenital transmission occurs much less readily (Dubey & Frenkel 1998).

Following ingestion of infected tissues by all nonimmune species, the cyst wall is dissolved by proteolytic enzymes in the small intestines (Dubey 1977), the released bradyzoites penetrate the local epithelial cells and infection then spreads to the mesenteric lymph nodes and other tissues. However, in cats the parasite also remains in the intestinal epithelial cells and commences a schizogonic cycle, followed by gametogeny, which gives rise to unsporulated oocysts which are then excreted in the faeces, from about the fourth day after infection until around the twelfth (Dubey & Frenkel 1972). These oocysts are not capable of initiating an infection until they have sporulated, usually between one and five days after excretion, and this depends on temperature, moisture and perhaps other factors (Dubey 1977). Oocysts, once sporulated and deposited in the environment, can survive in soil and water at ambient temperatures for over 500 days, although factors such as sunlight, dry conditions or frost may considerably reduce this time (Dubey & Beattie 1988).

The ingestion of sporulated oocysts or tachyzoites by susceptible cats also causes infection, but there is a very much smaller output of oocysts and shedding occurs only for a day or so about 20 days after infection, and even then only in a minority of cases (Dubey & Frenkel 1976). Following infection, cats seroconvert and develop immunity. Although they normally remain persistently infected, clinical illness is rare and they do not normally excrete oocysts again. Recrudescence of infection may occur if a cat is stressed (Dubey & Frenkel 1974), thereby causing re-excretion of oocysts, albeit in smaller numbers and for a shorter time than in a primary infection. There is accumulating evidence that some feline viruses, such as feline immunodeficiency virus (FIV), may also be capable of reactivating latent toxoplasma infections in cats (Witt et al. 1989; Heidel et al. 1990; Lappin et al. 1992) and that cats with clinical FIV infection may persistently excrete toxoplasma oocysts, in association with intractable diarrhoea (personal communication, Arvid Uggla, National Veterinary Institute, Uppsala, Sweden).

Thus the ingestion of tissue cysts by recently infected cats is greatly significant, because they produce large numbers of oocysts (one cat can shed 200 million, Dubey & Beattie 1988) which spread into the environment where they may be a primary source of human infection, as well as the principal source of infection for meat-producing animals, rodents and birds. Usually not more than 2% of cats may be expected to be shedding oocysts at any time (Dubey & Beattie 1988), and relatively more of them will be young cats as shedding follows a primary infection following the ingestion of small mammals and birds infected with *T. gondii*.

Cats are widespread in many countries throughout the world. For example in the UK there is a large population of domestic, farm and feral cats (cats living wild). Female cats can produce two to three litters a year, each up to eight kittens, and farm and feral cats may rear their young communally (Macdonald 1980). In rural areas male cats may have territories of 60 to 80 hectares (250 to 200 acres), while females usually occupy only a tenth of this area (Macdonald 1980). In an urban environment these territories are considerably smaller (Tabor 1980). The area occupied by feral cats is influenced by the supply of food, which includes mice, voles, shrews, rats, rabbits and small birds (Macdonald 1980), all potential reservoirs of infection (Jackson & Hutchison 1989; Peach et al. 1989; Literak et al. 1997; Dubey & Frenkel 1998). Oocysts may also be shed by felidae in zoos (Lukesova & Literak 1998).

Evidence from seroepidemiological and surveillance studies

In this section, information on the descriptive epidemiology (distribution by geography, age, sex, season, ethnic and socio-economic group) of toxoplasma infection is reviewed to determine what can be learned about risk factors for acquisition of the organism.

Geographical distribution

Climatic studies

If environmental oocysts are an important reservoir, toxoplasma infection should be more prevalent in regions of the world where the climate is moist and humid than in colder, drier climates. There is in fact a high seroprevalence in the Caribbean, Central America and in tropical West Africa (Table 3.1). Moreover a study in the French West Indies (La Guadelope) (Barbier et al. 1983) demonstrated a statistically significant increase in the proportion of *T. gondii*-antibody-positive individuals who lived in areas of higher rainfall (48% of those in areas of 200 cm/year). A study of pregnant women in Norway in 1992 (Jenum et al. 1998) found a significantly lower prevalence (6.7%) of *T. gondii* IgG in those from northern, dry, cold regions compared to those from southern counties (13.4%), where a mild coastal climate prevails. This difference was independent of other risk factors.

In Panama (Sousa et al. 1988) statistically significant differences in prevalence were associated with altitude, with the lowest occurring at the highest altitude (27% at 1820 metres) and the highest near sea level (60% at 215 metres). However, low altitude is not consistently associated with higher levels of positivity – higher rainfall and more humid conditions may better explain the observed variation. For example, in Burundi (Excler et al. 1988), where the highest *T. gondii* antibody prevalence rates were found at higher than at lower altitudes (58% at 1700–2200 m), the humidity and rainfall at these altitudes were also higher. In Iran, *T. gondii* antibody prevalence ranged from 2.9% in the southern, dry provinces to 20.5% in the more humid north (Assmar et al. 1997).

These data suggest that environmental conditions may affect the viability of the oocyst and thus not only modulate the risk of ingestion via soil but also indirectly affect disease transmitted via meat by increasing or reducing the prevalence of toxoplasma infection in the intermediate host population.

'Island' studies

There have been a number of studies in particular locales relating the prevalence of *T. gondii* antibody among humans and other intermediate hosts to the presence of cats in these areas.

Wallace et al. (1972) showed that antibody to the parasite was present in Man, domestic cats, pigs and rats on one Pacific Island. On an adjacent island, where there were cats but no people, the infection was present in the rats. On a further island without people or cats, toxoplasma infection was not detected in rats (however, the authors question the validity of their finding because only one species of rat was present, unlike the other islands, and the sample was very small). In further studies of island communities it was demonstrated that rats, mice and certain birds acted as intermediate hosts for *T. gondii*. The authors concluded that human infection was more common when the cat population was large, due in turn to an abundance of intermediate hosts as a supply of food, coupled with a warm, humid climate and plentiful shade to permit survival of infectivity in excreted oocysts (Wallace 1973, 1976). In other studies, Munday (1972) found only two *T. gondii* antibody-positive island-bred sheep out of 300 on a cat-free island in the Bass Strait (compared with over 30% of sheep *T. gondii* antibody positive on nearby cat-infested islands) and Dubey and colleagues demonstrated a low prevalence of *T. gondii* antibody in feral pigs on a remote island lacking cats (Dubey et al. 1997). Etheredge and Frenkel (1995) surveyed 760 children living on nine islands in Panama. The prevalence of *T. gondii* antibody ranged from 0% to 45%. The uninfected group came from three islands where, unlike the others, the cats also showed no serological evidence of infection.

These island studies illustrate how the presence of cats can influence the likelihood of intermediate host infection. It may in fact be the latter that is the principle source of human infection rather than direct ingestion of oocysts: Wallace and colleagues (1972) determined that there was some consumption of lightly cooked meat by humans in their Pacific atoll study. Similarly, the prevalence of *T. gondii* antibody among various tribes of New Guinea paralleled the presence or absence of cats in their environment – both domestic and wild (Wallace et al. 1974*b*); however, the particularly high prevalence in one tribe was ascribed to their eating neotropical felidae as much as to environmental oocyst ingestion.

Urban–rural studies

Conflicting theories exist as to the relative risk of acquiring toxoplasma infection from environmental oocysts among country compared to city dwellers. The former could be more likely to be exposed to soil on farms or when gardening (Stray-Pederson and Lorentzen-Styr 1980; Decavalas et al. 1990); the latter might be more exposed because of the limited environment available to domestic and particularly to feral cats for defaecation (Ades et al. 1993). Yet others point to the lower risk of city cats contaminating the environment, compared to their country counterparts, because owners are less likely to allow them outdoors, thus reducing both their chances of acquiring *T. gondii* from hunting and their opportunity to defaecate outside (Pereira et al. 1992).

Since all such statements are based on conjecture, it is not surprising that,

Table 3.4. *Toxoplasma gondii* serology in urban and periurban/rural areas

Country	Test (+ve Titre)	Urban %+ve	Peri-urban/ Rural %+ve	References
UK (1957)	DT (16)	22.5	36.0	Beattie 1957
UK (1980–1986)	Elisa (12 IU/ml)	19.5	7.5	Gilbert et al. 1993
Czechoslovakia	CFT (8)	18.2	28.0	Sýkora et al. 1992
Somalia	ELISA (400)	40.0	56.0	Ahmed et al. 1988
Burundi	IFA (8 IU/ml)	40.0	46.4	Excler et al. 1988
Saudi Arabia	IHAT (64)	22.1	23.5	Ahmed 1992
Brazil	IHAT (256)	61.0	63.4	Ricciardi et al. 1975
Brazil	IHAT (25)	39.3	20.3	Lovelace et al. 1978
Panama	DT (2)	58.6	57.5	Sousa et al. 1988
Canada	IHAT (32)	1.1	5.2	Pereira et al. 1992
Greece	IFAT (>12 i.u./ml)	39	64	Decavalas et al. 1990
Costa Rica	IFAT (2)	66.8	50.9	Frenkel & Ruiz 1980
Ireland (1990s)	LAT (1–4)	10.2	16.6	Taylor et al. 1997

although urban–rural differences in *T. gondii* antibody prevalence have been demonstrated in many different surveys, there is no consistent pattern, with rural predominance in some and urban in others (Table 3.4). In one Central American study in Costa Rica, city dwellers had a higher seroprevalence than those in surrounding areas. This was ascribed to the high density of feral cats, lack of adequate areas for cats to defaecate and subsequent contamination within houses or on hard surfaces, and also to poorer living standards, washing and toilet facilities and hygiene (Frenkel & Ruiz 1980). However, a later study from Costa Rica and a similar study in Panama showed no urban–rural difference in *T. gondii* antibody prevalence (Arias et al. 1996; Sousa et al. 1988). By contrast, a study in the 1990s of Irish schoolchildren showed that significantly more of those living in the country had *T. gondii* IgG compared to city children (16.6% versus 10.2%) (Taylor et al. 1997). In the UK a survey in 10 areas in 1957 demonstrated *T. gondii* antibody prevalences of 36% and 22.5% in rural and urban dwellers respectively (Beattie 1957). By contrast a more recent investigation showed a higher *T. gondii* antibody prevalence in UK born women living in inner and suburban London compared to those living in nonmetropolitan areas (12.7%, 7.5% and 5.5% respectively, Ades et al. 1993). However, Allain et al. (1998) found no difference in *T. gondii* antibody prevalence between pregnant women living in urban versus rural areas in East Anglia in 1992. Ljungstrom et al. (1995) also found no urban–rural differences in Sweden in the 1980s.

Stray-Pedersen and Lorentzen-Styr (1980) compared locales of both current and childhood residence among three groups of Norwegian pregnant women examined serologically and found to be uninfected, to have 'old' infection, or to be newly infected. There was no difference between the three groups regarding current residence but a significantly higher proportion of those with 'old' infection had lived on farms in rural areas in their childhood. A survey in Somalia (Ahmed et al. 1988) showed higher rates of toxoplasma antibody among village inhabitants than among residents of Mogadishu (Table 3.1). The rural excess was ascribed to the higher density of cats (kept to kill rats) in conjunction with the custom of all household activities, including food preparation, eating and sleeping, taking place on the ground. Apparently this was not the custom of city dwellers.

A problem with all these studies is that there is no consistency of definition of what constitutes an urban as against a rural area, or whether subjects both live *and* work in these environments. Furthermore, many do not take account of factors which might influence both the likelihood of toxoplasma infection and living in a particular area (confounding variables).

Age distribution

Age-specific *T. gondii* antibody prevalence surveys from a wide range of countries show two distinct patterns – 'type I' in which rates are high in childhood and very high proportions of the population have been infected by adult life; the other, 'type II', where the antibody prevalence is relatively low in children, but increases gradually with age such that approximately one-half of all adults show evidence of infection.

In general, the first pattern is seen in less developed countries; for example, Costa Rica (Arias et al. 1996); Panama (Sousa et al. 1988); the Pacific Islands (Wallace 1976); Somalia (Ahmed et al. 1988); Madagascar (Lelong et al. 1995); and Ghana (Anteson et al. 1979). The second is observed mainly in industrialized nations; for example, the UK (Jackson et al. 1987; Ades & Nokes 1993); Italy (Moschen et al. 1991); Japan (Suzuki et al. 1988); Sweden (Huldt et al. 1979); and the United States (Lamb & Feldman 1968).

It is widely believed that the first pattern indicates acquisition of toxoplasma infection principally from the ingestion of environmental oocysts. The justification of this is threefold. First, socioeconomic conditions are such that infants and toddlers are exposed to the ground in conditions of inadequate hygiene; second, domestic and feral cats are prevalent and defaecate in living areas; third, meat is 'usually' or 'always' eaten well cooked in that society, so viable toxoplasma tissue cysts are unlikely to be ingested. It is thought that the second age pattern reflects acquisition principally from ingestion of tissue cysts (further details in the section on tissue cysts below).

The hypotheses regarding exposure to oocysts do have some supportive evidence from carefully conducted studies, particularly those in Costa Rica (described further below: Frenkel & Ruiz 1980, 1981). However, it is important not to make generalizations – almost certainly risk factors for acquiring toxoplasma infection are multiple, even in the same area and will also vary from place to place. Thus some communities in developing countries have the 'Type II' age pattern of toxoplasma *T. gondii* antibody prevalence; for example, parts of India (Bowerman 1991; Mittal et al. 1995); Bangladesh (Samad et al. 1997); Rwanda (Gascon et al. 1989); Nigeria (Osiyemi et al. 1985); and Niger (Julvez et al. 1996). By contrast, some European countries, for example France and The Netherlands, have the 'Type I' pattern (Papoz et al. 1986; Conyn van Spaendonck 1991) although it may have changed recently. Moreover, the sophisticated mathematical modelling techniques referred to above revealed a previously unreported higher incidence (as against prevalence) of toxoplasma infection in children compared to adults, in a region of England (Ades & Nokes 1993; Marschner 1997).

Some surveys that have concluded that environmental oocysts play a major role in *T. gondii* transmission in a given community, because of the age distribution of antibody, have been less than rigorous in excluding other possibilities. When some authors have further investigated the claim that only well cooked meat is eaten in a particular culture, exceptions have been found. For example in Somalia, although meat was always reportedly eaten well cooked, goats' liver was sometimes consumed lightly cooked (Ahmed et al. 1988). These authors also referred to goats' milk consumption by the community – a neglected risk factor in most studies, but one known to be a vehicle for *T. gondii* (see below). In another study, from Ghana, it was stated that, although 'all' meat was well cooked before consumption in that culture, there were ceremonial occasions when meat was consumed partially cooked; furthermore, there were customs among young adults to buy partially cooked meat 'kebabs' from roadside vendors, and among young children to capture rodents during hunting expeditions and 'roast them hurriedly' (Anteson et al. 1979).

These small points emphasize the need for rigorous, detailed studies, geared to local customs, in order to elucidate relevant local risks for acquiring toxoplasma. They are not academic because they will inform local strategies for primary prevention.

Sex distribution

It has been consistently observed in series of cases of toxoplasma lymphadenopathy that males are over-represented among child and adolescent patients, whereas there is an excess of females among adult cases (McCabe et al. 1987). Furthermore, Ryan et al. (1995) observed statistically highly significant differences between the

Table 3.5. *Toxoplasma gondii* antibody prevalence in males and females

Country	n	% Males +ve	% Females +ve	References
Burundi	622	49.6	39.2	Excler et al. 1988
Kenya (Nairobi)	127	27	59	Bowry et al. 1986
South Africa	3,379	21	17	Jacobs & Mason 1978
Sudan (Gezira)	386	39.1	44.8	Abdel-Hameed 1991
Gabon	1,448	56.8	43.2	Beauvais et al. 1978
Niger	400	22.5	14	Develoux et al. 1988
Niger Delta	1,650	53	64.8	Arene 1986
Ivory Coast	2,000	67.6	56.6	Dumas et al. 1989
Nigeria	99	26.7	18.8	Osiyemi et al. 1985
Saudi Arabia	274	21.2	27	Ahmed 1992
Hong Kong	67	5.7	0	Ludlam et al. 1969
Malaysia	728	14.8	10.3	Tan & Zaman 1973
Indonesia (Central Java)	695	17.3	17.9	Cross et al. 1975
Indonesia (Paniai)	188	39.4	31.6	Gandalhusada & Endardjo 1980
India (Kumaon)	200	37	77	Singh & Nautiyal 1991
Singapore	803	48	40	Chew et al. 1982
Canada (Nova Scotia)	998	4	2.7	Pereira et al. 1992
Italy	1,494	18.2	17.5	MacKnight & Robinson 1992
Chile (Regions I,II,III)	19,798	33.9	32.9	Schenone et al. 1986a
Costa Rica (1970s)	883	66.4	57.5	Frenkel & Ruiz 1980
Costa Rica (1990s)	1,234	42.8	57.2	Arias et al. 1996
Ireland	1,276	12.7	12.8	Taylor et al. 1997

age distribution of males and females in reports of laboratory-confirmed toxoplasma lymphadenopathy in England and Wales, 1981–1992. The difference was
particularly marked among 15–19 years olds among whom there were twice as
many males.

Many *T. gondii* antibody prevalence studies show a slight excess of positivity
among males; others show no difference and a few show a striking female excess
(Table 3.5). In a study of Kenyan schoolchildren (Bowry et al. 1986) 27% of boys
were *T. gondii* antibody-positive compared with 59% of girls. However, just over
12% of both boys and girls had *T. gondii* IgG in Ireland (Taylor et al. 1997). In the
Kumaon region of India 77% of women were *T. gondii* antibody positive compared
with 37% of males (Singh & Nautiyal 1991). In Malaysia (Saleha 1984) a study of
728 healthy people demonstrated seropositivity in 14.8% of males and 10.3% of

females. When those of Indian origin were examined the ratios reversed with 10.8% of males being *T. gondii* antibody-positive compared with 28% of females.

It is difficult to interpret these conflicting findings in terms of risk factors for acquiring *T. gondii* infection. Age, local culture and environment are all likely to be interacting. However, it is suggested that the consistent observation of an increased risk among males at young ages is because boys have a tendency to undertake activities that expose them to soil and to be less fastidious about hand hygiene than girls (McCabe et al. 1987). It has further been suggested that the excess among adult women, compared to men, may be related to domestic exposure – both to oocysts, via gardening or handling the pet cat's litter tray, and to tissue cysts during the preparation of meat for meals (see below). It must, however, be emphasized that all these suggestions are conjectural – at least part of the female excess may be artefactual, representing increased rates of diagnosis because of cosmetic concern about lumps in the neck and because of concern about possible toxoplasma infection in pregnancy.

Seasonal distribution

It has been suggested that the incidence of acute toxoplasma infection is likely to decline during warmer, drier seasons because of a reduction in the number of viable oocysts in the environment. Indeed, two surveys in England and Wales and in Scotland did show summer dips (Bannister 1982; Chatterton et al. 1988). However, a similar Canadian survey showed a decline in September to November with high levels during the rest of the year (Tizard et al. 1976) and surveillance data on toxoplasmic lymphadenopathy for England and Wales, 1989–1991, showed no seasonal pattern at all (Ryan et al. 1995).

As with age and sex distributions, predictions about seasonal trends supporting the importance of environmental oocysts in toxoplasma transmission are likely to be too simplistic. It is not surprising that findings are conflicting, because of confounding variables such as the upsurge in overseas travel in summer months (which has also been found to be a risk factor, Stray-Pederson & Lorentzen-Styr 1980; Kapperud et al. 1996) and the increased likelihood of eating lightly cooked meat at barbecues during this season.

Ethnic and socioeconomic distributions

Patterns of prevalence of *T. gondii* antibody vary with ethnic groups sometimes even when these groups live closely together. In studies in Malaysia, native Malays had consistently higher *T. gondii* antibody prevalence rates compared with Indians and Chinese (Thomas et al. 1980; Saleha 1984; Yahaya 1991). In Hawaii (Wallace 1976) people of Japanese origin had rates of 14% compared with Caucasians (24%), Filipino (45%) and Portuguese (67%). In South Africa (Jacobs & Mason

1978) 34% of blacks were found to be *T. gondii* antibody-positive compared to 12% of whites and 9% of San (bushmen). Amongst pregnant women in London *T. gondii* antibody prevalence ranged from 7.6% (Asian women born in India and Sri Lanka) to 71.4% (white European women born in France; Gilbert et al. 1993). A survey of pregnant women in Norway in 1992 showed that women with foreign names had a higher prevalence (22.6%) of toxoplasma infection than women with Norwegian names (10%) (Jenum et al. 1998).

In Stockholm in 1987, *T. gondii* antibody prevalence among pregnant women who were immigrants mainly from Southern Europe was more than twice that among indigenous Swedish women; moreover, it had not declined over the 20-year study period among the immigrants, whereas it had among local women (Forsgren et al. 1991). The reverse has been observed in France. In the Toulouse area, 1980–1986, 73% of pregnant women who were both white French and born in France had antibody compared to 58% of North African, 52% of sub-Saharan African and 22% of south-east Asian immigrants. It was observed that the Asians were recent arrivals whereas the Africans were second-generation immigrants (Espeillac et al. 1989). Clearly, the pattern among immigrants will reflect both the serological pattern in their country of origin and the duration of their residence in the new country. Espeillac et al. speculated that second-generation immigrants had begun to take on the culture of France with its attendant increased risk of acquiring toxoplasma infection.

The ethnic differences described above probably do not reflect inherent differences in susceptibility to toxoplasma infection. For example low *T. gondii* antibody prevalence rates noted in the Chinese population in China and Hong Kong do not occur in Tahiti where the prevalence of infection in Chinese was found to be 86% (Wallace et al. 1974a). These Chinese had lived in Tahiti all their lives. The differences are likely to be cultural and may be due to different patterns of hygiene, cat density/ownership, food preparation and socioeconomic status or other factors not yet elucidated.

Yahaya (1991) speculated that the high *T. gondii* antibody prevalence they observed among Malays was due to the high density of cats (and therefore oocysts in their environment) caused, apparently, by the absence of dogs, which are not kept for religious reasons. They had no explanation for the low rate in Malaysian Chinese, but suggested that the intermediate rate among Indians was explained by their agricultural life style and use of hands for tilling oocyst-contaminated soil and for collecting produce. Gilbert et al. (1993) speculated that the ethnic distributions they observed may have reflected differences in the preparation and consumption of meat, unpasteurized milk and use of freezers (see below). Differences in exposure to oocysts was not cited as an explanation and they emphasized that there were no data to support their speculations.

One difficulty with studies of immigrant populations is the potential confounding variable of socioeconomic status which may be different (usually lower) in immigrants compared to the local population. Various indices of socioeconomic status have been used to study this factor in relation to *T. gondii* antibody prevalence. Of note is the observation that where environmental oocysts are thought to be the major source of infection, people of lower socioeconomic status have the highest *T. gondii* antibody prevalence rates. In Panama (Sousa et al. 1988), rates of *T. gondii* antibody-positivity of 66% were observed in those with a monthly income of $0–$75 compared with 56% in those earning $1000 or more. The possession of a private bathroom or an inside water supply were also associated with lower *T. gondii* antibody prevalence rates. In the French West Indies (Barbier et al. 1983), *T. gondii* antibody prevalence amongst white collar workers was 59% compared to 69% in blue collar workers. In Burundi (Excler et al. 1988) *T. gondii* antibody prevalence amongst urban people of low and high socioeconomic groups was 45% and 22% respectively. In Spain, low socioeconomic status was strongly associated with the presence of *T. gondii* antibody in pregnant women in 1993 (Guerra & Fernandez 1995).

Thus as with the findings on geographical, age, sex and seasonal distributions, patterns of toxoplasma infection among different ethnic and socioeconomic groups show interesting, often marked, variations which are likely to provide clues about transmission risks. However, the interaction of numerous confounding variables once again emphasizes the need for local risk factor studies informed by knowledge of local cultural practices so that locally appropriate preventive strategies can be devised (this may include different strategies for different cultural groups in the same locale).

Evidence from *T. gondii* antibody prevalence risk factor studies

In this type of epidemiological study a serological survey (measuring *T. gondii* IgG) is undertaken, and at the same time the study subjects are questioned about exposure to a variety of risk factors for toxoplasma infection. The histories of *T. gondii* antibody-positive and -negative subjects are then compared.

The problem with this approach is that the timing of the toxoplasma infection in *T. gondii* IgG antibody-positive subjects is unknown, so exposure histories cannot be related reliably to the event. Furthermore, the same observation about different assays and different cut-offs for positivity referred to above applies equally to most published *T. gondii* antibody prevalence risk factor studies. Other problems are that the antibody-negative group is not always comparable in age, there is frequently no simultaneous assessment of other risk factors and the questions asked of subjects are too vague.

It is, therefore, not surprising that conflicting results have been obtained. Ganley and Comstock (1980) reviewed ten such studies published, 1963–1977, of which eight (like their own) showed no association between tests positive for *T. gondii* and cat exposure, while two did. An eleventh study found no association with ordinary pet cats, but did with the ownership of pedigree cats. This illustrates the complexity of assessing the risk because the pedigree animals were fed raw meat significantly more often than the ordinary cats, thus their owners would have been more exposed to this vehicle than the comparison group (Ulmanen & Leinikki 1975). A later study also found a significant association between being a cat breeder and having *T. gondii* antibody (Woodruff et al. 1982). However, the possibility of raw meat exposure was not considered and the comparison group was not only not matched for age, but came from a different country.

The conflicting findings continue in studies published in the 1990s: Di Giacomo et al. (1990) found no association between exposure to cats at home or work and the prevalence of *T. gondii* antibodies in a university population in Seattle, USA. A study of Irish children aged 4–18 years found no association between toxoplasma infection and the presence of a cat in the home in the past two years (Taylor et al. 1997). By contrast, Decavalas et al. (1990), Seuri and Koskela (1992) and Pereira et al. (1992) all concluded from their studies (in south west Greece, Finland and Nova Scotia, respectively) that a combination of rural living and cat ownership, especially two or more cats, was a significant risk for human toxoplasma infection. The Canadian study may have been more valid than many because the subjects were children and adolescents (thus reducing recall and infection timing problems); unfortunately, no information on lightly cooked meat exposure was collected in any of these last four studies.

MacKnight and Robinson (1992) did collect detailed information from their *T. gondii* antibody-positive and -negative subjects, not only on lightly cooked meat exposure and gardening activity, but also on the feeding and defaecation behaviour of their cats. They concluded that past and present cat ownership was a risk factor for toxoplasma infection as was frequent gardening and the consumption of lightly cooked beef. However, neither this nor other studies have looked in detail at the precise gardening activities which might be risky (for example, weeding provides more exposure to soil than, say, pruning). It was, however, the first to note a lack of association between litter tray use by the pet and *T. gondii* antibody in the owner. Nevertheless, this study, like the others, suffered from having to relate risk factors to infection acquired at unknown times in the past.

Some of the most convincing seroepidemiological studies linking toxoplasma infection to environmental oocysts were those conducted in Costa Rica in the 1970s. Frenkel and Ruiz (Frenkel & Ruiz 1980, 1981; Ruiz & Frenkel 1980a, b) showed that infection occurred most commonly in children, the more so if there was individual cat contact, if there were large numbers of cats and if the family lived either in houses with wooden floors over a crawl space or in houses with cement floors and cats. They concluded that transmission to people was most likely to occur if, outside, the ground was covered in asphalt and concrete and there was little soil available for cat defaecation. The infection rate amongst intermediate hosts, such as mice, rats and sparrows, was 3.5%, 12.5% and 16% respectively and the authors concluded that a cat might eat an infected animal every 7–33 days. In these studies a human 'soil contact index' was devised; this correlated negatively with infection – possibly because cat density was greater in cities. The authors suggested that because the animals were mostly feral and not kept as pets, children did not acquire toxoplasma infection from direct contact with the cats, but from contaminated floor surfaces. A survey from Panama came to similar conclusions (Etheredge & Frenkel 1995), but a later study from Costa Rica showed no significant correlation between *T. gondii* antibody prevalence and 'cat contact', whereas there was an association with consumption of raw meat (Arias et al. 1996). The authors speculated that there had been a change in the pattern of transmission previously described for Costa Rica.

Evidence from studies of recent infections

In these studies the timing of the subjects' infections is known with greater precision than in those cited in the previous section; risk factor associations are therefore more valid. There are two types of study: investigations of outbreaks of toxoplasmosis and risk factor studies in which subjects with serological evidence of recent infection (seroconversion or presence of *T. gondii* IgM antibody) are compared with those who have no antibody or evidence of past infection.

There are four well documented outbreak investigations implicating *T. gondii* oocyst ingestion.

In the first, in 1977, 37 patrons of a riding stable in Atlanta, Georgia, developed acute toxoplasmosis. *Toxoplasma gondii* was recovered from the tissues of the stables' kittens and the older cats had antibody. Dietary history eliminated meat as the source of the outbreak, but patrons who spent most of their time eating sandwiches at the end of the indoor arena where one of the cats defaecated had the highest incidence of infection. It was postulated that environmental oocysts were dispersed by the movement of the horses, although oocysts were not recovered from this environment (Teutsch et al. 1979).

In a large family outbreak in 1976 which mainly affected preschool age children, an association between illness and both playing in a garden and geophagia was demonstrated. The *T. gondii* antibody-positive family cat had had kittens which had died of an undiagnosed nonspecific illness a month before. No oocysts were isolated from the garden soil, but it was presumed that this was the likely source as there was no history of ingestion of lightly cooked meat (Stagno et al. 1980).

In the third outbreak, 31 soldiers on a training course in the Panamanian jungle in 1979 developed toxoplasma infection. There was a strong epidemiological association between illness and drinking water from one particular source. No attempts were made to isolate oocysts from the water – it was assumed to have been contaminated by jungle cats (Benenson et al. 1982). It was, however, subsequently shown by Kasper and Ware (1985) that the sera of the infected soldiers contained antibodies to stage-specific oocyst sporozoite antigens.

In 1995 there was a sudden increase of serologically confirmed cases of acute toxoplasmosis and of toxoplasmic retinochoroiditis in the Greater Victoria area of British Columbia, Canada (Bowie et al. 1997). Case–control and mapping studies showed significant associations between acute infection and residence in the distribution system of one municipal reservoir supplying water to Greater Victoria. The outbreak had been preceded by a period of excessive rainfall associated with increased turbidity in the implicated reservoir. It was suggested that runoff from the surrounding land may have contaminated the reservoir with T. gondii oocysts, because domestic and feral cats, including cougars, were present in the watershed. Four of seven cats trapped in the watershed had antibody to T. gondii as did all five cougars from a nearby locale. A subsequent study of local cougars demonstrated T. gondii oocysts in the faeces of one animal captured within the implicated reservoir's watershed (Aramini et al. 1998). The water treatment system was considered inadequate to cope with the period of contamination (see below).

Six risk factor studies of serologically confirmed recent infections have examined the possibility of acquisition via oocyst ingestion. One, from Norway, involved newly delivered women (Stray-Pedersen & Lorentzen-Styr 1980). The criteria for recent infection were T. gondii seroconversion, significant rises in T. gondii antibody titre, or T. gondii IgM detected during the pregnancy. No association, compared with uninfected women or those with 'old' infection, was demonstrated with recent 'cat contact' or current residence either in the country or in a house with a garden.

Similarly, in another study of pregnant women in the Naples area of Italy between 1991 and 1994, women with recent infection were not, on multivariate analysis, significantly more likely to have ever owned a cat, lived on a farm, or gardened, than seronegative subjects (Buffolano et al. 1996).

Another more recent Norwegian study of pregnant women between 1992 and 1994 used similar methodology except that control subjects not only had no T. gondii antibody, but were also matched to cases for age, gestational stage and geographical area of residence (Kapperud et al. 1996). Subjects were questioned in detail about a range of risk factors for acquiring T. gondii. Although other factors contributed larger fractions to the attributable risk (see next section), an independent association between infection and cleaning the cat litter tray was found on multivariate analysis. Washing the hands after cleaning the box was not protective. By contrast, when no association with soil contact was found, the authors comment that because such activity was followed by handwashing in almost all subjects, or they used gloves, these measures were protective. There is no explanation for these conflicting findings.

The authors also found an independent association between infection and the consumption of unwashed raw vegetables and fruits, commenting that this was a major factor contributing to maternal infection in Norway, presumably because of *T. gondii* oocyst-contaminated soil on these foodstuffs. On univariate analysis there was no association between infection and living in a household with an adult cat, although there was an association with living with a kitten under one year old. This study illustrates the importance of asking the subjects of risk factor surveys detailed questions about their association with cats.

Frenkel et al. (1995) studied a cohort of 571 Panama City children prospectively over a 5-year period for acquisition of antibody to *T. gondii*. Risk factors were compared between the 72 (12%) who seroconverted and those who remained uninfected. High relative risks of transmission were predicted by contact histories with unweaned cats, 6- to 12-month-old cats and nursing cats. There was also a highly significant association with contact with nursing dogs, weaned dogs, 'many flies', 'much garbage' and 'many roaches'. The authors hypothesize that dogs, by eating and rolling in cat faeces, may, like some insects, aid in the mechanical transmission of *T. gondii*. This is interesting in view of the association between toxoplasma infection and both recently whelping bitches and toxocara seropositivity described by Taylor et al. (1997). Frenkel et al.'s (1995) Panamanian study supports both their theories about *T. gondii* transmission in their earlier Costa Rican studies and the evidence that a lower socioeconomic status is a risk for toxoplasma infection in some communities.

The fifth study followed up *T. gondii* antibody-negative, HIV-positive individuals every 6 months to detect seroconversion (Wallace et al. 1993). There was no association between this event and cat ownership or litter tray exposure. Moreover there appeared to be a protective effect of cat possession! Unfortunately, no information on other possible sources of infection was gathered, so neither oocyst ingestion via, say, gardening nor tissue cyst ingestion could be excluded. However, the authors concluded that HIV-positive patients could be reassured about cat ownership providing reasonable hygiene precautions were taken.

In the sixth study, set in large European cities, Cook et al. (2000) determined risk factors for acquiring toxoplasma infection by comparing two groups of pregnant women: those with acute infection detected by seroconversion or the presence of specific IgM, and those who had no antitoxoplasma antibody. No significant associations were found between infection and the presence of either adult cats or kittens, the diet and hunting habits of pet cats, or cleaning litter trays. However, there was an association with working in fields or gardens 'with hands in the soil'.

This section has presented the evidence, from both descriptive and analytical epidemiological studies, that ingestion of environmental oocysts plays an important role in human toxoplasma infection. Most authors who attempt to make the distinction agree that actual physical contact with cats is not a risk factor. This is not surprising given the usually clean habits of these animals in terms of grooming and disposal of faeces. All the evidence suggests that an environment heavily contaminated with cats' faeces – be it garden soil or solid ground in urban areas where soil is unavailable to feral cats – is an important risk factor for human toxoplasma infection either directly or indirectly via consumption of locally reared animals.

In spite of all the research, however, little is known about precisely how human beings ingest oocysts. The extent of the risk and the routes of transmission are likely to vary considerably from place to place according to climate, cultural practices and socioeconomic conditions. In countries or areas where cats are prevalent, hygienic conditions are poor and where all activities take place on the ground, contamination of fingers and food by oocysts is easy to imagine. Spread in such conditions may also be facilitated by dogs acting as transport hosts and by coprophagous insects such as flies and cockroaches, which have been shown experimentally to be effective transport hosts of oocysts (Smith 1991). However, the role of insects and dogs in the epidemiology of human toxoplasma infection is unknown. The roles of gardening and of litter tray emptying as risk factors in more wealthy societies are still conjectural and undefined. Such evidence as there is, is conflicting.

The recent decline in toxoplasma infection observed in several countries and noted in the first part of this chapter is often hypothesized as being due to changes in meat production and storage practices (see below). However, there could be an oocyst-related explanation. In recent decades there has been a marked change in the western world in the retailing of vegetables and salads such that the heavy soil contamination that used to be brought into the kitchen is rarely seen nowadays. Exceptions would be home-grown and some 'organic' produce. Indeed the increasing popularity of 'pick your own' vegetables may re-introduce soil into the kitchen.

Very little work on isolation of oocysts from soil has been undertaken. Such as there is, has examined the environment rather than soil contaminating food at the retail outlet. For example, Coutinho et al. (1982) found oocysts in vegetable garden soil near the houses of farm workers, among whom there had been cases of toxoplasmosis. Frenkel et al. (1995) in their Panama City study found that 1.1% of soil samples tested in mice resulted in *T. gondii* antibody seroconversion.

Similarly, the role of contaminated water as a vehicle for ingestion of oocysts has been under-investigated. It was certainly the cause of two outbreaks of toxoplasma infection (Benenson et al. 1982; Bowie et al. 1997) and has been suggested as an important factor in societies where meat is not eaten, but toxoplasma antibody is prevalent (Rawal 1959; Hall et al. 1999).

Bowie et al. (1997) point out that many communities may have a water supply sharing the features of that in the Canadian outbreak which makes them at risk – a surface water supply susceptible to direct or indirect contamination, access to the supply by domestic and feral cats, a short retention time in the intake reservoir, use of weak chemicals for primary disinfection and lack of filtration for water treatment. There have been a number of waterborne cryptosporidium and giardia outbreaks in England and Wales in recent years (Stanwell-Smith 1999). The conditions which permitted contamination by these organisms could well also allow the presence of toxoplasma oocysts. One source might be run-off from pastureland, which has been spread with manure from the farmyard dung heap – a common defaecation site for farm cats (see below).

T. gondii transmission via ingestion of tissue cysts

Evidence from the lifecycle of T. gondii

Following the ingestion of environmental T. gondii oocysts by a nonimmune warm-blooded vertebrate, infection will occur and persist for months, or even years, in the form of bradyzoites in cysts in various tissues, including skeletal muscle, brain, heart and liver. In this form the parasite is a potential source of infection for any animal – including Man – that ingests such tissues raw or partially cooked. In only a minority of instances does infection with the parasite cause clinical illness in domestic or wild animals. Infection of sheep, goats and pigs can, however, precipitate abortion and neonatal mortality, while severe illness and death may occur in certain peculiarly susceptible wild animals when kept in zoological collections (Innes 1997).

Spread of infection to farm livestock

As well as contaminating the soil, cats will, given the opportunity, bury their faeces in stores of uncovered grain (Plant et al. 1974). Fifty grams of infected cat faeces may contain as many as 10 million oocysts (Dubey & Frenkel 1972) which, if evenly dispersed throughout 10 tonnes of concentrated animal feed, would result in each kilogram containing between 5 and 25 sheep infective doses (McColgan et al. 1988). Contamination of this nature can therefore create a considerable reservoir of infection for livestock.

Farm cats often rear young in the farm steading and in barns of hay and straw, where they may deposit infected faeces. Thus cattle, sheep, goats, pigs and farmed deer are frequently maintained in an environment harbouring T. gondii oocysts and may therefore receive contaminated food (Blewett 1983; Blewett & Watson 1983, 1984). Still or slowly moving water may also be a source of infection if it is draining rain water run-off from contaminated pastures. The latter can be a common source of infection, particularly if the fields have been treated with manure and bedding from farm buildings where cats live (Faull et al. 1986).

Clinicopathological findings in animals

Sheep and goats

A primary infection of pregnant sheep and goats with *T. gondii* results in infection of the placenta and foetus. Infection in midgestation may be fatal for the foetus, in which case partial resorption will lead to mummification and subsequent expulsion alongside a live sibling, although the latter may sometimes be too weak to survive. Infection in late gestation does not normally cause any mortality although the lambs or kids will be infected (Buxton 1991). However, in all cases the placenta is infected and shows characteristic white necrotic foci 2–3 mm in diameter in the placental cotyledons (Beverley et al. 1971). Infected ewes and nanny goats do not normally show any other clinical signs, apart from abortion (Buxton 1991). Histopathological lesions, which are largely confined to the brains of stillborn and weak offspring, consist of focal leukomalacia in the cerebrum and widespread foci of microglial clusters often surrounding foci of necrosis (Buxton 1989).

Pigs

The incidence of clinical toxoplasma infection in pigs following exposure to infection is variable (reviewed by Dubey 1986a). Primary infection during pregnancy may or may not result in congenital infection. When infection of the developing foetus does occur, piglets may be stillborn and live piglets may or may not be infected. Infected piglets may remain healthy or may die in the first few weeks of life. Prior to death, fever, ataxia and diarrhoea may be evident and, at necropsy, hepatitis, lymphadenitis and pneumonia may be present. Pulmonary oedema, fibrinonecrotic alveolitis, nonsuppurative encephalitis, granulomatous nephritis and necrotizing hepatitis have all been recorded histologically (reviewed by Dubey 1986a).

Cattle

Natural toxoplasma infection appears to be rare in cattle; older serological tests to detect *T. gondii* antibodies in bovines gave false positives and greatly overestimated its incidence. A wide range of symptoms has been reported (Dubey 1986b) and in a few instances naturally acquired toxoplasma has been associated with abortion in cattle (Gottstein et al. 1998).

Wild animals

Toxoplasma gondii can infect many animal species in the wild and in captivity without precipitating clinical illness, but certain species in zoos are especially susceptible. For example, infection in New World monkeys may manifest as sudden death or acute illness of a few days followed by death. Clinical signs include dyspnoea, neurological symptoms and sometimes diarrhoea, while the consistent pathological change is necrosis, particularly in the liver, spleen and lungs but also in the lymph nodes, cardiac muscle and brain (McKissock et al. 1968; Cunningham et al. 1992; Juan-Salles et al. 1998). Old World monkeys, in contrast, are relatively resistant to *T. gondii* (McKissock et al. 1968). Marsupials, particularly wallabies and kangaroos, may also develop acute, disseminated, fatal infection (Obendorf & Munday 1983; Patton et al. 1986; Dubey et al. 1988; Canfield et al. 1990).

Persistence of infection

Sheep, goats and pigs remain persistently infected for months and probably life (Dubey & Beattie 1988), with tissue cysts in muscles, brain and other tissues. Cattle and deer, however, appear not to remain persistently infected to the same extent. The reason for this apparent host-species difference is not known.

Evidence from surveys of meat animals and meat

Lamb or mutton, goat meat and pork probably present the greatest risk of being contaminated, but beef (Dubey 1992; Dubey & Thulliez 1993) horsemeat and wild game may also harbour the parasite (Smith 1991). Table 3.6 summarizes the findings of some often-cited surveys of meat animals. Poultry are not included because they have been studied relatively little, although all birds can be intermediate hosts for *T. gondii*. Cysts have been found in the edible tissues of chickens (Dubey 1986c), although not in the eggs of experimentally inoculated birds (Biancifiori et al. 1986). Intensively reared poultry is likely to be clear of infection because the diet and environment are not usually contaminated with *T. gondii* oocysts, but free-range poultry may ingest the parasite and so their meat may present a risk to humans if consumed inadequately cooked. Meat animals infrequently eaten in western countries are not shown in Table 3.6. In Bangladesh 13% of slaughtered goats had significant titres of *T. gondii* antibody (Samad et al. 1997). Wild animals may be an important source of *T. gondii* in some cultures since hunters may handle and eviscerate them in unhygienic conditions and may eat them lightly cooked (Sacks et al. 1983).

The decline in *T. gondii* antibody prevalence among pigs observed in both The Netherlands and Scotland (Table 3.6) has been ascribed to changing farming practice away from free-range grazing to more intensive and controlled production. Geographical and seasonal variations in *T. gondii* antibody prevalence in both

Table 3.6. Prevalence of *T. gondii* in meat animals and retail meat

	Animals			Meat		
	Antibody prevalence %	Place	Reference	% samples infected	Place	Reference
Sheep	37	USA	Dubey 1990	5 (estimated)	USA	Dubey 1986c
	15	Glasgow (1974)	Jackson & Hutchison 1992			
	25	Glasgow (1984)	Jackson & Hutchison 1992			
	10–15 (lambs)	Norway	Waldeland 1976	8	Romania	Pop et al. 1989
	25–37 (sheep)	Norway	Waldeland 1976			
	31 (range 0–96)	Worldwide	Fayer 1981			
Pigs	29 (range 1–98)	Worldwide	Fayer 1981	10	USA	Dubey 1986a
	9	Glasgow (1974)	Jackson & Hutchison 1992	5	Germany	Jackson & Hutchison 1992
	4	Glasgow (1984)	Jackson & Hutchison 1992			
	69	The Netherlands (1970s)	Van Knapen et al. 1995	9	Romania	Pop et al. 1989
	1	The Netherlands (1990s)	Van Knapen et al. 1995	4	Portugal	Fortier et al. 1990
	32	USA	Dubey 1986a			
Cattle	22	The Netherlands	Jackson & Hutchison 1992	5	USA	Dubey 1986b
	3	Glasgow (1974)	Jackson & Hutchison 1992			
	8	Glasgow (1984)	Jackson & Hutchison 1992			
	25 (range 0–99)	Worldwide	Fayer 1981	10	Romania	Pop et al. 1989

sheep and cattle have been related to dampness of the pasture, proximity to the farmstead with its cats and to indoor *versus* outdoor housing (Jackson & Hutchinson 1992). Furthermore, the prevalence of *T. gondii* antibody, as with humans, increases with age and this may explain the risk associated with cured meats (see below) (Blewett 1983; Dubey 2000).

Few studies have been performed to determine the prevalence of *T. gondii* tissue cysts in retail meat, mainly because of the difficulty of the bioassay. In one study in the United States of an epizootic of toxoplasma infection among a flock of pregnant ewes, 40% of liveborn lambs had serological evidence of congenital infection. Viable *T. gondii* cysts were found in edible muscles of all of a random sample of *T. gondii* antibody-positive lambs tested; the remainder went to market and their meat must be assumed to have been equally infected (Dubey & Kirkbride 1989). It is also interesting that the degree of infectivity in sheep meat may be influenced by the initial infective dose ingested (Esteban-Redondo & Innes 1998).

In another study of edible tissues of experimentally infected pigs, it was shown that *T. gondii* could be isolated from a range of muscles and internal organs from almost all of them and that it persisted for well beyond the life of pigs raised for market (Dubey 1988). The author pointed out that other surveys had shown that retail minced beef was sometimes contaminated with pork; thus although beef is generally not considered to be such a risk for toxoplasma infection as pork and lamb, when purchased as mince it might pose an increased threat. Further work is needed to determine the prevalence of *T. gondii* in a range of retail meats and to monitor trends, so that preventive measures can be better targeted and evaluated. The newer laboratory molecular assays may facilitate such studies. For example, Warnekulasuriya et al. (1998), using polymerase chain reaction, detected viable *T. gondii* in one of 67 ready-to-eat samples of cured meat in the UK.

Evidence from descriptive human seroepidemiological and surveillance studies
Secular, seasonal, cultural and socioeconomic patterns of toxoplasma infection

The roles of oocysts and tissue cysts in most human toxoplasma infection are closely interrelated; therefore, much of this work has already been reviewed in the previous section. However, some extra points can be made.

The decline in toxoplasma infection observed in a number of western countries is explained by almost all authors as due to two factors: first, increasing use of meat which has been deep frozen, a process which kills *T. gondii* during subsequent thawing (Dubey 1974; Lunden & Uggla 1992). Second, a decline in the prevalence of infection in meat, particularly pork, associated with more hygienic production. Both these statements are true, but their relationship to trends in human toxoplasma infection remains conjectural.

Another 'meat trend' in the UK and elsewhere which might be relevant is that of changing patterns of consumption of different types. Thus between 1966 and 1989 annual total UK supplies of beef fell by 9.4%, of lamb fell by 25%, of bacon and ham fell by 29%, of offal fell by 9.5%, of pork rose by 23%, and of poultry rose by 62%. Furthermore, annual imports of beef and lamb fell by about 50% over the same period whereas imports of pork rose by nearly 9% (personal communication, P. Sockett, 1993).

Changing patterns of source of meat animals and the reduction in lamb and beef consumption accompanied by an increase in poultry consumption could both alter the exposure of the population to *T. gondii* tissue cysts. It is, therefore, regrettable that so little is known about the prevalence of the organism in market meats. It has been remarked that poultry is unlikely to be an important vehicle because it is 'always eaten well done' (Smith 1992). However, that is not the case in the UK, as evidenced by the extensive problem of poultry-associated salmonellosis.

Data on UK household meat purchase by month of the year also support the difficulties outlined in an earlier section, of drawing inferences from seasonal trends in toxoplasma infection. Thus if a decline in summer months is observed it might equally be associated with the 20–30% decline in red meat consumption, which also occurs in the UK at that time (personal communication, P. Sockett, 1993), as with a reduction in environmental oocysts. We have already mentioned that the ethnic and socioeconomic patterns of *T. gondii* antibody prevalence may reflect differing cultural habits regarding the consumption of meat and/or its hygienic handling. The high *T. gondii* antibody prevalence in France is ascribed by many authors to that nation's fondness for consuming lightly cooked or even raw meat as in the French speciality dish 'steak tartare'. A food survey completed in 1988 showed that, in relation to other European countries, Britain was one of the lowest meat consumers (kg *per capita*) whereas France was the highest (Ho Yen & Joss 1992). Presumably even young children in France consume lightly cooked meat if the high *T. gondii* antibody prevalence among children in that country is related to tissue cyst rather than oocyst ingestion.

Different national habits were strikingly evident in the 71% prevalence of *T. gondii* antibody among pregnant white women who had been born in France compared to the 13% among native born British women observed by Gilbert et al. (1993). National differences have also been ascribed to different types of meat favoured; thus, much more mutton and lamb is eaten in France than in the United States (Dupouy-Camet et al. 1993). In 1984 lamb constituted only 0.8% of American red meat consumed (Dubey 1986*c*) compared to 13% in the UK in the same year (personal communication, P. Sockett, 1993). Gilbert et al. also noted a striking difference in *T. gondii* antibody prevalence between Asian women born in India and Sri Lanka and those born in Pakistan and Bangladesh. They hypothesized that the former would have been largely vegetarian Hindu, whereas the latter would have been Muslim women who may have been infected while eating or preparing meat which, in this culture, does not include pork, whereas sheep meat is favoured.

In countries where lightly cooked meat consumption is thought to be a common route of infection, the relationship between socioeconomic factors and *T. gondii* antibody prevalence may differ. For example in Oslo, Norway, *T. gondii* antibody prevalence was highest amongst subjects living in wealthier districts of the city (Stray-Pederson & Lorentzen-Styr 1980). The authors speculated that such people, having a high income, visited other countries more often and adopted such 'foreign' food cultures as consumption of lightly cooked meat. By contrast, Moschen et al. (1991) found the highest rates of antibody among Italian children whose fathers had the fewest years of schooling. They hypothesized that a poor life-style might be associated with an increased risk of consuming lightly cooked meat, presumably due to economizing on fuel.

Evidence from *T. gondii* antibody prevalence risk factor studies

There have been a number of studies which have already been cited above in the oocyst section, but which have also enquired about possible exposure to *T. gondii* tissue cysts. The same criticisms apply as already outlined, so it is not surprising that the results are again conflicting.

Sacks et al. (1983) found a significant association between the presence of *T. gondii* IgG antibody and a history of eating raw or rare venison in a study of 62 wildlife workers. Their investigation was prompted by three patients with acute toxoplasmosis who were all deer hunters who had recently consumed raw venison.

MacKnight and Robinson (1992) found an association between *T. gondii* anti-body-positivity and consumption of rare–medium cooked beef, but not well cooked beef or rare–medium cooked lamb or pork. Unfortunately the actual data were not presented, so it was not possible to assess whether small numbers of subjects eating pork and lamb might have affected the validity of the statistics. Di Giacomo et al. (1990) found a slight, but nonsignificant excess of subjects who preferred eating rare meat (type unspecified) among their *T. gondii* antibody-positives compared to negative subjects. In a survey of occupationally acquired toxoplasma infection, involving farmers in Finland, there was no difference in the proportion with *T. gondii* antibody between a group who tasted raw minced meat while preparing food and a group who did not (Seuri & Koskela 1992). By contrast, there was an association between *T. gondii* antibody positivity and raw meat consumption in a study of Japanese farmers (Kominishi & Takahashi 1987). Broadbent et al. (1981), in an antenatal serological survey, found no difference in rates of consumption of lightly cooked or raw meat between *T. gondii* antibody-positive and -negative London women. However, Jeannel (1988) did find such an association among pregnant women in Paris in the mid 1980s.

Evidence from studies of recent infections

There have been a number of outbreaks of toxoplasma infection recorded in the literature in which meat has been implicated as the vehicle of infection. In four of these, involving households or families, there was a possible association with the consumption of lightly cooked lamb but the evidence was anecdotal (Hall 1986). In another outbreak, among five college students in the United States in 1969, there was good epidemiological evidence that the vehicle was lightly cooked beefburger. There was, however, no microbiological confirmation of this and it was noted that the same grinding machine which produced the minced beef was also used for pork, so there could have been cross-contamination (Kean et al. 1969). Two outbreaks of acute human toxoplasmosis in Korea in 1994 and 1995, in which three patients had retinochoroiditis, were linked to the ingestion of uncooked pig meat and viscera (Choi et al. 1997). There was a cultural belief that such food had special nutritional value. In Brasil, a party in 1993 at which raw mutton was eaten resulted in 17 cases of acute symptomatic toxoplasmosis, including one case of retinochoroiditis (Bonametti et al. 1996).

A further outbreak was the first reported among pregnant women and it occurred in an Inuit community in Northern Quebec in 1987. There were only four cases, all were asymptomatic seroconversions detected as part of a screening programme (McDonald et al. 1990). Seroconversion was significantly associated with the skinning of animals for fur and frequent consumption of raw caribou meat and seal liver. There was no association with cats or cat litter handling.

Five of the six risk factor studies of patients with serologically confirmed recent toxoplasma infection, described in the section above on toxoplasma transmission via ingestion of oocysts, also examined exposure to tissue cysts. Stray-Pedersen and Lorentsen-Styr (1980) demonstrated that raw meat was consumed significantly more often among recently infected pregnant women than those who were uninfected. The authors commented on recent changes in meat consumption preference in Norway towards eating meat that is raw or semi-raw. The later Norwegian study (Kapperud et al. 1996) also demonstrated that the greatest independent risk, on multivariate analysis, was with eating raw or undercooked minced meat products – cases were four times more likely than controls to report this behaviour. Mutton, poultry, pork and minced meat purchased in Norway were all implicated. Infrequent washing of kitchen knives after preparation of raw meat was also an independent risk factor.

Buffolano et al. (1996) showed that recent toxoplasma infection in pregnant women in Naples in the early 1990s was strongly associated with frequency of consumption of cured pork and raw meat. Eating these foods at least once a month increased the risk threefold. This was the first report to identify cured meat as a source of toxoplasma infection. Cook et al. (2000) subsequently also found an association between infection and consumption of cured meats, as well as undercooked lamb, beef or game. These meats accounted for between 30% and 63% of infections in the six different study centres. By contrast to the other studies, Frenkel et al. (1995) found no association between recent infection and consumption of raw or lightly cooked meat in their study of children in Panama City.

Other evidence

Two 'classic' studies are often quoted as evidence for transmission of *T. gondii* by meat (Weinman & Chandler 1955; Desmonts et al. 1965). In the first, in 1956, it was shown that the prevalence of *T. gondii* antibody was significantly higher among patients with trichinosis (who presumably had consumed lightly cooked pork) than amongst the 'normal' population. However, the control group was not matched for age, making these results difficult to interpret. In the second, in 1965, it was found that children in a French tuberculosis sanatorium who were fed lightly cooked meat (mainly beef or horse meat) developed *T. gondii* antibodies at a rate five times that in the general population. When a subgroup was fed lightly cooked mutton the yearly rate of antibody acquisition doubled in comparison with the other patients.

Thus there is substantial and convincing evidence from a range of descriptive and analytical epidemiological studies that ingestion of tissue cysts present in raw and lightly cooked meat plays an important role in human toxoplasma infection. It is also clear that tissue cysts have more importance in some locales than others – depending on cultural food habits and on the practice of rearing meat animals. Unfortunately, many of the published studies are not appropriately designed to define precisely how humans ingest tissue cysts; for example, subjects are often not questioned about the different types of meat consumed or about opportunities for cross-contamination in the kitchen. Furthermore, little is known about the extent of, and trends in, *T. gondii* contamination of the range of retail meats most commonly eaten today.

Toxoplasma transmission via ingestion of tachyzoites

Ingestion of tachyzoites probably plays little role in the acquisition of human toxoplasma infection, because they are a relatively transient phase of the lifecycle of the parasite and because they are not adapted for prolonged survival outside the body of a living host. Moreover they are destroyed by gastric juice (unlike the bradyzoites and sporozoites protected within tissue cysts and oocysts respectively). Nevertheless, tachyzoites have been found in the milk, urine and saliva of experimentally infected goats, mice and rabbits (Terragna et al. 1984; Petterson 1984; Vitor et al. 1990) and in the colostrum of a naturally infected cow (Sanger et al.

1953). Furthermore, the infection has been experimentally transmitted to offspring via milk in mice and pigs. In explanation it was suggested that some strains of *T. gondii* are relatively acid resistant or that penetration through oropharyngeal mucosa can occur.

Transmission of infection in blood, sweat, tears, milk or semen to normal, healthy human individuals is considered unlikely (Frenkel 1979). There is little epidemiological evidence that milk is an important vehicle for human toxoplasma infection. Nevertheless, its role has not been as widely studied as that of meat and cats and there are some convincing reports: one of a baby who probably acquired toxoplasma infection from raw goat's milk (Riemann et al. 1975*a*); and another of a family outbreak also associated with raw goat's milk (Sacks et al. 1982). In neither report, however, was the incriminated goat or its milk available for examination. More recently, two children in a family that owned goats in which an epizootic of toxoplasma infection had occurred were serologically confirmed to have acute toxoplasma infection at the same time. The whole family had a variety of risk factors for toxoplasma infection, but only the children were infected and only they drank unheated raw milk from the herd. The organism was also isolated from a milk sample (Skinner et al. 1990). Cook et al. (2000), in their case–control study of European pregnant women, found an association between toxoplasma infection and consumption of unpasteurized milk or milk products. They speculated that oocyst contamination caused by unhygienic production techniques, or tissue cyst infection associated with the eating habits of subjects whose lifestyle included drinking raw milk, was just as likely an explanation as ingestion of tachyzoites.

Nonoral acquisition of *T. gondii* (including occupational risk)

The most important routes of nonorally transmitted *T. gondii* are transplacental (tachyzoites) and via transplanted organs (tissue cysts). The epidemiological aspects of materno–foetal and transplant-acquired toxoplasma infection have already been discussed in this chapter and are also reviewed elsewhere (in Chapters 6, 7, 8, 9 and 10).

The contribution of other nonoral routes to the size of the problem of human toxoplasma infection is unknown. They include blood product transfusions and laboratory accidents where personnel handle infected animals or contaminated needles and glassware (Ho Yen and Joss 1992). These two routes are unlikely to constitute an important public health problem, but others in which toxoplasma infection may be acquired occupationally (other than in diagnostic laboratories) may be more significant.

People occupationally at risk of exposure to *T. gondii* include those who work with animals suffering from clinical toxoplasma infection and those handling raw meat and offal from persistently infected farm livestock. They may of course acquire the organism orally via contaminated hands, but there is also the possibility of direct inoculation through broken skin or even of inhalation (Smith 1991). There are no published studies which have assessed the relative risks of these different routes, although a number of authors have investigated whether workers in these occupations have increased prevalence rates of *T. gondii* antibody.

Those specifically at risk include stockmen, veterinary surgeons and others who come into contact with aborted lambs, kids and piglets and their placentas. Equally, those who handle raw meat or dead animals, such as slaughtermen, butchers, food processing workers, caterers and zoo workers, should be aware of the risks involved. At postmortem examination, tachyzoites may be present in large numbers in the tissues of animals such as marsupials and New World monkeys that die with severe disseminated toxoplasma infection.

Sero-epidemiological studies of occupation as a risk factor for toxoplasma infection have mainly concentrated on those professions that have direct contact with animals and/or meat. They are subject to the same criticisms as those outlined earlier in this chapter and it is therefore not surprising that results are conflicting. The effects, for example, of age and socioeconomic group as confounding variables for associations observed with different occupations are rarely examined.

In 1954 a study in the UK (Beverley et al. 1954) demonstrated that abattoir workers and veterinarians had higher *T. gondii* antibody prevalence rates than the general population (43%, 12% and 2% respectively with dye test titres of 16 or greater). In 1961 a study in Japan (Komiya et al. 1961) also showed that abattoir workers had higher *T. gondii* antibody prevalence with 68% positive compared to 30% of three control groups. There were also differences between butchers (40%) and a comparison general population (25%). Samad et al. (1997) found that 50% of butchers in a district of Bangladesh had *T. gondii* antibody compared to 12% of blood donors and 11% of pregnant women.

In a Brazilian abattoir *T. gondii* antibody prevalence varied with the particular job undertaken (Riemann et al. 1975b). The *T. gondii* antibody prevalences for employees who handled meat in the deboning and sausage departments were 80% and 79% with geometric mean titres (GMT) of 412 and 340 respectively. These levels exceeded the *T. gondii* antibody prevalences of 60% and 65% and GMTs of 168 and 120 for employees who worked with cattle in the corrals and who worked on the killing floor respectively. Cook et al. (2000) found a significant association between acute toxoplasma infection in pregnant women and working with animals in farms, in an abattoir, or with meat as a butcher or cook.

Pig farmers in Finland (Seuri & Koskela 1992) were shown to have much higher *T. gondii* antibody prevalence rates than either abattoir workers or grain/berry farmers (37%, 25% and 23% respectively). The authors commented that the lack of excess risk among abattoir workers in their study probably reflected the high level of hygiene in modern Finnish slaughterhouses compared to those investigated in earlier studies. They also noted that workers were put on sick leave for even minor hand scratches and concluded that handling raw meat with intact skin carried no risk of infection from T. gondii. A study in the United States which found that regular handling of deer viscera did not increase the risk of toxoplasma infection substantiates this (Sacks et al. 1983). The significant association between infection and skinning animals trapped for fur (McDonald et al. 1990) does, however, emphasize the potential risk in conditions of poor hygiene. All these findings have implications for the much larger, but unresearched occupational group of people preparing meat in the domestic kitchen for family and pet consumption. A positive correlation between handling pet food (usually raw offal) and a positive dye test was found in one family-based study (Price 1969).

In the Finnish study the excess risk for pig farmers held even after age and cat ownership standardization. The authors hypothesized that these workers could have been exposed to oocysts in the dust of the farm environment, especially in swine confinement buildings. The risk of exposure to the products of conception of sheep with toxoplasma infection has been little studied. Following an epizootic among a flock in the United States, the only persons who had high titres of T. gondii antibody were those who had been involved with lambing (Behymer et al. 1985). Similarly a Scottish farmer was surmised to have acquired toxoplasma infection from his aborting sheep; however, the evidence was unconvincing (Baijail & Holt 1989).

Veterinary students have been shown to have higher rates of positive responses to skin testing than medical students (19.4% and 14.9% respectively) (McCulloch et al. 1963). Another study demonstrated differences in T. gondii antibody prevalence between personnel at a veterinary research institute and veterinary students (33.3% versus 20.4%) and also a relationship between length of time at veterinary college and presence of antibody (class of 1975, 31%; class of 1976, 13.1%) (Zimmerman 1976). However, other studies do not reproduce these findings. In India, veterinary students, veterinarians and other campus residents had similar T. gondii antibody prevalence rates (24.5%, 28.3% and 28.1% respectively). A Californian study found similar serological evidence of exposure to T. gondii among veterinarians (43.7%) as among nonveterinarians (44%) (Behymer et al. 1973) and small-animal practitioners in Canada (Tizard & Caoili 1976) had no more T. gondii antibodies than a control group.

Five occupational groups in Malaysia were examined for T. gondii antibodies (Tan & Zaman 1973). Padi-planters (who have extensive soil contact) were found to have the highest prevalence (22.2%) followed by veterinarians (20.2%), workers in oil palm and rubber estates (13.5%), antimalarial workers (10.1%) and underground tin miners (3.7%). Another study in Malaysia found that zoo workers had the highest prevalence rates (51.25%) followed by medical students (41.7%) and housewives (25%) (Yahaya 1991). The risk of toxoplasma infection from close, daily occupational cat exposure as occurs in breeders and cattery workers has been little studied. The two studies already cited in this chapter (Ulmanen & Leinikki 1975; Woodruff et al. 1982) both suggested that there was an excess risk; however, both had flaws which made the conclusions tenuous.

Thus acquisition of *T. gondii* via routes such as broken skin or the respiratory tract is theoretically a risk for certain occupational groups whose work brings them into contact with live or dead animals. The oral route is also a hazard for such persons. The epidemiological evidence is conflicting and many studies are unsatisfactory; however, it appears that such occupations may pose an excess risk, particularly under conditions of poor hygiene. There is no information on the relative hazards of nonoral routes of transmission except that intact skin is probably protective.

Strategies for prevention

Two major purposes of epidemiology are to produce strategies for prevention and to evaluate such strategies. The general principles of disease prevention are summarized in Table 3.7. Secondary and tertiary prevention involve specific screening strategies such as those aimed at pregnant women, potential transplant recipients and organ donors and persons infected with HIV. These, as well as specific primary prevention strategies in transplant recipients, are covered in detail in other chapters and will not be considered further here. The options for primary prevention of toxoplasma infection (which clearly will always be better than secondary or tertiary prevention) are summarized in Table 3.7; details are provided below.

Primary prevention strategies

Preventing infection in the definitive and intermediate (meat animal) hosts

Toxoplasma infection will never be an infection suitable for global eradication (like smallpox or polio) because of the widespread infection of the equally widespread definitive host – all members of the cat family (domestic, feral, large). This problem is magnified by the self-maintaining reservoir in small rodents. Thus recommendations to minimize the risk of domestic cats becoming infected and also of contaminating the environment are, unfortunately, likely to contribute little to the overall prevention of human toxoplasma infection.

Such recommendations include keeping pet cats indoors to prevent hunting, or wearing bells to reduce their success; avoiding feeding raw meat or offal; encouraging them to use a litter tray rather than defaecating outside. Any or all of these can

Table 3.7. Primary prevention of human toxoplasmosis in outline*

Objective	Measure
• Prevent infection in the definitive host (Felidae)	Prevent consumption of tissue cysts, oocysts Vaccinate
• Prevent infection in intermediate (meat animal) hosts	As above
• Prevent human ingestion of tissue cysts, oocysts, tachyzoites	Health education to *avoid* • 'risky' food, milk and water* • 'risky' food-handling practices* • ingestion of soil and dirt to *promote* • hand hygiene • awareness of occupational risk* • production of clean water
Prevent human-to-human transmission	Match seronegative transplant recipients to seronegative donors Prophylactic chemotherapy for transplant recipients

*See text for details.

be encouraged but compliance may be poor especially among suburban and rural owners with gardens. Clearly, the prevention of soil contamination with oocysts is an unachievable goal. However, cats also have a predilection for burying their faeces in children's sandpits which should, therefore, be kept covered when not in use.

On farms, measures to reduce environmental contamination by oocysts should be aimed at reducing the number of cats capable of shedding oocysts. This would include attempts to limit the numbers of young cats. If male farm cats are neutered and returned to their colonies the stability of the colony is maintained; fertile male cats do not challenge the neutered males (Tabor 1980) and breeding is controlled. Thus the maintenance of a small, healthy population of mature cats will reduce oocyst excretion as well as help control rodents. Animal feed should be kept covered at all times to prevent its contamination by cat faeces and rodents. Pigs and other dead animals should be removed promptly to prevent cannibalism by other pigs and scavenging by cats. Foetal membranes and dead foetuses should not be handled with bare hands and should be buried or incinerated to prevent infection of cats and other animals on the farm (Dubey 1991).

A vaccine to prevent ovine toxoplasma abortion is commercially available in the UK, Republic of Ireland and France (Toxovax, Intervet B. V.) (Buxton & Innes 1995). As it is a live tachyzoite vaccine it could not be used to prevent human disease caused by *T. gondii*. Control of feline toxoplasma infection by vaccination has been suggested but, for the reasons given above, is unlikely to be a practical proposition.

Prevention of human ingestion of toxoplasma

The two key messages are hand and kitchen hygiene and avoidance of consuming lightly cooked or raw meat or offal. Hands should be washed with soap and water after handling meat, soil or soil-covered produce and after cleaning cats' litter trays.

Much has been written about safe handling of cats' litter trays. In urban areas some cat owners dispose of soiled cat litter by flushing it down the toilet, so that if *T. gondii* oocysts are present in the faeces they might eventually find their way into water courses and the sea. Contaminated water can be a source of human infection (Benenson et al. 1982) and it is possible that heavily contaminated sea water may also be a risk. The observation that seals in the wild can become infected with *T. gondii* (Van Pelt & Dietricht 1973) indicates that oocysts can reach the sea to contaminate parts of the coast. Therefore, cat faeces should be disposed of within 24 hours, before the oocysts have sporulated and become infectious, preferably by carefully wrapping (in newspaper for example) and securely sealing in an appropriate plastic bag (a supermarket carrier bag is ideal) and disposal in the household rubbish, which normally goes for landfill.

Whenever practical, susceptible people such as pregnant women and immunocompromised patients should avoid emptying the litter tray. They should be aware of why cats' faeces may be a risk, that kittens which have just started hunting are particularly likely to develop the infection and that any pet cat with diarrhoea may be more of a hazard because of soiling outside the litter tray. If pregnant women and immunocompromised patients have to empty cat litter trays they should follow the above precautions, if practical wear gloves, but most importantly wash their hands thoroughly with soap and water afterwards.

Good kitchen hygiene should include washing food preparation surfaces and knives with detergent and water after cutting up meat and using separate preparation surfaces for foods that are to be eaten uncooked. The same applies to soil-covered vegetable and salads. Flies in food preparation and storage areas should be killed.

All the above measures are part of good general hygiene which is to be encouraged for many reasons, not just for prevention of toxoplasma infection. However, many people enjoy eating raw and lightly cooked meat and would not want to give it up. As toxoplasma infection is usually not a serious illness for people other than the pregnant and immunocompromised, it is neither practical nor desirable to advocate this measure generally (with the exception of poultry, because of the much greater risk of salmonellosis).

Tissue cysts are killed if meat is cooked thoroughly (at least 65°C throughout a joint), cured with salt and sugar, subjected to low temperature (50°C) smoking for 24–48 hours (Lunden & Uggla 1992) or frozen and then thawed (Jacobs et al. 1960; Hellesnes & Mohn 1977; Lunden & Uggla 1992). A simple guide for cooking red meat is to ensure that it changes colour, indicating that the temperature reached is likely to have killed any tissue cysts present. However, meat on the bone that is cooked in a microwave oven may give the appearance of having been heated sufficiently, but may still contain viable tissue cysts (Lunden & Uggla 1992).

The 'at risk' groups should avoid *any* meat that is pink or bloody. They should also be aware that microwaved meat may not be evenly cooked even when the cooking instructions have been followed. It is clear that minced meat may be a particular hazard, all the more so when it is made into hamburgers. Barbecued burgers (and other meat) and those from 'fast food outlets' are particularly likely to be lightly cooked – as evidenced from the recently recognized association with *Escherichia coli* O157 outbreaks. Although there is no evidence that they play an important role in human toxoplasma infection (except for the college student outbreak described above), 'at risk' subjects would be wise to avoid this foodstuff unless cooked to an internal temperature of 65°C (unfortunately this may also render it less palatable).

It has recently been shown that cured and fermented meats or sausages (which are uncooked) pose a risk of toxoplasma infection (Buffolano et al. 1996; Cook et al. 2000). Experimental work suggests that although curing with salt and smoke does kill the parasite (Lunden & Uggla 1992), this depends on the salt concentration used (Navarro et al. 1992) and on the temperature. Buffolano et al. (1996) observed that the conditions in which some pork products are cured are not necessarily lethal to *T. gondii*. 'At risk' groups should therefore be aware that there is a risk from these foodstuffs.

Another approach to primary prevention is to render meat free of *T. gondii* by irradiation (Song Chang-Cun et al. 1993). This has been approved in the United States (Smith 1991) but is unlikely to gain widespread public acceptance.

Regarding possible acquisition of *T. gondii* from milk and water: 'at risk' subjects should be advised to avoid unpasteurized milk of any type. The contribution that contaminated water – be it treated, or private untreated supplies – is unknown because it has been little studied. Kapperud et al. (1996) found no association between recent infection in pregnant women in Norway and drinking untreated water. However, Cook et al. (2000) found such an association in their study covering six European centres. There could be scope for further primary prevention if there were increased awareness of this risk among water companies and public

health officials; there is a need for more sensitive microbiological and clinical surveillance for waterborne outbreaks of toxoplasma infection (Bowie et al. 1997). A
technique for detecting *T. gondii* oocysts in drinking water has recently been developed (Isaac-Renton et al. 1998). In the meantime, untreated water is probably best
avoided by 'at risk' subjects, not least because of the hazards of other microbiological contaminants.

**Prevention for specific occupations – veterinary surgeons; stockmen; persons who may be in
contact with aborted lambs, kids or piglets; handlers of dead animals or raw meat; zoo and
cattery workers**

People in occupations likely to expose them to *T. gondii* should be aware of the
organism and its effects on the foetus and the immunocompromised. Unfortunately,
specific advice is difficult to formulate because so little research on risk factors has
been undertaken and because it has to be tempered with pragmatism. Hand hygiene
and avoidance of exposing broken skin are sensible general precautions. Pregnant
women should not assist with lambing as not only *T. gondii* but other hazardous
organisms such as *Chlamydia psittaci*, *Coxiella burnetii* and *Listeria monocytogenes*
may be encountered. During an outbreak of abortion or stillbirths, great care should
be taken by all farm staff and they should include measures to avoid infection being
introduced into the home, for example on boots or clothing.

Cattery and zoo workers should know about toxoplasma infection so that 'at
risk' subjects can avoid exposure to the parasite. The following precautions represent good advice for all workers: individuals undertaking necropsies on marsupials and New World monkeys that die of disseminated toxoplasma infection should
pay special attention to hand hygiene and wearing of masks as *T. gondii* may
survive for several days in certain tissues (Raisanen & Saari 1978); if large cats are
fed raw meat, preferably it should have been frozen and should be beef (Dubey
1991); brooms and shovels and other equipment used to clean cat cages should be
heated to 70°C for at least ten minutes; while cleaning cages, animal caretakers
should wear masks and protective clothing; feline faeces should be removed daily
(Dubey 1991).

Putting prevention into practice and its evaluation

It is clear from the preceding section that the primary prevention of human toxoplasma infection depends heavily on effective health education. It is not difficult to
decide on the content of such education, but packaging the message into an acceptable format, delivering it in a sustained fashion and evaluating it are all problematic. The problems include determining the target audience and the 'where',
'when' and 'how' of delivery. Two obvious groups are *T. gondii* antibody-negative
immunocompromised persons and pregnant women. The latter could be educated

at antenatal clinics (Department of Health 1996) but, given that first attendance usually occurs at the end of the first trimester, this may be too late for some.

In contrast to the 1980s, when popular literature for expectant mothers in the UK and even the Health Education Authority's Pregnancy Book contained no mention of toxoplasma infection (Hall 1986), most of such literature now does contain information. However, one survey (Newton & Hall 1994) showed that only just over a half of health districts in England and Wales had a policy to promote the primary prevention of materno–foetal toxoplasma infection. Furthermore, a review of the content of a variety of booklets and leaflets given to pregnant women showed that much of the information was inadequate, conflicting and sometimes erroneous (Newton & Hall 1995).

There are few published studies on the effectiveness of the primary prevention of toxoplasma infection (Conyn van Spaendonck 1991) and such as there are have related to 'one-off' specific studies rather than ongoing national programmes. One survey in France, a country where there is prenatal screening and a 'high profile' for toxoplasma infection in pregnant women, showed that even there pregnant women were not well informed: only half of susceptible pregnant women knew of more than one risk factor for toxoplasma infection and 11% could not cite any (Wallon et al. 1994). In their multicentre European study, Cook et al. (2000) found that the proportion of women who could not cite any risk factors ranged from 2% in Brussels to 51% in Naples. Furthermore, knowledge did not necessarily lead to avoidance of exposure. A similar survey in a London hospital antenatal clinic also showed that 30% of women in the second and third trimester had never heard of toxoplasma infection. Furthermore, knowledge was associated with being white and with increasing age (personal communication, E. Hall, 1993).

It is clear that while theoretically congenital toxoplasma infection is a preventable disease, little sustained high quality effort is going into primary prevention in any country. Even less is known about the extent and effectiveness of primary prevention of systemic toxoplasma infection in immunosuppressed persons. It is noted earlier in this chapter that monitoring such programmes by national surveillance schemes is also fraught with difficulty.

Conclusion

There has been a wealth of epidemiological study of human and animal toxoplasma infection throughout the world since the first reported case in the early 1900s. Much has been learned but there are still large gaps in our knowledge of precisely how humans acquire the infection and of the size of the clinical problem. Probably for these reasons, efforts at preventing its serious effects – especially in pregnancy – have been disappointing and have attracted little commitment from health authorities. The means are available now, and we now require resources and action, which should not necessarily be standardized across all countries, but should be based on information about risk factors for toxoplasma infection derived from local epidemiological studies.

Summary

Epidemiology is the study of the distribution and determinants of disease in populations in order to inform strategies for prevention. Epidemiological studies of human and animal toxoplasma infection are reviewed in this chapter to demonstrate both what has been learned about the magnitude of its effects on human health and also about risk factors for acquiring *T. gondii*.

First, we review studies of the prevalence and incidence of toxoplasma infection worldwide, as well as attempts to assess the size of the clinical burden. Trends over time suggest that the overall incidence may be falling in western countries although that of severe manifestations is on the increase because of the underlying increase in numbers of immunocompromised patients. We then review what evidence there is – from both human and animal studies – to support the hypothesis that most toxoplasma infection is acquired from the ingestion of oocysts or tissue cysts.

The clinical and epidemiological animal studies we review involve both the definitive and the intermediate hosts of *T. gondii*. Studies of humans are usually based on subjects whose *T. gondii* antibody status has been determined. They include assessment of infection status by age, sex, geographic locality, ethnic and socioeconomic group – this is 'descriptive' epidemiology. We also review analytical studies of risk factors for acquiring toxoplasma infection. In many of these the subjects being compared are those with or without *T. gondii* IgG, so the precise timing of acquisition of infection is unknown. More valid, therefore, are studies of patients with documented recent infection. These are of two types. Those ascertained during an outbreak and those with antibody evidence, such as specific IgM or seroconversion, are measured in a special survey.

We conclude that there is good evidence that oral ingestion of both tissue cysts and oocysts plays a major role in human toxoplasma infection. However, the contribution and risks of transmission of each varies from place to place according to local social, economic, cultural and, probably, climatic conditions.

We also review the evidence for acquisition of infection via tachyzoites of *T. gondii* and for nonoral portals of entry. For both, the evidence is scanty but this partly reflects the fact that relatively little research has been done in this area. This section includes occupational risk for persons in contact with animals and animal products. Although findings are often conflicting, it appears that such occupations may pose an excess risk, particularly under conditions of poor hygiene.

Finally, we review strategies for primary prevention of infection both in animals and in humans. For the latter this depends largely on health education directed at appropriate 'target' groups such as immunocompromised persons and pregnant women. The key messages centre on hand and kitchen hygiene and avoidance of consuming lightly cooked or raw meat. We also highlight measures to reduce the risk of contamination of meat by *T. gondii* and under-researched areas such as the risks from water and untreated milk.

Putting the theories of prevention into practice requires appropriate allocation of health-care resources and sustained commitment both to the programme and to its evaluation. Because risk factors for human toxoplasma infection vary from place to place, it is essential that efforts at prevention are tailored to local risks and therefore informed by local studies.

REFERENCES

Abdel-Hameed, A. A. (1991). Sero-epidemiology of toxoplasmosis in Gezira, Sudan. *Journal of Tropical Medicine and Hygiene*, 94, 329–32.

Ades, A. E. (1992). Methods for estimating the incidence of primary infection in pregnancy: a reappraisal of toxoplasmosis and cytomegalovirus data. *Epidemiology and Infection*, 108, 367–75.

Ades, A. E. & Nokes, D. J. (1993). Modeling age- and time-specific incidence from seroprevalence: toxoplasmosis. *American Journal of Epidemiology*, 137, 1022–34.

Ades, A. E., Parker, S., Gilbert, R., Tookey, P. A., Berry, T., Hjelm, M., Wilcox, A. H., Cubitt, D. & Peckham, C. S. (1993). Maternal prevalence of Toxoplasma antibody based on anonymous neonatal serosurvey: a geographical analysis. *Epidemiology and Infection*, 110, 127–33.

Ahmed, H. J., Mohammed, H. H., Yusuf, M. W., Ahmed, S. F. & Huldt, G. (1988). Human toxoplasmosis in Somalia. Prevalence of Toxoplasma antibodies in a village in the lower Scebelli region and in Mogadishu. *Transactions of the Royal Society of Tropical Medicine and Hygiene*, 82, 330–2.

Ahmed, M. M. (1992). Seroepidemiology of Toxoplasma infection in Riyadh, Saudi Arabia. *Journal of the Egyptian Society of Parasitology*, 22, 407–13.

Al-Nakib, W., Ibrahim, M. E., Hathout, H. et al. (1983). Seroepidemiology of viral and toxoplasmal infections during pregnancy among Arab women of child-bearing age in Kuwait. *International Journal of Epidemiology*, 12, 220–3.

Allain, J. P., Palmer, C. R. & Pearson, G. (1998). Epidemiological study of latent and recent infection by *Toxoplasma gondii* in pregnant women from a regional population in the U. K. *Journal of Infection*, 36, 189–96.

Anteson, R. K., Yoshida, T. & Nyonator, M. A. (1979). Studies on Toxoplasmosis in Ghana. III. Some observations on the epidemiology of the disease. *Ghana Medical Journal*, 18, 11–14.

Aramini, J. J., Stephen, C. & Dubey, J. P. (1998). *Toxoplasma gondii* in Vancouver Island cougars: serology and oocyst shedding. *Journal of Parasitology*, 84, 438–40.

Arene, F. (1986). The prevalence of toxoplasmosis among inhabitants of the Niger Delta. *Folia Parasitol*, 33, 311–14.

Arias, M. L., Chinchilla, M., Reyes, L. & Linder, E. (1996). Seroepidemiology of toxoplasmosis in humans: possible transmission routes in Costa Rica. *Revista de Biologia Tropical*, 44, 377–81.

Assmar, M., Amirkhani, A., Piazak, N., Hovanesian, A., Kooloobandi, A. & Etessami, R. (1997). [Toxoplasmosis in Iran. Results of a seroepidemiological study]. [French]. *Bulletin de la Societe de Pathologie Exotique*, 90, 19–21.

Baijail, E. & Holt, K. (1989). Toxoplasmosis in sheep and shepherd. *Communicable Diseases Scotland*, 89/01, 4–5.

Bannister, B. (1982). Toxoplasmosis 1976–80: review of laboratory reports to the Communicable Disease Surveillance Centre. *Journal of Infection*, 5, 301–6.

Barbier, D., Ancelle, T., Martin-Bouyer, G. (1983). Seroepidemiological survey of toxoplasmosis in La Guadeloupe, French West Indies. *American Journal of Tropical Medicine and Hygiene*, 32, 935–42.

Beattie, C. P. (1957). Clinical and epidemiological aspects of toxoplasmosis. *Transactions of the Royal Society of Tropical Medicine and Hygiene*, 51, 96–103.

Beauvais, B., Garin, Y., Languillat, G. & Lariviere, M. (1978). Toxoplasmosis in Eastern Gabon. Results of a serologic survey. *Bulletin de la Societe de Pathologie Exotique et de ses Filiales*, 71, 172–81.

Behymer, D. E., Ruppanner, R., Davis, E. W., Franti, C. E. & Les, C. M. (1985). Epidemiologic study of toxoplasmosis on a sheep ranch. *American Journal of Veterinary Research*, 46, 1141–4.

Behymer, R. D., Harlow, D. R., Behymer, D. E. & Franti, C. E. (1973). Serologic diagnosis of toxoplasmosis and prevalence of *Toxoplasma gondii* antibodies in selected feline, canine and human populations. *Journal of the American Veterinary Association*, 162, 526–32.

Benenson, M. W., Takafuji, E. T., Lemon, S. M., Greenup, R. L. & Sulzer, A. J. (1982). Oocyst-transmitted toxoplasmosis associated with ingestion of contaminated water. *New England Journal of Medicine*, 307, 666–9.

Beverley, J. K. A. (1959). Congenital transmission of toxoplasmosis through successive generation of mice. *Nature*, 183, 1348–9.

Beverley, J. K. A., Beattie, C. P. & Roseman, C. (1954). Human toxoplasma infection. *Journal of Hygiene*, 52, 32–46.

Beverley, J. K. A., Watson, W. A. & Payne, J. M. (1971). The pathology of the placenta in ovine abortion due to toxoplasmosis. *Veterinary Record*, 88, 124–8.

Biancifori, F., Rondini, D., Grellori, V. & Frescura, T. (1986). Avian toxoplasmosis, experimental infection of chickens and pigeons. *Comparative Immunology, Microbiology and Infectious Disease*, 9, 337–46.

Blewett, D. A. (1983). The epidemiology of ovine toxoplasmosis. I. The interpretation of data for the prevalence of antibody in sheep and other host species. *British Veterinary Journal*, 139, 537–45.

Blewett, D. A. & Watson, W. A. (1983). The epidemiology of ovine toxoplasmosis. II. Possible sources of infection in outbreaks of clinical disease. *British Veterinary Journal*, 139, 546–55.

Blewett, D. A. & Watson, W. A. (1984). The epidemiology of ovine toxoplasmosis. III. Observations on outbreaks of clinical toxoplasmosis in relation to possible mechanisms of transmission. *British Veterinary Journal*, 140, 54–63.

Bonametti, A. M., Passos, J. D., da Silva, E. M. & Bortoliero, A. L. (1996). [Outbreak of acute tox-oplasmosis transmitted thru the ingestion of ovine raw meat]. [Portuguese]. *Revista Da Sociedade Brasileira de Medicina Tropical,* 30, 21–5.

Bowerman, R. J. (1991). Seroprevalence of *Toxoplasma gondii* in rural India: a preliminary study. *Transactions of the Royal Society of Tropical Medicine and Hygiene,* 85, 622.

Bowie, W. R., King, A. S., Werker, D. H., Isaac-Renton, J. L., Bell, A., Eng, S. B. & Marion, S. A. (1997). Outbreak of toxoplasmosis associated with municipal drinking water. The BC Toxoplasma Investigation Team. *Lancet,* 350, 173–7.

Bowry, T. R., Camargo, M. E. & Kinyanjui, M. (1986). Sero-epidemiology of *Toxoplasma gondii* infection in young children in Nairobi, Kenya. *Transactions of the Royal Society of Tropical Medicine and Hygiene,* 80, 439–41.

Broadbent, E. J., Ross, R. & Hurley, R. (1981). Screening for toxoplasmosis in pregnancy. *Journal of Clinical Pathology,* 34, 659–64.

Buffolano, W., Gilbert, R. E., Holland, F. J., Fratta, D., Palumbo, F. & Ades, A. E. (1996). Risk factors for recent toxoplasma infection in pregnant women in Naples. *Epidemiology and Infection,* 116, 347–51.

Buxton, D. (1989). Toxoplasmosis in sheep and other farm animals. *In Practice,* 11, 9–12.

Buxton, D. (1991). Toxoplasmosis. In *Diseases of sheep,* 2nd edn., ed. W. B. Martin & I. D. Aitken, pp. 49–58. London: Blackwell Scientific Publication.

Buxton, D. & Innes, E. A. (1995). A commercial vaccine for ovine toxoplasmosis. *Parasitology,* 110, S11–S16.

Canfield, P. J., Hartley, W. J. & Dubey, J. P. (1990). Lesions of toxoplasmosis in Australian mar-supials. *Journal of Comparative Pathology,* 103, 159–67.

Carney, W. P., Cross, J. H., Joseph, S. W., Van Peenen, P. F., Russell, D. & Sulianti Saroso, J. (1978). Serological study of amoebiasis and toxoplasmosis in the Malili area, South Sulawesi, Indonesia. *Southeast Asian Journal of Tropical Medicine and Public Health,* 9, 471–9.

Catar, G., Giboda, M., Gutvirth, J. & Hongvanthong, B. (1992). Seroepidemiological study of toxoplasmosis in Laos. *Southeast Asian Journal of Tropical Medicine and Public Health,* 23, 491–2.

Chatterton, J. M. W., Skinner, L. J., Moir, I. L. et al. (1988). Toxoplasmosis 1983–1987: season, sex, and behaviour. *Communicable Diseases Scotland,* 12, 5–7.

Chew, L. K., Pillai, R. & Singh, M. (1982). A study of the prevalence of antibodies to *Toxoplasma gondii* in Singapore. *Southeast Asian Journal of Tropical Medicine and Public Health,* 4, 547–50.

Choi, W. Y., Nam, H. W., Kwak, N. H. et al. (1997). Foodborne outbreaks of human toxoplasmo-sis. *Journal of Infectious Diseases,* 175, 1280–2.

Clarke, M. D., Cross, J. H., Carney, W. P., Hadidjaja, P., Joesoef, A., Putrali, J. & Sri Oemijati, N. (1975). Serological study of amebiasis and toxoplasmosis in the Lindu Valley, Central Sulawesi, Indonesia. *Tropical Geographical Medicine,* 27, 274–8.

Clumeck, N. (1991). Some aspects of the epidemiology of toxoplasmosis and pneumocystosis in AIDS in Europe. *European Journal of Clinical Microbiology and Infectious Diseases,* 10, 177–8.

Cochereau-Massin, I., LeHoang, P., Lautier-Frau, M., Zerdoun, E., Zazoun, L., Robinet, M., Marcel, P., Girard, B., Katlama, C., Leport, C. et al. (1992). Ocular toxoplasmosis in human immunodeficiency virus-infected patients. *American Journal of Ophthalmology,* 114, 130–5.

Contreras, M., Schenone, H., Salinas, P. et al. (1996) Seroepidemiology of human toxoplasmosis in Chile. *Revista do Instituto do Instituto de Medicina Tropical de Sao Paulo*, **38**, 431–5.

Conyn van Spaendonck, C. (1991). *Prevention of congenital toxoplasmosis in the Netherlands*, pp. 13–144. Bilthoven: National Institute of Public Health and Environmental Protection.

Cook, A. J. C., Gilbert, R. E., Buffolano, W. et al. (2000). Sources of toxoplasma infection in pregnant women: European multicentre case–control study. *British Medical Journal*, **321**, 142–7.

Coutinho, S. G., Lobo, R. & Dutra, G. (1982). Isolation of Toxoplasma from the soil during an outbreak of toxoplasmosis in a rural area in Brazil. *Journal of Parasitology*, **68**, 866–8.

Cross, J. H., Irving, G. S. & Gunawan, S. (1975). The prevalence of *Entamoeba histolytica* and *Toxoplasma gondii* antibodies in Central Java, Indonesia. *Southeast Asian Journal of Tropical Medicine and Public Health*, **6**, 467–71.

Cunningham, A. A., Buxton, D. & Thomson, K. M. (1992). An epidemic of toxoplasmosis in a captive colony of squirrel monkeys (*Saimiri sciureus*). *Journal of Comparative Pathology*, **107**, 207–19.

De Roever-Bonnet, H. (1969). Congenital toxoplasma infections in mice and hamsters infected with avirulent and virulent strains. *Tropical and Geographical Medicine*, **21**, 443–50.

Decavalas, G., Papapetropoulou, M., Giannoulaki, E., Tzigounis, V. & Kondakis, X. G. (1990). Prevalence of *Toxoplasma gondii* antibodies in gravidas and recently aborted women and study of risk factors. *European Journal of Epidemiology*, **6**, 223–6.

Department of Health. (1996). *While you are pregnant – how to avoid infection from food and contact with animals.* London: Department of Health.

Desmonts, G., Couvreur, J., Alison, F., Bandelot, J., Gerbeaux, J. & Lelong, M. (1965). Etude epidemiologique sur la toxoplasmose: de l'influence de la cuisson des viandes de boucherie sur la frequence de l'infection humaine. *Revue Francais Etudes Cliniques Biologiques*, **10**, 952–8.

Develoux, M., Candolfi, E., Hanga Doumbo, S. & Kien, T. (1988). Toxoplasmosis in Niger. A serological analysis of 400 subjects. *Bulletin de la Societe de Pathologie Exotique*, **81**, 253–9.

Di Giacomo, R. F., Harris, N. V., Huber, N. L. & Cooney, M. K. (1990). Animal exposures and antibodies to *Toxoplasma gondii* in a university population. *American Journal of Epidemiology*, **131**, 729–33.

Doehring, E., Reiter-Owona, I., Bauer, O., Kaisi, M., Hlobil, H., Quade, G., Hamudu, N. A. & Seitz, H. M. (1995). *Toxoplasma gondii* antibodies in pregnant women and their newborns in Dar es Salaam, Tanzania. *American Journal of Tropical Medicine and Hygiene*, **52**, 546–8.

Dubey, J. P. (1974). Effect of freezing on the infectivity of toxoplasma cysts to cats. *Journal of the American Veterinary Medical Association*, **165**, 534–536.

Dubey, J. P. (1977). *Toxoplasma, Hammondia, Besnoitia, Sarcocystis*, and other tissue cyst-forming coccidia of man and animals. In *Parasitic protozoa*, vol III, ed. J. P. Kreier, pp. 101–237. London: Academic Press.

Dubey, J. P. (1981). Isolation of encysted *Toxoplasma gondii* from musculature of moose and pronghorn in Montana. *American Journal of Veterinary Research*, **42**, 126–7.

Dubey, J. P. (1986a). A review of toxoplasmosis in pigs. *Veterinary Parasitology*, **19**, 181–223.

Dubey, J. P. (1986b). A review of toxoplasmosis in cattle. *Veterinary Parasitology*, **22**, 177–97.

Dubey, J. P. (1986c). Toxoplasmosis. *Journal of the American Veterinary Medical Association*, **189**, 166–70.

Dubey, J. P. (1988). Long-term persistence of *Toxoplasma gondii* in tissues of pigs inoculated with *T. gondii* oocysts and effect of freezing on viability of tissue cysts in pork. *American Journal of Veterinary Research*, **49**, 910–13.

Dubey, J. P. (1990). Status of toxoplasmosis in sheep and goats in the United States. *Journal of the American Veterinary Medical Association*, **196**, 259–62.

Dubey, J. P. (1991). Toxoplasmosis – an overview. *Southeast Asian Journal of Tropical Medicine and Public Health*, **22**, 88–92.

Dubey, J. P. (1992). Isolation of *Toxoplasma gondii* from a naturally infected beef cow. *Journal of Parasitology*, **78**, 151–3.

Dubey, J. P. (2000). Sources of *Toxoplasma gondii* infection in pregnancy. *British Medical Journal*, **321**, 127–8.

Dubey, J. P. & Beattie, C. P. (1988). *Toxoplasmosis of animals*. Boca Raton, FL: CRC Press.

Dubey, J. P. & Frenkel, J. K. (1972). Cyst-induced toxoplasmosis in cats. *Journal of Protozoology*, **19**, 155–77.

Dubey, J. P. & Frenkel, J. K. (1974). Immunity to feline toxoplasmosis: modification by administration of corticosteroids. *Veterinary Pathology*, **11**, 350–79.

Dubey, J. P. & Frenkel, J. K. (1976). Feline toxoplasmosis from acutely infected mice and the development of *Toxoplasma* cysts. *Journal of Protozoology*, **23**, 537–46.

Dubey, J. P. & Frenkel, J. K. (1998). Toxoplasmosis of rats: a review, with considerations of their value as an animal model and their possible role in epidemiology. *Veterinary Parasitology*, **77**, 1–32.

Dubey, J. P. & Kirkbride, C. A. (1989). Economic and public health considerations of congenital toxoplasmosis in lambs. *Journal of the American Veterinary Medical Association*, **195**, 1715–16.

Dubey, J. P. & Thulliez, P. H. (1993). Persistence of tissue cysts in edible tissues of cattle fed *Toxoplasma gondii* oocysts. *American Journal of Veterinary Research*, **54**, 270–3.

Dubey, J. P., Ott-Joslin, J., Torgerson, R. W., Topper, M. J. & Sundberg, J. P. (1988). Toxoplasmosis in Black-faced kangaroos (*Macropus fuliginosus melanops*). *Veterinary Parasitology*, **30**, 97–105.

Dubey, J. P., Rollor, E. A., Smith, K. et al. (1997). Low seroprevalence of *Toxoplasma gondii* in feral pigs from a remote island lacking cats. *Journal of Parasitology*, **83**, 839–41.

Dumas, N., Cazaux, M., Rivaillier, P. & Seguela, J. (1985). Toxoplasmosis in the African tropical zone. Preliminary studies. *Bulletin de la Societe de Pathologie Exotique*, **78**, 795–800.

Dumas, P. S., Cazaun, M., Perly-Therizol, M. & Seguela, J. P. (1989). The epidemiology of toxoplasmosis in Ivory Coast. *Bulletin de la Societe de Pathologie Exotique*, **82**, 513–19.

Duong, T. H., Dufillot, D., Martz, M., Richard-Lenoble, D. & Kombila, M. (1992). Etude sero-epidemiologique de la toxoplasmose a Libreville, Gabon. *Annals of the Belgian Society of Tropical Medicine*, **72**, 289–93.

Dupouy-Camet, J., Gavinet, M. F., Paugam, A. & Tourte Schaefer, C. (1993). Mode de contamination, incidence et prevalence de la toxoplasmose. *Medicin Maladies Infectieuses*, **23** (special), 139–47.

Durfee, P. T., Cross, J. H., Rustam & Susanto (1976). Toxoplasmosis in man and animals in South Kalimantan (Borneo), Indonesia. *American Journal of Tropical Medicine and Hygiene*, **23**, 42–7.

Durmaz, R., Durmaz, B., Tas, I. & Rafiq, M. (1995). Seropositivity of toxoplasmosis among reproductive-age women in Malatya, Turkey. *Journal of the Egyptian Society of Parasitology*, **25**, 693–8.

Dutton, G. N. (1989). Toxoplasmic retinochloroiditis – a historical review and current concepts. *Annals of the Academy of Medicine*, 18, 214–21.

Eichenwald, H. (1948). Experimental toxoplasmosis. 1. Transmission of the infection *in utero* and through the milk of lactating female mice. *American Journal of Diseases of Children*, 76, 307–15.

Espeillac, D., Malavaud, S., Bessieres, M. H. & Grandjean, H. (1989). Etude seroepidemiologique vis-a-vis de la toxoplasmose chez la femme enceinte dans la region toulousaine. *Medicin Maladies Infectieuses*, 19, 80–2.

Esteban-Redondo, I. & Innes, E. A. (1998). Detection of *Toxoplasma gondii* in tissues of sheep orally challenged with different doses of oocysts. *International Journal of Parasitology*, 28, 1459–66.

Etheredge, G. D. & Frenkel, J. K. (1995). Human Toxoplasma infection in Kuna and Embera children in the Bayano and San Blas, eastern Panama. *American Journal of Tropical Medicine and Hygiene*, 53, 448–57.

European Network on Congenital Toxoplasmosis Infection. (1993). *A concerted action under the BIOMED1 Programme of the Commission of the European Communities*. Newsletter no. 1.

Excler, J. L., Pretat, E., Pozzetto, B., Charpin, B. & Garin, J. (1988). Sero-epidemiological survey for toxoplasmosis in Burundi. *Tropical Medicine and Parasitology*, 39, 139–41.

Faull, W. B., Clarkson, M. J. & Winter, A. C. (1986). Toxoplasmosis in a flock of sheep: some investigations into its source and control. *Veterinary Record*, 119, 491–3.

Fayer, R. (1981). Toxoplasma update and public health implications. *Canadian Veterinary Journal*, 22, 344–52.

Feldman, H. A. (1956). Serological study of toxoplasmosis prevalence. *American Journal of Hygiene*, 64, 320–335.

Feldman, H. A. (1968). Toxoplasmosis. *New England Journal of Medicine*, 279, 1370–5.

Fisher, O. D. (1951). Toxoplasma infection in English chidren. *Lancet*, ii, 904–6.

Fleck, D. G. (1963). Epidemiology of Toxoplasmosis. *Journal of Hygiene*, 61, 61–5.

Fleck, D. G. (1965). Toxoplasmosis in Tristan da Cuhna. *Journal of Hygiene*, 63, 389–93.

Fleck, D. G. (1969). Toxoplasmosis. *Public Health, London*, 83, 131–5.

Forsgren, M., Gille, E., Ljungstrom, I. & Nokes, D. J. (1991). *Toxoplasma gondii* antibodies in pregnant women in Stockholm in 1969, 1979, and 1987 [Letter]. *Lancet*, 337, 1413–14.

Fortier, B., De Almeida, E., Pinto, I., Ajana, F. & Camus, D. (1990). Prevalence de la toxoplasmose porcine et bovine a porto. *Medicin Maladies Infectieuses*, 20, 551–4.

Frenkel, J. K. (1979). Transmission of toxoplasmosis by tachyzoites: possibility and probability. *Medical Hypotheses*, 5, 529–32.

Frenkel, J. K. & Ruiz, A. (1980). Human toxoplasmosis and cat contact in Costa Rica. *American Journal of Tropical Medicine and Hygiene*, 29, 1167–80.

Frenkel, J. K. & Ruiz, A. (1981). Endemicity of toxoplasmosis in Costa Rica Transmission between cats, soil, intermediate hosts and humans. *American Journal of Epidemiology*, 113, 254–69.

Frenkel, J. K., Hassanein, K. M., Hassanein, R. S., Brown, E., Thulliez, P. & Quintero-Nunez, R. (1995). Transmission of *Toxoplasma gondii* in Panama City, Panama: a five-year prospective cohort study of children, cats, rodents, birds, and soil. *American Journal of Tropical Medicine and Hygiene*, 53, 458–68.

Gandahusada, S. & Endardjo, S. (1980). Toxoplasma antibodies in Obano, Irian Jaya, Indonesia. *Southeast Asian Journal of Tropical Medicine and Public Health*, 11, 276–9.

Ganley, J. P. & Comstock, G. W. (1980). Association of cats and toxoplasmosis. *American Journal of Epidemiology*, 111, 238–46.

Gascon, J., Torres-Rodriguez, J. M., Soldevila, M. & Merlos, A. M. (1989). Sero-epidemiologia de la toxoplasmosis en dos comunidades de Rwanda (Africa Central). *Revue Instituto Medico Tropicano Sao Paulo*, 31, 399–402.

Gilbert, R. E., Tookey, P. A., Cubitt, W. D., Ades, A. E., Masters, J. & Peckham, C. S. (1993). Prevalence of toxoplasma IgG among women in west London according to country of birth and ethnic group. *British Medical Journal*, 306, 306.

Gilbert, R. E., Dunn, D. T., Lightman, S., Murray, P. I., Pavesio, C. E., Gormley, P. D., Masters, J., Parker, S. P. & Stanford, M. R. (1999). Incidence of symptomatic toxoplasma eye disease: aetiology and public health implications. *Epidemiology and Infection*, 123, 283–9.

Glasner, P. D., Silveira, C., Kruszon-Moran, D., Martins, M. C., Burnier Junior, M., Silveira, S., Camargo, M. E., Nussenblatt, R. B., Kaslow, R. A. & Belfort Junior, R. (1992). An unusually high prevalence of ocular toxoplasmosis in southern Brazil. *American Journal of Ophthalmology*, 114, 136–44.

Goldsmith, R. S., Kagan, I. G., Zarate, R., Reyes-Gonzalez, M. A. & Cedeno-Ferreira, J. (1991). Low Toxoplasma antibody prevalence in serologic surveys of humans in southern Mexico. *Archivos De Investigacion Medica*, 22, 63–73.

Gottstein, B., Hentrich, B., Wyss, R., Thur, B., Busato, A., Stark, K. D. C. & Muller, N. (1998). Molecular and immunodiagnostic investigations on bovine neosporosis in Switzerland. *International Journal of Parasitology*, 28, 679–91.

Grant, I. H., Gold, J. W., Rosenblum, M., Niedzwiecki, D. & Armstrong, D. (1990). *Toxoplasma gondii* serology in HIV-infected patients: the development of central nervous system toxoplasmosis in AIDS. *AIDS*, 4, 519–21.

Griffin, L. & Williams, K. A. B. (1983). Serological and parasitological survey of blood donors in Kenya for toxoplasmosis. *Transactions of the Royal Society of Tropical Medicine and Hygiene*, 77, 763–6.

Guerra, G. C. & Fernandez, S. J. (1995). [Seroprevalence of *Toxoplasma gondii* in pregnant women]. [Spanish]. *Atencion Primaria*, 16, 151–3.

Hall, S. M. (1983). Congenital toxoplasmosis in England, Wales, and Northern Ireland: some epidemiological problems. *British Medical Journal*, 287, 453–5.

Hall, S. M. (1986). Zoonoses in the '80s: new developments and prospects for control. *Journal of Small Animal Practice*, 27, 617–731.

Hall, S. M. (1992). Congenital toxoplasmosis [see comments] [Review]. *British Medical Journal*, 305, 291–7.

Hall, S. M., Pandit, A., Golwilkar, A. & Williams, T. S. (1999). How do Jains get toxoplasma infection? *Lancet*, 354, 486–7.

Heidel, J. R., Dubey, J. P., Blythe, L. L., Walker, L. L., Duimstra, J. R. & Jordan, J. S. (1990). Myelitis in a cat infected with *Toxoplasma gondii* and feline immunodeficiency virus. *Journal of the American Veterinary Medical Association*, 196, 316–18.

Hellesnes, I. & Mohn, S. F. (1977). Effects of freezing on the infectivity of *Toxoplasma gondii* cysts for white mice. *Zentralblatt fur Bakteriologie Parasitenkunde Infektionkrankheiten und Hygiene, Abteilung I, Originale A*, **238**, 143–8.

Henderson, J. B., Beattie, C. P., Hale, E. G. & Wright, T. (1984). The evaluation of new services: possibilities for preventing congenital toxoplasmosis. *International Journal of Epidemiology*, **13**, 65–72.

Ho Yen, D. O. & Joss, A. W. L. (1992). *Human Toxoplasmosis*. Oxford: Oxford University Press.

Holliman, R. E. (1990). Serological study of the prevalence of toxoplasmosis in asymptomatic patients infected with human immunodeficiency virus. *Epidemiology and Infection*, **105**, 415–18.

Holliman, R. E., Stevens, P. J., Duffy, K. T. & Johnson, J. D. (1991). Serological investigation of ocular toxoplasmosis. *British Journal of Ophthalmology*, **75**, 353–5.

Huldt, G., Lagercrantz, R. & Scheehe, P. R. (1979). On the epidemiology of human toxoplasmosis in Scandinavia, especially in children. *Acta Paediatrica Scandinavia*, **68**, 745–9.

Innes, E. A. (1997). Toxoplasmosis: comparative species susceptibility and host immune response. *Comparative Immunology Microbiology and Infectious Disease*, **20**, 131–8.

Isaac-Renton, J., Bowie, W. R., King, A., Irwin, G. S., Ong, C. S., Fung, C. P., Shokeir, M. O. & Dubey, J. P. (1998). Detection of *Toxoplasma gondii* oocysts in drinking water. *Applied and Environmental Microbiology*, **64**, 2278–80.

Jackson, M. H. & Hutchison, W. M. (1989). The prevalence and source of *Toxoplasma* infection in the environment. In *Advances in Parasitology*, vol. 28, ed. J. R. Baker & R. Muller, pp. 55–105. London: Academic Press.

Jackson, M. H. & Hutchison, W. M. (1992). Toxoplasma infection. *Environmental Health*, June, 160–162.

Jackson, M. H., Hutchison, W. M. & Siim, J. C. (1987). A seroepidemiological survey of toxoplasmosis in Scotland and England. *Annals of Tropical Medicine and Parasitology*, **81**, 359–65.

Jacobs, L., Remington, J. S. & Melton, M. L. (1960). The resistance of the encysted form of *Toxoplasma gondii*. *Journal of Parasitology*, **46**, 11–21.

Jacobs, M. R. & Mason, P. (1978). Prevalence of Toxoplasma antibodies in Southern Africa. *South African Medical Journal*, **53**, 619–21.

Jeannel, D., Niel, G., Costagliola, D., Danis, M., Traore, B. M. & Gentilini, M. (1988). Epidemiology of toxoplasmosis among pregnant women in the Paris area. *International Journal of Epidemiology*, **17**, 595–602.

Jenum, P. A., Kapperud, G., Stray-Pedersen, B., Melby, K. K., Eskild, A. & Eng, J. (1998). Prevalence of *Toxoplasma gondii* specific immunoglobulin G antibodies among pregnant women in Norway. *Epidemiology and Infection*, **120**, 87–92.

Joss, A. W., Chatterton, J. M. & Ho-Yen, D. O. (1990). Congenital toxoplasmosis: to screen or not to screen? *Public Health*, **104**, 9–20.

Joynson, D. H. (1992). Epidemiology of toxoplasmosis in the U. K [Review]. *Scandinavian Journal of Infectious Diseases – Supplementum*, **84**, 65–9.

Juan-Salles, C., Prats, N., Marco, A. J. et al. (1998). Fatal acute toxoplasmosis in three golden lion tamarins. *Journal of Zoo and Wildlife Medicine*, **29**, 55–60.

Julvez, J., Magnaval, J. F., Meynard, D., Perie, C. & Baixench, M. T. (1996). [Seroepidemiology of toxoplasmosis in Niamey, Niger]. [French]. *Medecine Tropicale*, **56**, 48–50.

Kapperud, G., Jenum, P. A., Stray-Pedersen, B., Melby, K. K., Eskild, A. & Eng, J. (1996). Risk factors for *Toxoplasma gondii* infection in pregnancy. Results of a prospective case–control study in Norway. *American Journal of Epidemiology,* **144**, 405–12.

Kasper, L. H. & Ware, P. W. (1985). Recognition and characterisation of stage-specific oocyst/sporozoite antigens of *Toxoplasma gondii* by human antisera. *Journal of Clinical Investigation,* **75**, 1570–7.

Kean, B. H., Kimball, A. C. & Christenson, W. N. (1969). An epidemic of acute toxoplasmosis. *Journal of the American Medical Association,* **208**, 1002–4.

Khan, E. A. & Correa, A. G. (1997). Toxoplasmosis of the central nervous system in non-human immunodeficiency virus-infected children: case report and review of the literature. *Pediatric Infectious Disease Journal,* **16**, 611–18.

Ko, R. C., Wong, F. W., Todd, D. & Lam, K. (1980). Prevalence of *Toxoplasma gondii* antibodies in the Chinese population of Hong Kong. *Transctions of the Royal Society of Tropical Medicine and Hygiene,* **74**, 351–4.

Komiya, Y., Kobayashi, A. & Koyama, T. (1961). Human toxoplasmosis, particularly on the possible source of its infection in Japan. *Japanese Journal of Medical Sciences and Biology,* **14**, 157–72.

Kominishi, E. & Takahashi, J. (1987). Some epidemiological aspects of Toxoplasma infections in a population of farmers in Japan. *International Journal of Epidemiology,* **16**, 277–81.

Lamb, G. A. & Feldman, H. A. (1968). Risk in acquiring toxoplasma antibodies. *Journal of the American Medical Association,* **206**, 1305–6.

Lappin, M. R., Gasper, P. W., Rose, B. J. & Powell, C. C. (1992). Effect of primary phase feline immunodeficiency virus infection on cats with chronic toxoplasmosis. *Veterinary Immunology and Immunopathology,* **35**, 121–31.

Lebech, M., Joynson, D. H., Seitz, H. M., Thulliez, P., Gilbert, R. E., Dutton, G. N., Ovlisen, B. & Petersen, E. (1996). Classification system and case definitions of *Toxoplasma gondii* infection in immunocompetent pregnant women and their congenitally infected offspring. European Research Network on Congenital Toxoplasmosis [see comments]. *European Journal of Clinical Microbiology and Infectious Diseases,* **15**, 799–805.

Lelong, B., Rahelimino, B., Candolfi, E., Ravelojaona, B. J., Villard, O., Rasamindrakotroka, A. J. & Kien, T. (1995). [Prevalence of toxoplasmosis in a population of pregnant women in Antananarivo (Madagascar)]. [French]. *Bulletin de la Societe de Pathologie Exotique,* **88**, 46–9.

Literak, I., Pinowski, J., Anger, M., Juricova, Z., Kyu-Whang, H. & Romanowski, J. (1997). *Toxoplasma gondii* antibodies in house sparrows and tree sparrows. *Avian Pathology,* **26**, 823–7.

Ljungstrom, I., Gille, E., Nokes, J., Linder, E. & Forsgren, M. (1995). Seroepidemiology of *Toxoplasma gondii* among pregnant women in different parts of Sweden. *European Journal of Epidemiology,* **11**, 149–56.

Lovelace, J. K., Moraes, M. A. & Hagerby, E. (1978). Toxoplasmosis among the Ticuna Indians in the state of Amazonas, Brazil. *Tropical and Geographical Medicine,* **30**, 295–300.

Ludlam, G. B., Wong, S. K. & Field, C. E. (1969). Toxoplasma antibodies in sera from Hong Kong. *Journal of Hygiene,* **67**, 739–41.

Luft, B. J. & Castro, K. G. (1991). An overview of the problem of toxoplasmosis and pneumocystosis in AIDS in the USA: implication for future therapeutic trials. *European Journal of Clinical Microbiology and Infectious Diseases,* **10**, 178–81.

Luft, B. J. & Remington, J. S. (1984). Acute Toxoplasma infection among family members of patients with acute lymphadenopathic toxoplasmosis. *Archives of Internal Medicine*, 144, 53–6.

Luft, B. J. & Remington, J. S. (1985). Toxoplasmosis of the central nervous system. *Current Clinical Topics in Infectious Disease*, 6, 315–58.

Lukesova, D. & Literak, I. (1998). Shedding of *Toxoplasma gondii* oocysts by Felidae in zoos in the Czech Republic. *Veterinary Parasitology*, 74, 1–7.

Lunden, A. & Uggla, A. (1992). Infectivity of *Toxoplasma gondii* in mutton following curing, smoking, freezing or microwave cooking. *International Journal of Food Microbiology*, 15, 357–63.

Luyaso, V., Robert, A., Lissenko, D., Bertrand, M., Bohy, E., Wacquez, M. & De Bruyere, M. (1997). A seroepidemiological study on toxoplasmosis [published erratum appears in *Acta Clinica Belgica* 1997; 52, 68]. *Acta Clinica Belgica*, 52, 3–8.

Macdonald, D. (1980). The behaviour and ecology of farm cats. In *The Ecology and Control of Feral Cats*, pp. 23–9. Potters Bar, Herts: University Federation for Animal Welfare.

MacKnight, K. T. & Robinson, H. W. (1992). Epidemiologic studies on human and feline toxoplasmosis. *Journal of Hygiene, Epidemiology, Microbiology and Immunology*, 36, 37–47.

Marschner, I. C. (1997). A method for assessing age-time disease incidence using serial prevalence data. *Biometrics*, 53, 1384–98.

McCabe, R. E., Brooks, R. G., Dorfman, R. F. & Remington, J. S. (1987). Clinical spectrum in 107 cases of toxoplasmic lymphadenopathy [Review]. *Reviews of Infectious Diseases*, 9, 754–74.

McColgan, C., Buxton, D. & Blewett, D. A. (1988). Titration of *Toxoplasma gondii* oocysts in non-pregnant sheep and the effects of subsequent challenge during pregnancy. *Veterinary Record*, 123, 467–70.

McCulloch, W. F., Braun, J. L., Heggen, D. W. & Top, F. H. (1963). Studies on medical and veterinary students skin tested for toxoplasmosis. *Public Health Reports*, 78, 689–98.

McDonald, J. C., Gyorkos, T. W., Alberton, B. et al. (1990). An outbreak of toxoplasmosis in pregnant women in northern Quebec. *Journal of Infectious Diseases*, 161, 769–74.

McKissock, G. E., Ratcliffe, H. L. & Koestner, A. (1968). Enzootic toxoplasmosis in caged squirrel monkeys *Saimiri sciureus*. *Pathologica Veterinaria*, 5, 538–60.

Mittal, V., Bhatia, R., Singh, V. K. & Sehgal, S. (1995). Prevalence of toxoplasmosis in Indian women of child bearing age. *Indian Journal of Pathology and Microbiology*, 38, 143–5.

Monjour, L., Niel, G., Palminteri, R., Sidatt, M., Daniel Ribeiro, C., Alfred, C. & Gentilini, M. (1983). An epidemiological survey of toxoplasmosis in Mauritania. *Tropical and Geographical Medicine*, 35, 21–5.

Moschen, M. E., Stroffolini, T., Arista, S., Pistoia, D., Giammanco, A., Azara, A., De Mattia, D., Chiaramonte, M., Rigo, G. & Scarpa, B. (1991). Prevalence of *Toxoplasma gondii* antibodies among children and teenagers in Italy. *Microbiologica*, 14, 229–34.

Munday, B. L. (1972). Serological evidence of toxoplasma infection in isolated groups of sheep. *Research Veterinary Science*, 13, 100–2.

Navarro, I. T., Vidotto, O., Giraldi, N. & Mitsuka, R. (1992). [Resistance of *Toxoplasma gondii* to sodium chloride and condiments in pork sausage]. [Portuguese]. *Boletin de la Oficina Sanitaria Panamericana*, 112, 138–43.

Newton, L. H. & Hall, S. M. (1994). Survey of local policies for prevention of congenital toxoplasmosis. *Communicable Disease Report*, 4 (review no. 10), R121–R124.

Newton, L. H. & Hall, S. M. (1995). A review of health education material for primary prevention of congenital toxoplasmosis. *Communicable Disease Report*, 5, R21–R27.

Obendorf, D. L. & Munday, B. L. (1983). Toxoplasmosis in wild Tasmanian wallabies. *Australian Veterinary Journal*, 60, 62.

Omland, T., Tonjum, A. & Frentzel Beyme, R. (1977). Prevalence of *Toxoplasma gondii* antibodies in different populations of native Liberians. *Tropenmed Parasitol*, 28, 372–6.

Osiyemi, T. I., Synge, E. M., Agbonlahor, D. E. & Agbavwe, R. (1985). The prevalence of
Toxoplasma gondii antibodies in man in Plateau State and meat animals in Nigeria.
Transactions of the Royal Society of Tropical Medicine and Hygiene, 79, 21–3.

Owen, M. R. & Trees, A. J. (1998). Vertical transmission of *Toxoplasma gondii* from chronically
infected house and field mice determined by polymerase chain reaction. *Parasitology*, 116,
299–304.

Papoz, L., Simondon, F., Saurin, W. & Sarmini, H. (1986). A simple model relevant to toxoplasmosis applied to epidemiologic results in France. *American Journal of Epidemiology*, 123,
154–61.

Patton, S., Johnson, S. L., Loeffler, D. G., Wright, B. G. & Jensen, J. M. (1986). Epizootic of toxoplasmosis in kangaroos, wallabies and potaroos: possible transmission via domestic cats.
Journal of the American Veterinary Medical Association, 189, 1166–9.

Peach, W., Fowler, J. & Hay, J. (1989). Incidence of *Toxoplasma* infection in a population of
European starlings *Sternus vulgaris* from central England. *Annals of Tropical Medicine and
Parasitology*, 83, 173–7.

Peña, E., Sandoval, L., Quinteros, M. A., Assar, A. M., Vidal, S., Contreras, M. C. & Schenone, H.
(1986). Seroepidemiological study on human toxoplasmosis and hydatidosis in blood donors
and delivering mothers at the Regional Hospital of Talca, VII Region, Chile. 1985–1986. *Bol
Chil Parasitol*, 41, 87–99.

Pereira, L. H., Staudt, M., Tanner, C. E. & Embil, J. A. (1992). Exposure to *Toxoplasma gondii* and
cat ownership in Nova Scotia. *Pediatrics*, 89, 1169–72.

Pettersen, E. K. (1984). Transmission of toxoplasmosis via milk from lactating mice. *Acta
Pathologica, Microbiologica, et Immunologica Scandinavica – Section B, Microbiology*, 92, 175–6.

Plant, J. W., Richardson, N. & Moyle, G. G. (1974). *Toxoplasma* infection and abortion in sheep
associated with feeding grain contaminated with cat faeces. *Australian Veterinary Journal*, 50,
19–21.

Pomeroy, C. & Filice, G. A. (1992). Pulmonary toxoplasmosis: a review. *Clinical Infectious
Diseases*, 14, 863–70.

Pop, A., Oprisan, A., Cerbu, A., Stavarache, M. & Nitu, R. (1989). Toxoplasmosis prevalence parasitologically evaluated in meat animals. *Archives Roumaines de Pathologie Experimentale et de
Microbiologie*, 48, 373–8.

Price, J. H. (1969). Toxoplasma infection in an urban community. *British Medical Journal*, 4,
141–3.

Raccurt, C. P., Mojon, M. & Boncy, J. (1986). *Toxoplasma gondii* in Haiti. Results of a sero-
epidemiologic survey in a rural area. *Bulletin de la Societe de Pathologie Exotique et de Ses
Filiasles*, 79, 721–9.

Raisanen, S. A. & Saari, K. M. (1978). The importance of trophozoites in transmission of toxoplasmosis: survival and pathogenicity of *Toxoplasma gondii* trophozoites in liquid media. *Medical Hypotheses*, **4**, 367–75.

Rawal, B. D. (1959). Toxoplasmosis: a dye list survey on sera from vegetarians and meat eaters in Bombay. *Transactions of the Royal Society of Tropical Medicine and Hygiene*, **53**, 61–3.

Remington, J. S. & Desmonts, G. (1990). *Toxoplasmosis – In Infectious Diseases of the Fetus and Newborn Infant*, pp. 89–193. Philadelphia: WB Saunders.

Ricciardi, I. D., Sandoval, E. F. & Mayrink, W. (1975). Preliminary notes on the prevalence of human toxoplasmosis in Brazil. *Transactions of the Royal Society of Tropical Medicine and Hygiene*, **69**, 516–17.

Riemann, H. P., Meyer, M. E., Theis, J. H., Kelso, G. & Behymer, D. E. (1975a). Toxoplasmosis in an infant fed unpasteurized goat milk. *Journal of Pediatrics*, **87**, 573–6.

Riemann, H. P., Brant, P. C., Behymer, D. E. & Franti, C. E. (1975b). *Toxoplasma gondii* and *Coxiella burnetti* antibodies among Brazilian slaughterhouse employees. *American Journal of Tropical Medicine and Hygiene*, **102**, 386–93.

Rifaat, M. A., Salem, S. A., Khalil, H. M., Khaled, M. L. M., Sadek, M. S. M. & Azab, M. E. (1975). Toxoplasmosis serological surveys among inhabitants of some governorates of Egypt. *Transactions of the Royal Society of Tropical Medicine and Hygiene*, **69**, 118–20.

Ruiz, A. & Frenkel, J. K. (1980a). *Toxoplasma gondii* in Costa Rican cats. *American Journal of Tropical Medicine and Hygiene*, **29**, 1150–60.

Ruiz, A. & Frenkel, J. K. (1980b). Intermediate and transport hosts of *Toxoplasma gondii* in Costa Rica. *American Journal of Tropical Medicine and Hygiene*, **29**, 1161–6.

Ruoss, C. F. & Bourne, G. L. (1972). Toxoplasmosis in pregnancy. *Journal of Obstetrics and Gynaecology of the British Commonwealth*, **79**, 1115–18.

Ryan, M. J., Hall, S. M., Barrett, N., Balfour, A. H., Holliman, R. E. & Joynson, D. H. M. (1995). Toxoplasmosis in England and Wales 1981–1992. *Communicable Disease Report*, **5**, 13–21.

Sacks, J. J., Roberto, R. R. & Brooks, N. F. (1982). Toxoplasmosis infection associated with raw goat's milk. *Journal of the American Medical Association*, **248**, 1728–32.

Sacks, J. J., Delgado, D. G., Lobel, H. O. & Parker, R. L. (1983). Toxoplasmosis associated with eating undercooked venison. *American Journal of Epidemiology*, **118**, 832–8.

Saleha, A. (1984). Observations on some epidemiological aspects of toxoplasmosis in Malaysia. *International Journal of Zoonoses*, **11**, 75–83.

Samad, M. A., Dey, B. C., Chowdhury, N. S., Akhtar, S. & Khan, M. R. (1997). Sero-epidemiological studies on *Toxoplasma gondii* infection in man and animals in Bangladesh. *Southeast Asian Journal of Tropical Medicine and Public Health*, **28**, 339–43.

Sanger, V. L., Chamberlain, D. M., Chamberlain, K. W., Cole, C. R. & Farrell, R. L. (1953). Toxoplasmosis. V. Isolation of toxoplasma from cattle. *Journal of the American Veterinary Medical Association*, **123**, 87–91.

Schenone, H., Contreras, M. C., Salinas, P. et al. (1986a). Epidemiology of toxoplasmosis in Chile. I. Prevalence of human infection, studied by the indirect hemagglutination reaction, in the 1st 3 regions. 1982–1985. *Bol Chil Parasitol*, **41**, 36–39.

Schenone, H., Contreras, M. C., Salinas, P. et al. (1986b). Epidemiology of toxoplasmosis in Chile. II. Prevalence of human infection, studied by means of indirect hemagglutination reaction, in Regions IV, V and VI. 1982–1986. *Bol Chil Parasitol*, **41**, 82–86.

Schenone, H., Contreras, M. C., Salinas, P., Tello, P., Sandoval, L., Pena, A. M., Villarroel, F. & Rojas, A. (1987). Epidemiology of toxoplasmosis in Chile. III. Prevalence of the human infection, studied by means of indirect hemagglutination reaction, in the Metropolitan region of Santiago. 1982–1987. *Bol Chil Parasitol*, 42, 28–32.

Seuri, M. & Koskela, P. (1992). Contact with pigs and cats associated with high prevalence of Toxoplasma antibodies among farmers. *British Journal of Industrial Medicine*, 49, 845–9.

Shen, L., Zhichung, L., Biaucheng, Z. & Huayuan, Y. (1990). Prevalence of *Toxoplasma gondii* infection in man and animals in Guangdong, Peoples Republic of China. *Veterinary Parasitology*, 34, 357–60.

Singh, S. & Nautiyal, B. L. (1991). Seroprevalence of toxoplasmosis in Kumaon region of India. *Indian Journal of Medical Research*, 93, 247–9.

Skinner, L. J., Timperley, A. C., Wightman, D., Chatterton, J. M. & Ho-Yen, D. O. (1990). Simultaneous diagnosis of toxoplasmosis in goats and goatowner's family. *Scandinavian Journal of Infectious Diseases*, 22, 359–61.

Smith, J. L. (1991). Foodborne toxoplasmosis. *Journal of Food Safety*, 12, 17–57.

Smith, J. L. (1992). *Toxoplasma gondii* in meats – a matter of concern? *Dairy, Food and Environmental Sanitation*, 12, 341–5.

Song Chang-Cun, Yuang Xing-Zheng, Shen Li-Ying, Gan Xiao-Xian, Ding Jiang-Zu (1993). The effect of cobalt-60 irradiation on the infectivity of *Toxoplasma gondii*. *International Journal of Parasitology*, 23, 89–93.

Sousa, O. E., Saenz, R. E. & Frenkel, J. (1988). Toxoplasmosis in Panama: a 10-year study. *American Journal of Tropical Medicine and Hygiene*, 38, 315–22.

Stagno, S., Dykes, A. C., Amos, C. S., Head, R. A., Juranek, D. D. & Walls, K. (1980). An outbreak of toxoplasmosis linked to cats. *Pediatrics*, 65, 706–12.

Stanwell-Smith, R. (1999). Public health and waterborne diseases. *Public Health Medicine*, 2, 53–60.

Stray-Pedersen, B. & Lorentzen-Styr, A. M. (1980). Epidemiological aspects of Toxoplasma infections among women in Norway. *Acta Obstetrica et Gynecologica Scandinavica*, 59, 323–6.

Sun, R. G., Liu, Z. L. & Wang, D. C. (1995). [The prevalence of Toxoplasma infection among pregnant women and their newborn infants in Chengdu]. [Chinese]. *Chung-Hua Liu Hsing Ping Hsueh Tsa Chih Chinese Journal of Epidemiology*, 16, 98–100.

Suzuki, H., Aso, T., Yamamoto, Y. & Matsumoto, K. (1988). Seroepidemiology of toxoplasma infection in two islands of Nagasaki by ELISA. *Tropical Medicine*, 30, 129–39.

Sykora, J., Zastera, M. & Stankova, M. (1992). Toxoplasmic antibodies in sera of HIV-infected persons. *Folia Parasitologica*, 39, 177–80.

Tabor, R. (1980). General biology of feral cats. In *The Ecology and Control of Feral Cats*, pp. 5–11. Potters Bar, Herts: University Federation for Animal Welfare.

Tan, S. K. & Zaman, V. (1973). Toxoplasma antibody survey in West Malaysia. *Medical Journal of Malaysia*, 27, 188.

Taylor, M. R., Lennon, B., Holland, C. V. & Cafferkey, M. (1997). Community study of toxoplasma antibodies in urban and rural schoolchildren aged 4 to 18 years. *Archives of Disease in Childhood*, 77, 406–9.

Terragna, A., Morandi, N., Canessa, A. & Pellegrino, C. (1984). The occurrence of *Toxoplasma gondii* in saliva. *Tropenmedizin und Parasitologie*, 35, 9–10.

Teutsch, S. M., Juranek, D. D., Sulzer, A., Dubey, J. P. & Sikes, R. K. (1979). Epidemic toxoplasmosis associated with infected cats. *New England Journal of Medicine*, 300, 695–9.

Thomas, V., Sinniah, B. & Yap, P. (1980). Prevalence of antibodies including IgM to *Toxoplasma gondii* in Malaysians. *Southeast Asian Journal of Tropical Medicine and Public Health*, 11, 119–25.

Tizard, I. R. & Caoili, F. A. (1976). Toxoplasmosis in veterinarians: an investigation into possible sources of infection. *Canadian Veterinary Journal*, 17, 24–5.

Tizard, I. R., Fish, N. A. & Quin, J. P. (1976). Some observations on the epidemiology of toxoplasmosis in Canada. *Journal of Hygiene (Cambridge)*, 77, 11–21.

Ulmanen, I. & Leinikki, P. (1975). The role of pet cats in the seroepidemiology of toxoplasmosis. *Scandinavian Journal of Infectious Diseases*, 7, 67–71.

Vaage, L. & Midtvedt, T. (1975). Epidemiological aspects of toxoplasmosis. II. The prevalence of positive toxoplasmin reactions in naval recruits from different parts of Norway. *Scandinavian Journal of Infectious Diseases*, 7, 218–21.

Valcavi, P. P., Natali, A., Soliani, L., Montali, S., Dettori, G. & Cheezi, C. (1995). Prevalence of anti-*Toxoplasma gondii* antibodies in the population of the area of Parma (Italy). *European Journal of Epidemiology*, 11, 333–7.

Van Knapen, F., Kremers, A. F., Franchimont, J. H. & Narucha, U. (1995). Prevalence of antibodies to *Toxoplasma gondii* in cattle and swine in the Netherlands: towards an integrated control of livestock production. *Veterinary Quarterly*, 17, 87–91.

Van Pelt, R. W. & Dietricht, R. A. (1973). Staphylococcal infection and toxoplasmosis in a young harbor seal. *Journal of Wildlife Diseases*, 9, 258–61.

Velasco-Castrejon, O., Salvatierra-Izaba, B., Valdespino, J. L. et al. (1992). [Seroepidemiology of toxoplasmosis in Mexico.] [Spanish]. *Salud Publica De Mexico*, 34, 222–9.

Vitor, R. W. A., Pinto, J. B. & Chiari, C. A. (1990). *Toxoplasma gondii* in urine, saliva and milk of infected goats. *Mem Inst Oswaldo Cruz*, 85 [Suppl. 1], 146.

Waldeland, H. (1976). Toxoplasmosis in sheep. The prevalence of toxoplasma antibodies in lambs and mature sheep from different parts of Norway. *Acta Veterinaria Scandinavica*, 17, 432–4.

Walker, J., Nokes, D. J. & Jennings, R. (1992). Longitudinal study of Toxoplasma seroprevalence in South Yorkshire. *Epidemiology and Infection*, 108, 99–106.

Wallace, G. D. (1973). Intermediate and transport hosts in the natural history of *Toxoplasma gondii*. *American Journal of Tropical Medicine and Hygiene*, 22, 446–56.

Wallace, G. D. (1976). The prevalence of toxoplasmosis on Pacific islands, and the influence of ethnic group. *American Journal of Tropical Medicine and Hygiene*, 25, 48–53.

Wallace, G. D., Marshall, I. & Marshall, M. (1972). Cats, rats and toxoplasmosis on a small Pacific island. *American Journal of Tropical Medicine and Hygiene*, 95, 475–82.

Wallace, G. D., Laigret, J. & Kaeuffer, H. A. (1974a). Comparison of the prevalences of toxoplasma antibody in Tahitians and Chinese living in Tahiti. *Southeast Asian Journal of Tropical Medicine and Public Health*, 5, 350–2.

Wallace, G. D., Zigas, V. & Gajdusek, D. C. (1974b). Toxoplasmosis and cats in New Guinea. *American Journal of Tropical Medicine and Hygiene*, 23, 8–14.

Wallace, M. R., Rossetti, R. J. & Olson, P. E. (1993). Cats and toxoplasmosis risk in HIV-infected adults. *Journal of the American Medical Association*, **269**, 76–7.

Wallon, M., Mallaret, M. R., Mojon, M. & Peyron, F. (1994). Congenital toxoplasmosis, assessment of prevention policy. *Presse Medicale*, **23**, 1467–70.

Warnekulasuriya, M. R., Johnson, J. D. & Holliman, R. E. (1998). Detection of *Toxoplasma gondii* in cured meats. *International Journal of Food Microbiology*, **45**, 211–15.

Weinman, D. & Chandler, A. H. (1955). Toxoplasmosis in man and swine – an investigation of the possible relationship. *Journal of the American Medical Association*, **161**, 229–32.

Williams, K. A. B., Scott, J. M., MacFarlane, D. E. et al. (1981). Congenital toxoplasmosis: a prospective study in the West of Scotland. *Journal of Infection*, **3**, 219–29.

Witt, C. J., Moench, T. R., Gittelsohn, A. M., Bishop, B. D. & Childs, J. E. (1989). Epidemiologic observations on feline immunodeficiency virus and *Toxoplasma gondii* coinfection in cats in Baltimore, Md. *Journal of the American Veterinary Medical Association*, **194**, 229–30.

Woodruff, A. W., De Savigny, D. H. & Hendy-Ibbs, P. M. (1982). Toxocaral and toxoplasmal antibodies in cat breeders and in Icelanders exposed to cats but not to dogs. *British Medical Journal*, **284**, 309–10.

Yahaya, N. (1991). Review of toxoplasmosis in Malaysia. *Southeast Asian Journal of Tropical Medicine and Public Health (Supplement)*, **22**, 102–6.

Zadik, P. M., Kudesia, G. & Siddons, A. D. (1995). Low incidence of primary infection with toxoplasma among women in Sheffield: a seroconversion study. *British Journal of Obstetrics and Gynaecology*, **102**, 608–10.

Zardi, O., Adorisio, E., Harare, O. & Nuti, M. (1980). Serological survey of toxoplasmosis in Somalia. *Transactions of the Royal Society of Tropical Medicine and Hygiene*, **74**, 577–81.

Zigas, V. (1976). Prevalence of toxoplasma antibodies in New Britain, Papua New Guinea. *Papua New Guinea Medical Journal*, **19**, 225–30.

Zimmerman, W. J. (1976). Prevalence of *Toxoplasma gondii* antibodies among veterinary college staff and students, Iowa State University. *Public Health Reports*, **91**, 526–32.

4

Infection in the immunocompetent

D. O. Ho-Yen

Toxoplasma Reference Laboratory, Raigmore Hospital, Inverness, Scotland

Introduction

Infection with *Toxoplasma gondii* in the immunocompetent individual has generally been regarded as being of little significance. This is probably because many clinicians are influenced by the normally favourable outcome of toxoplasmic lymphadenopathy, the most characteristic clinical presentation. However, toxoplasma infection has a world-wide distribution and since the vast majority of infections are usually not diagnosed (Ho-Yen 1992), the true importance of toxoplasma in the immunocompetent individual is unknown.

A vast amount of information is now available on toxoplasma infection, and the possible outcomes in the immunocompetent individual are shown in Figure 4.1. In those who have not been infected with toxoplasma, significant exposure to the organism usually results in a primary infection. However, there is some evidence that in a few immune individuals and where there is significant strain variation, a second infection is possible (Abdul-Fattah et al. 1992). Reactivated infections are probably more common than second infections, especially in individuals with immune dysfunction that may result from concomitant viral infections, for example human immunodeficiency virus (HIV) or immunosuppressive therapy. Acute toxoplasma infections can be primary, reactivated or second infections (Figure 4.1) and have a wide variety of clinical presentations. In the 1970s, it was generally regarded that acquired toxoplasmosis in the immunocompetent individual resulted in infection rather than disease (Feldman 1974). Now, this belief is being questioned. A greater awareness of the infection and better diagnostic techniques have increased the recognition of acquired toxoplasmosis. Yet, acquired toxoplasmosis is subtle in its clinical presentations, and clinicians still have to demonstrate great acumen to establish the true importance of this infection.

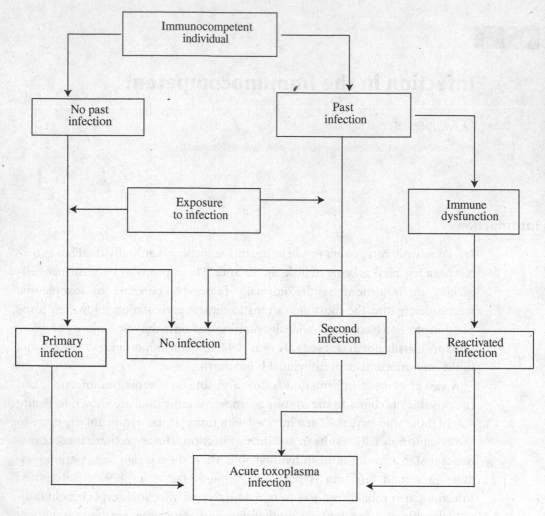

Figure 4.1   Toxoplasma infection in the immunocompetent individual

Infection

Exposure of a susceptible individual to toxoplasma will not necessarily result in infection. Infection will occur only if the stage of the parasite, the route of infection, the virulence of the strain and the infectious dose have occurred in the right individual. Much of the initial work on the relative importance of these factors (Figure 4.2) was done using animal models (Frenkel 1973), but the information appears to be relevant to human infections. These factors also determine the incubation period, the period between exposure to infection and clinical symptoms. Although precise data are not available for acquired toxoplasmosis, it is

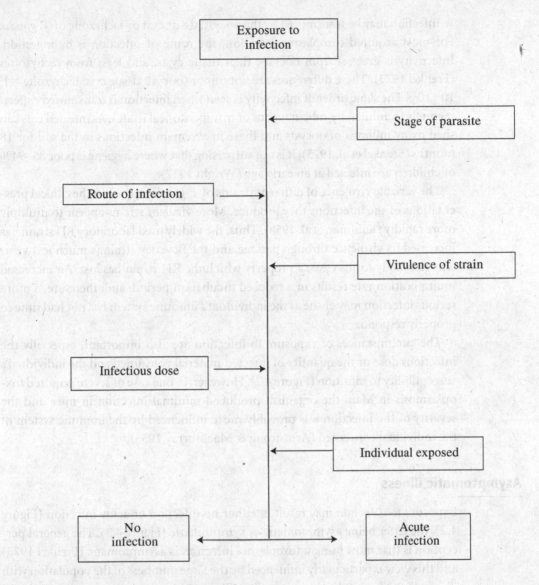

Figure 4.2   Factors influencing toxoplasma infection

believed that the incubation period is 4–21 days with most illness in the second
week after exposure (Ho-Yen 1992). When outbreaks of infection are examined,
it is obvious that a wide range of incubation times is possible (Ho-Yen 1992).
However, this should not be too surprising as the influential factors in Figure 4.2
may have positive or negative effects. These factors determine whether infection
occurs, its incubation period, its seriousness and perhaps even its clinical presentation.

Infection may be transmitted by the oocyst, tissue cyst or tachyzoite of *T. gondii*. For most acquired toxoplasma infection, the route of infection is by ingestion. Infectivity is greatest from oocysts, then tissue cysts, and least from tachyzoites (Frenkel 1973). These differences are not minor (oocyst: tissue cyst: tachyzoite = 1: 10^2: 10^5). The same order of infectivity is seen when infection is transmitted experimentally to animals by subcutaneous or intraperitoneal routes. As infected cats can shed many millions of oocysts and these may remain infectious in the soil for 18 months (Frenkel et al. 1975), it is not surprising that where hygiene is poor 85–94% of children are infected at an early age (Wright 1957).

The variable virulence of different strains of *T. gondii* may affect the clinical presentations of the infections they produce. More virulent strains appear to multiply more rapidly (Kaufman et al. 1958). Thus, the widely used laboratory RH strain has increased its virulence through passage and the Beverley strain is much less virulent and easily forms cysts, a property which the RH strain has lost. An increased multiplication rate results in a reduced incubation period, and, therefore, a more serious infection may ensue as the individual's immune system has not had time to properly respond.

The circumstances of exposure to infection are also important, especially the infectious dose or the quantity of infected material consumed and the individual's susceptibility to infection (Figure 4.2). However, in one case of severe acquired toxoplasmosis in Man, the organism produced minimal infection in mice and the severity of the infection was probably more influenced by the immune system of the individual concerned (Armstrong & MacMurray 1953).

Asymptomatic illness

Exposure to *T. gondii* may result in either no infection or acute infection (Figure 4.2), the latter being asymptomatic or symptomatic (Figure 4.3). The general perception is that most human toxoplasma infection is asymptomatic (Frenkel 1973) and this view is particularly influenced by the large numbers of the population with *T. gondii* antibody who do not recall an illness with relevant symptoms. Recently, outbreaks of toxoplasmosis have been examined (Ho-Yen 1992) and although it was recognized that the information from outbreaks may be particularly influenced by the virulence of the toxoplasma strain involved, it was concluded that only about 25% of toxoplasma infections are asymptomatic. Thus, the failure to recognize nonspecific symptoms caused by *T. gondii* is responsible for the previously held view that the majority of infections are asymptomatic.

There are several possible outcomes after acute *T. gondii* infection (Figure 4.3), the terminology of which can be misleading. It has been suggested that the state after acute infection where the parasite has encysted and the individual is asymp-

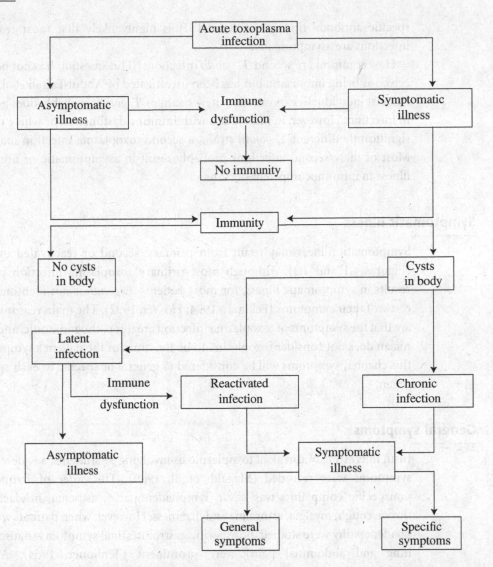

Figure 4.3   Results of acute toxoplasma infection

tomatic should be labelled 'chronic infection'. This is probably more correctly called 'latent infection' (Figure 4.3), and the term 'chronic infection' should be reserved for the patients with continuing symptoms. Reactivation of latent infection can occur following the release of encysted parasites, locally or systemically (Ho-Yen 1992). This situation may result from the periodic immune dysfunction that may accompany concomitant infections. The advantage to the individual is that the body's immune system becomes periodically stimulated, and a significant specific antibody titre is maintained. It is highly likely that most reactivated infections are asymptomatic.

How common are second *T. gondii* infections? This question has not been perceived as being important, but has been investigated by Abdul-Fattah et al. (1992). In most individuals, exposure to a new strain of *T. gondii* probably does not result in infection. However, in individuals with immune dysfunction or where there is a significantly different *T. gondii* strain, a second toxoplasma infection may result. Most of these second infections probably result in asymptomatic or nonspecific illness in immunocompetent persons.

Symptomatic illness

Symptomatic illness may result from primary, second or reactivated infections (Figures 4.1 and 4.3). Although most primary toxoplasma infection probably results in symptomatic illness, for most patients *T. gondii* is not identified as the cause of their symptoms (Feldman 1974; Ho-Yen 1992). The main reasons for this are that the symptoms of toxoplasma infection are not pathognomonic, and the clinician does not consider toxoplasma to be the cause of the patient's symptoms. In this chapter, symptoms will be considered as general or specific to each system or organ.

General symptoms

In an interesting outbreak of toxoplasmosis involving 99 students, a wide variety of symptoms were recorded (Magaldi et al. 1969). The order of frequency of nonspecific complaints was: fever, lymphadenopathy, asthenia, headache, sore throat, cough, myalgia, arthralgia and dizziness. However, when patients with lymphadenopathy were studied, nonspecific gastrointestinal symptoms (nausea, vomiting and abdominal pain) were prominent (Tenhunen 1964). A better understanding of nonspecific symptoms may result from looking at outbreaks as these patients are usually questioned more closely about their complaints. When the best-documented outbreaks of toxoplasma infection were considered, nonspecific complaints were shown to be very common (Ho-Yen 1992). When all of the patients in the outbreaks were aggregated, the frequency of major nonspecific symptoms was: pyrexia (70%), lymphadenopathy (64%), malaise (54%) and myalgia (43%). These complaints are schematically represented in Figure 4.4. Pyrexia is usually low grade (38–40°C) and persistent, but may be intermittent. As symptoms such as pyrexia, malaise and myalgia are extremely common, most clinicians would not investigate such patients, but simply describe their complaints as being a result of a 'viral' infection.

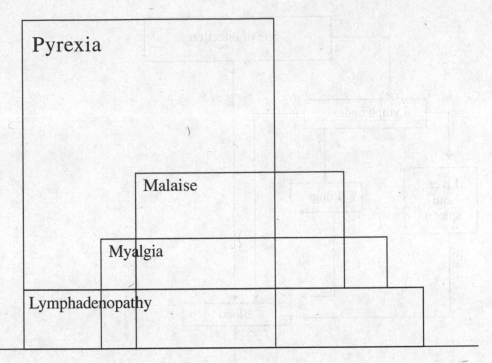

Figure 4.4   Schematic representation of general symptoms in toxoplasma infection

Specific symptoms

Most immunocompetent patients with toxoplasma infection are either asymptomatic or have general symptoms. This, however, should not make a clinician complacent about an acute toxoplasma infection, since fatal and serious infections have occurred in immunocompetent individuals. In spite of a remarkably large amount of literature on the systematic clinical presentations of this infection, the medical profession's awareness of toxoplasmosis is low. In the rest of this chapter, the body's systems and individual organs will be considered in order of the usual spread of infection: reticulo-endothelial, respiratory, haemopoietic, central nervous, heart, muscle, skin and others (Figure 4.5). The pathological changes of acquired toxoplasmosis show that extraneural viscera are more frequently involved than the central nervous system (Sexton et al. 1953), unlike congenital infection or infection in the immunocompromised.

Reticulo-endothelial system

Toxoplasma infection principally affects the lymph nodes, liver and spleen in the reticulo-endothelial system (Figure 4.5).

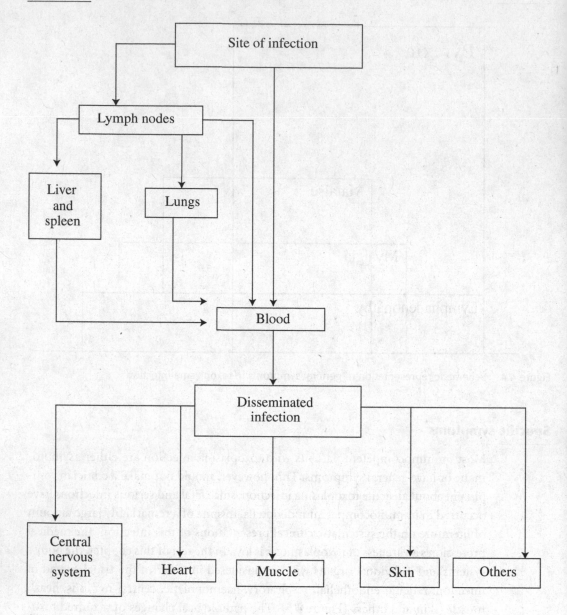

Figure 4.5   Potential spread of toxoplasma infection

Lymph nodes

Lymphadenopathy can be caused by infection with many organisms and may be regarded as a general symptom. However, the clinical presentation of *T. gondii* associated lymphadenopathy has special characteristics and warrants more detailed consideration, especially as this is the most commonly recognized form of acquired toxoplasmosis. The frequency of lymphadenopathy varies with age in the different sexes: there are more boys than girls under 15 years of age, and more women than men among adults (Beverley et al. 1976). For both sexes, the peak age group involved is 21–25 years (Miettinen et al. 1980). These results are probably real and not due to sampling errors. These groups of individuals are those most exposed to infection: young boys playing in the dirt; women preparing food and caring for cats; and young adults being adventurous in their choices of travel and food.

Any group of lymph nodes in the body may be affected. When the information from three large studies was amalgamated (Ho-Yen 1992), the most common sites were: neck (65%), axillae (24%) and groin (11%). Anterior cervical lymphadenopathy appears to be twice as common as posterior cervical lymphadenopathy. Although lymphadenopathy is much more frequent at single sites, multiple sites are usually found in children.

The clinical characteristics of the enlarged lymph nodes are that they are firm, discrete and unattached to the overlying skin. The nodes are rarely painful, but may be initially tender. The majority of nodes are 1–2 cm in diameter (Tenhunen 1964), but may occasionally be three times this size. Lymphadenopathy may occur without other general symptoms or with the patient feeling completely well. Alternatively, lymphadenopathy may be accompanied by general symptoms such as pyrexia, malaise or myalgia (Figure 4.4); this scenario probably occurs in the majority of cases. General symptoms may also be present without lymphadenopathy.

An unexpected finding in acquired toxoplasmic lymphadenopathy is its persistence in many patients. When details from three large studies were combined (Ho-Yen 1992), the persistence of lymphadenopathy could be determined for 185 patients. In most patients (60%) lymphadenopathy lasted less than 2 months, usually less than 1 month. However, lymphadenopathy lasted 2–4 months in 25%; 4–6 months in 8%; and more than 6 months in 6%. The persistence of lymphadenopathy can result in both the patient and the doctor becoming worried about a more sinister cause. Therefore, it is not too surprising that in many cases of acquired toxoplasmosis, the diagnosis is made on a lymph node biopsy sample.

The differential diagnosis of patients with toxoplasmic lymphadenopathy, with or without systemic symptoms, encompasses many medical conditions. When systemic symptoms are present, especially pyrexia, infections are first considered. Many viral and bacterial infections produce lymphadenopathy, but most are not investigated. Among those patients who are investigated, Epstein–Barr virus and cytomegalovirus are probably the most common other causes of a similar illness (Ho-Yen 1992). However, other infections must be considered, especially other herpes and respiratory viruses, streptococcal infection and tuberculosis.

In the differential diagnosis, apart from infection, malignancy and autoimmune disease have to be considered. In many of these cases, the persistence of the lymphadenopathy, the absence of general symptoms, and the concern of the patient or doctor are the main reasons why a lymph node biopsy is performed. In such circumstances, the most common malignancies are Hodgkin's disease and nonHodgkin's lymphoma (Miettinen & Franssila 1982). The diagnosis of toxoplasmosis was made in 2–4% of patients who had lymphadenopathy and a biopsy sample taken (Miettinen et al. 1980). Nevertheless, in patients with lymphadenopathy for which the clinician is contemplating lymph node biopsy, good clinical practice should dictate that toxoplasma serology should first be performed.

In a smaller group of patients, symptoms may suggest the possibility of infectious mononucleosis. First, it is important to recognize that 'glandular fever' is any illness with enlarged glands and pyrexia, whereas infectious mononucleosis is a definite illness with specific clinical, haematological and serological characteristics (Ho-Yen 1992). Many infectious agents may cause glandular fever, but Epstein–Barr virus is the accepted cause of infectious mononucleosis. However, toxoplasmosis may produce an illness that fulfils the clinical and haematological criteria of infectious mononucleosis (Ho-Yen 1992). In toxoplasmic lymphadenopathy, the clinical picture differs from that of infectious mononucleosis: pyrexia is less persistent, the sore throat is not as prominent, there is less generalized lymphadenopathy and hepatosplenomegaly is not as common. Laboratory tests also show great differences. In toxoplasmic lymphadenopathy, liver function tests are abnormal in only a few patients and atypical lymphocystosis is uncommon. Thus, toxoplasmosis is a rare cause of an infectious mononucleosis-like illness in Britain. However, this may not be the case in countries where most of the population has Epstein–Barr virus infections in childhood. In such countries, for example in Malaysia, Epstein–Barr virus infection is rare in adolescence, and individuals with an infectious mononucleosis-like illness in this age group are more likely to have acquired toxoplasmosis (Tan et al. 1978).

Liver

The liver is probably involved early in the infective process (Figure 4.5). However, abnormal liver function tests and jaundice are usually uncommon in toxoplasmosis. The most probable explanation of this apparent conundrum is that infection spreads to the liver early in the illness, but is not severe enough to produce laboratory or clinical abnormalities. This view is supported by the finding that hepatic involvement of *T. gondii* can present in three ways: initial lymphadenopathy followed by hepatitis several months later; hepatitis without lymphadenopathy; and simultaneous lymphadenopathy and hepatitis (Weitburg et al. 1979). These various clinical presentations may be influenced by the circumstances of the exposure to infection (Figure 4.2).

The frequency of hepatitis in individuals with toxoplasma infection varies between 11% and 89% (Ho-Yen 1992). This finding is difficult to explain. It may be related to the fact that when 89% of patients were found to have had hepatitis, a particular virulent strain of toxoplasma was present. A reasonable explanation of the pathophysiology is that most strains of toxoplasma spread slowly and detectable hepatitis (abnormal liver function tests or jaundice) is uncommon; when infection is particularly virulent, hepatitis is more common. This hypothesis would explain two of the three situations (Weitberg et al. 1979) previously described, and the explanation of lymphadenopathy preceding hepatitis by some months could be that the initial low grade infection has a greater effect with time, either because of passage of the organism or prolonged infection reducing the patient's immunity.

In the immunocompetent individual, the place of specific antitoxoplasma therapy remains to be defined. Individuals with acute hepatitis caused by toxoplasma-induced infection can recover quickly without specific treatment (Weitberg et al. 1979). Most patients with hepatitis should not have specific antitoxoplasma therapy. Such therapy should be reserved for those individuals whose significantly impaired immune system is unlikely to function.

Spleen

The spleen appears to be involved early in toxoplasma infection (Sexton et al. 1953), but palpable splenomegaly is uncommon. The spleen plays an important role in the phagocytic function of the body, so early involvement would be expected (Figure 4.5). It is probable that most acquired toxoplasma infections are not severe enough to produce clinical splenomegaly, the absence of which could be useful in clinically differentiating toxoplasma infection from Epstein–Barr virus infection.

Studies of toxoplasmic lymphadenopathy have shown that palpable splenomegaly is rare (Tenhunen 1964; Miettinen et al. 1980). In many of these patients, abdominal complaints were common, but it is likely that mesenteric lymphadenopathy or hepatitis rather than splenomegaly was the cause of the abdominal symptoms. By contrast, two other studies with good clinical information showed splenomegaly to be more common: in Britain, five of 30 (17%) patients (Beverley & Beattie 1958) and in Greece, five of 23 (22%) patients (Thomaidis et al. 1977). Although splenomegaly is more common in tropical countries because of chronic infections, these two studies suggest that the differences between tropical and temperate countries are not great. However, the most important finding is that age is a critical factor. In the Greek group, all of the patients were 16 years or younger. The British study was of patients aged 3–50 years, but of the five patients with splenomegaly, four were 14 years or younger. Therefore, splenomegaly is probably be more common in those aged 16 years or younger. It is also more likely that individuals with systemic manifestations have splenomegaly, as in three of the five cases in the Greek study (Thomaidis et al. 1977). Treatment is probably not indicated in most cases.

Respiratory system

The frequency of toxoplasma infection of the respiratory system is unknown. In animal models, lung involvement appears early in the infection, and pulmonary toxoplasmosis is frequent in the immunocompromised patient or in congenital infection (Catterall et al. 1986). Among the immunocompetent, pulmonary toxoplasmosis would appear to be uncommon. However, 30 years ago, it was suggested that toxoplasma was a cause of atypical pneumonia, but that problems in diagnosis and the lack of awareness of the condition explained why pulmonary toxoplasmosis was rarely identified (Ludlam & Beattie 1963). The subsequent discovery of *Mycoplasma pneumoniae* as an important cause of atypical pneumonia further reduced interest in pulmonary toxoplasmosis.

There is little doubt that *T. gondii* can produce pneumonia in immunocompetent individuals (Candolfi et al. 1993) and patients are often breathless, pyrexial and may have a cough. Although pneumonia is sometimes found, the more common finding is pulmonary pneumonitis. Radiological changes are usually bilateral with diffuse infiltrates, but occasionally one lobe alone may be involved. More rarely, toxoplasma infection may be a cause of multiple nodular radiographic densities in the lungs (Prosmanne et al. 1984).

Pulmonary toxoplasmosis is rarely diagnosed even though the organism probably involves the lungs early in the infection (Figure 4.5). In most cases infection does not produce significant symptoms, and is, therefore, not investigated; many patients probably have a cough without significant sputum production and are diagnosed as having 'atypical pneumonia'. These cases may resolve with time or following the usual tetracycline treatment for atypical pneumonias. Tetracycline may also have an antitoxoplasma effect (Joss 1992), and many toxoplasma infections may resolve because of presumed treatment of other infections.

The diagnosis of respiratory toxoplasmosis is difficult because sputum production is poor. The parasite can be detected in bronchoalveolar lavage fluid (Candolfi et al. 1993), but most patients are probably not ill enough to warrant such procedures. It is also unlikely that toxoplasma will be looked for in sputum. In the majority of cases, the diagnosis will be made serologically as in other causes of atypical pneumonia.

Haemopoietic system

Parasitaemia is a feature of acute *T. gondii* infection (Derouin & Garin 1991). The degree and duration of the parasitaemia probably depends on the circumstances of the infection, especially the virulence of the organism and the infectious dose. In one study, apparent parasitaemia (detected by polymerase chain reaction, PCR) could be demonstrated for up to 12–16 weeks in some patients after the development of lymphadenopathy (Guy & Joynson 1995). From the blood, the parasite can spread to other organs (Figure 4.5), but not all organs are equally affected. In a study of disseminated toxoplasmosis, the brain was affected in 86.5%, the heart in 86.5% and the lungs in 72.9% (Yermakov et al. 1982). Although this latter study was mainly of immunocompromised patients, two (5%) of the 37 patients studied appeared to be immunocompetent. A feature of disseminated infection is the absence of lymphadenopathy (Yermakov et al. 1982). In another report of disseminated infection in an immunocompetent patient, the brain and skin were mainly involved (Bach & Armstrong 1983), and lymphadenopathy was not present.

While parasitaemia is the main mode of dissemination of infection, there are also individual effects on the haemopoietic system. In most patients, the total white cell count is normal, but leucocytosis is present in 20% of cases (Beverley & Beattie 1958). By contrast, lymphocytosis is found in 50–84% of cases (Beverley & Beattie 1958; Miettinen et al. 1980). Although eosinophilia has been described in acquired toxoplasmosis, it is a rare occurrence (Ho-Yen 1992). Of greater importance is the finding that toxoplasmosis may produce atypical lymphocytosis, a characteristic feature of infectious mononucleosis. In patients with toxoplasmic lymphadenopathy, atypical lymphocytosis varies between 8% (Miettinen et al. 1980) and 17% (Beverley & Beattie 1958). These differences may be partly strain-dependent, as in a large outbreak of toxoplasmosis due to ingestion of contaminated drinking water 39% of patients had atypical lymphocytosis (Benenson et al. 1982). In a large study of patients with atypical lymphocytosis and lymphadenopathy, the majority of patients had Epstein–Barr virus infection; nevertheless, it was found that 5% of patients had acquired toxoplasmosis (Ho-Yen & Martin 1981). Thus, acquired toxoplasmosis should be remembered as a cause of an infectious mononucleosis-like illness.

Profound anaemia, leucopaenia and hepatosplenomegaly with erythroid hyperplasia of the marrow has been described in severe cases of toxoplasmosis (Kalderon et al. 1964). Other associations with toxoplasma infection have been less frequently documented. Thus the relationship between toxoplasmosis and thrombocytopaenic purpura or acquired haemolytic anaemia is difficult to evaluate. Although both of these conditions are frequently described as idiopathic, toxoplasmosis is unlikely to be a major cause.

Central nervous system

It had been recognized for some time that acquired toxoplasma infection can readily involve the central nervous system (Sexton et al. 1953). Animal studies also confirm that acquired toxoplasmosis involves the central nervous system as a major target of infection (Derouin & Garin 1991). Although this system is more likely to be involved in infections among immunocompromised individuals or those with congenital infection, there is also significant infection in the immunocompetent. There are three main clinical presentations: encephalitis, ocular disease and a myalgic encephalomyelitis-like illness. These conditions may present as part of disseminated infection with the other organs involved, or the central nervous system may be involved on its own. In the latter case, it is postulated that the sequence of events is as in Figure 4.5, but that the blood–brain barrier allows preferential progression of infection in the brain (Ghatak et al. 1970). Some cases of central nervous system infection may result from the reactivation of a previous infection, but in the immunocompetent this is unlikely to be as common as acquired infection. Ocular disease is considered in Chapter 11.

Encephalitis

In the past, cerebral toxoplasmosis was diagnosed infrequently before the patient died (Townsend et al. 1975). During the last decade there has been a dramatic increase in this condition because of the greater use of immunosuppressive therapy and increasing HIV infection. The increased prevalence of toxoplasmic encephalitis has heightened clinicians' awareness in immunocompromised patients. However, among immunocompetent individuals the condition is seldom considered in the differential diagnosis of encephalitis of unknown cause. This can be particularly unfortunate as patients who are treated with appropriate antibiotics often have a favourable outcome (Townsend et al. 1975).

In a review of toxoplasmic encephalitis in 1975 (Townsend et al. 1975) 22 of 45 (49%) patients were believed to be immunocompetent. This contrasts with a more recent study (incorporating the results of the first study) whereby 48 of 200 (24%) such patients were identified (Luft & Remington 1985). A consistent clinical picture emerged, with immunocompetent patients having three main presentations: diffuse encephalitis in about 20%, meningoencephalitis in about 25% and localized encephalitis in the remainder (Townsend et al. 1975).

Cases of diffuse encephalitis often have a complicated clinical picture. Patients are often confused, delirious or even comatosed. In these patients, the encephalitis may be accompanied by seizures. As well as encephalitis, the presence of meningitis (pleocytosis in the cerebrospinal fluid) is common; however, not all of the patients have the classic signs of meningitis. Localized encephalitis can present as single or multiple lesions. The clinical impression may be that of an expanding tumour (Luft & Remington 1985), and it is not surprising that a large toxoplasmic granuloma containing pseudocysts, an inflammatory response and oedema may mimic a neoplasm.

Acute toxoplasmic retinochoroiditis may happen before or at the same time as involvement of the central nervous system (Luft & Remington 1985). This may be because the eye is protected from the immune response, allowing easier proliferation of the organism. Nevertheless, it should be remembered that toxoplasmic encephalitis is probably a result of disseminated infection (Figure 4.5), and so other specific complaints (for example vestibular dysfunction) may accompany the encephalitis (Luft & Remington 1985).

Myalgic encephalomyelitis

This condition is known by many names (Royal Free disease, post-viral fatigue syndrome, chronic fatigue syndrome). There have been several suggestions that the illness is all in the mind, but a clear definition has been established (Sharpe et al. 1991). The characteristic findings are: generalized, relapsing fatigue for at least 6 months with muscle weakness on exercise, complaints of prominent disturbance of concentration and/or short-term memory impairment and the exclusion of any obvious organic cause of a similar illness. The vast majority of patients have been previously well, and remember an initiating illness with malaise and pyrexia (Ho-Yen 1999). Although the syndrome is a frequent complication of infectious mononucleosis, the association with toxoplasmosis has been only recently made (Ho-Yen 1992). This is probably because toxoplasma is an infrequent cause of an infectious mononucleosis-like illness, and there is a general lack of knowledge of toxoplasmosis among medical practitioners. Nevertheless, the association between acquired toxoplasmosis and a prolonged illness has been well-documented (Beverley & Beattie 1958; Tenhunen 1964).

In a study of patients with myalgic encephalomyelitis, acquired toxoplasmosis was believed to be a cause in 4% of patients (Ho-Yen 1992). The symptoms are believed to persist more in patients with lymphadenopathy (17%) (Beverley & Beattie 1958). This may be because patients with lymphadenopathy may have more severe disease or an exaggerated immune response (Ho-Yen 1999). Patients fall into two groups: those with high toxoplasma IgG antibodies without IgM antibodies, and those with high IgG and IgM antibodies. It has been postulated that the polymerase chain reaction may be a useful discriminator. In patients whose specimens have evidence of *T. gondii* infection by polymerase chain reaction, there is evidence of parasitaemia and so specific antitoxoplasma therapy is indicated (Ho-Yen et al.

1992). Those patients with negative results are best managed conservatively, as are most patients with myalgic encephalomyelitis (Ho-Yen 1999). The good news is that among patients with myalgic encephalomyelitis, the prognosis appears better in patients with acquired toxoplasmosis (Ho-Yen 1992) compared to those with a viral infection.

Cases of chronic active toxoplasmosis are being recognized in which there is chronic or recurrent lymphadenopathy, myalgia and fatigue in immunocompetent individuals (O'Connell et al. 1993). The diagnosis is made by persistence of IgM, polymerase chain reaction positivity and acute pattern IgG immunoblots. Although there may initially be a response to toxoplasma antimicrobial agents, adverse drug reactions may limit long-term use (O'Connell et al. 1993).

The heart

In cases of fatal disseminated toxoplasmosis, the postmortem examination shows that the heart is almost always involved (Sexton et al. 1953). The progression of infection is probably as in Figure 4.5. Infection of the heart may be due to primary or reactivated infection. The most frequent cardiac presentations are probably myocarditis or pericarditis (Theologides & Kennedy 1969). Often the clinical picture of myocarditis is obscured by the more obvious signs and symptoms of disseminated infection; however, arrhythmias and cardiomegaly are common findings. Myocarditis may also present on its own without evidence of systemic infection (Theologides & Kennedy 1969) and then the usual clinical presentation is of chronic cardiomyopathy. Pericarditis may present as part of a generalized, acute infection or on its own with a chronic pericardial effusion (Sagrista-Sauleda et al. 1982). The pericardial effusion is invariably haemorrhagic. As toxoplasmic pericardial effusions may last for many years, the organism must be considered before chronic pericardial effusions are designated as 'idiopathic' (Sagrista-Sauleda et al. 1982). Acute, acquired toxoplasmosis may also present as a pancarditis (Cunningham 1982), but such presentations are very uncommon.

There are problems in making the diagnosis of toxoplasmosis in patients with cardiac involvement. Many of these patients have reactivated infection and dye test titres are not suggestive of recent infection (Theologides & Kennedy 1969). If *T. gondii* is cultured from biopsy material, it may represent detection of dormant cysts rather than acute infection. In cases where specific IgM is present and there is a response to antitoxoplasma therapy, the diagnosis is acceptable; however, in other cases tests need to be developed for diagnosing reactivated infection. Treatment is also problematic. In some cases, antitoxoplasma treatment has no effect until corticosteroids are added (Cunningham 1982); in other cases, pericardiectomy may be required (Sagrista-Sauleda et al. 1982). It is suggested that corticosteroids, because of their anti-inflammatory effects, are indicated in cases of arrhythmias and conduction defects (Theologides & Kennedy 1969).

In general, with appropriate treatment, cardiac toxoplasmosis has a favourable outcome. However, as might be expected, the organism may encyst in cardiac muscle and can subsequently reactivate to produce a relapse (Cunningham 1982).

Muscle

Myalgia is a frequent symptom in acute, acquired toxoplasmosis (Figure 4.4), and is probably caused by the body's immune reaction to the infection rather than to the direct action of toxoplasma on skeletal muscle. Nevertheless, in a small number of patients, elevated muscle enzymes and an abnormal muscle biopsy may accompany the acute illness (Adams et al. 1984). This acute myositis may be more common in children (Behan et al. 1983). In the majority of patients with polymyositis, the infection appears to be due to reactivated toxoplasmosis, with patients having no serological evidence of acute infection (Behan et al. 1983). Many of these patients were immunosuppressed, having received steroids, and so may have been predisposed to a reactivated infection.

Specific antitoxoplasma therapy may produce a dramatic improvement in some patients; however, in most cases there is little or no improvement (Behan et al. 1983). The explanation may lie in there being two mechanisms causing the polymyositis: either a direct action of *T. gondii* on muscle or *T. gondii* producing an indirect immune action on muscle. In the latter case, there may be *T. gondii* immune complex deposition in muscle (Behan et al. 1983); alternatively, *T. gondii* may produce antigenic changes in muscle to which the body's immune system has reacted (Adams et al. 1984). Obviously, in cases where there is immune damage to muscle, antitoxoplasma therapy would be expected to have limited effects.

Patients may have an acute *T. gondii* infection, recover and then develop polymyositis years later (Adams et al. 1984). Such a presentation is reminiscent of toxoplasmic ocular disease, where the diagnosis of reactivated infection is difficult and serological tests can only support the diagnosis. Until better tests are developed, many cases of toxoplasmic polymyositis will not be definitively diagnosed. However, it seems reasonable to test for evidence of past *T. gondii* infection in symptomatic patients, as this would exclude the diagnosis in the majority of the population in Britain. Patients with evidence of acute infection may benefit from treatment (Behan et al. 1983) but those with a more chronic infection may benefit less from specific treatment.

Skin

In acute acquired toxoplasmosis in immunocompetent individuals, a variety of skin lesions have been reported. The spectrum of clinical findings is wide: erythema multiforme-like, papular-urticarial, purpuric, telangiectatic, vesicular and bulbous rashes have been associated with *T. gondii* infection (Binazzi 1986). As the skin is frequently involved in disseminated infection (Figure 4.5), this wide spectrum is not too surprising. However, it is probably more likely that skin involvement does not produce signs and symptoms. In a large series of patients with toxoplasmic lymphadenopathy, none had a rash (Beverley & Beattie 1958). Though *T. gondii* can be frequently found in the skin, pathological changes in this tissue may not occur.

Cutaneous toxoplasmosis may accompany muscle involvement as in dermatomyositis (Harland et al. 1991). This report described periorbital oedema, with transient erythematous scaly plaques over knuckles, wrists, elbows and knees, as well as muscle involvement. Specific antitoxoplasma therapy was successful. There was serological evidence of reactivated *T. gondii* infection and retinochoroiditis accompanied the dermatomyositis.

An excellent review of the literature reveals that the clinical presentation differs according to the age group (Binazzi 1986). Among adults, a chronic, treatment-resistant prurigo can be found which may be cured with antitoxoplasma treatment. In the elderly, cyanotic, hard, painless nodules with or without a follicular horny plug can be found. Fleshy, ulcerative, vegetating numular lesions have also been described, especially on the limbs.

Rarer conditions, such as lichen spinulosus, dermohypodermitis, lichen parapsoriasis and pityriasis rubra pilaris, have also been associated with toxoplasma infection. Other conditions, such as erythema chronicum migrans (now known to be caused by *Borrelia burgdorferi*) or Behçet disease may have occurred by chance. Nevertheless, skin manifestations of toxoplasmosis have been convincingly demonstrated, and may be particularly related to certain strains of *T. gondii* and may be more likely when there is systemic infection (Figure 4.5) or when patients are immunocompromised.

Other conditions

Toxoplasma gondii infection has been infrequently linked with other illnesses. Although in some cases *T. gondii* may rarely cause some of these conditions, in most cases the linkage has probably occurred by chance. The situation may be further complicated as illness may present many years after the acute infection, such as ocular disease caused by congenital toxoplasmosis. Patients with renal disease also highlight some of the problems. A case of acute nephritis with nephrotic syndrome has been described in a 10-week-old baby with congenital toxoplasmosis (Wickbom & Winberg 1972). If this illness had presented later in life, diagnosis may have been more difficult. In another report it was possible to link nephritis to toxoplasma infection by demonstrating immune complexes containing *T. gondii* antigen in renal biopsy material (Ginsberg ct al. 1974). Biopsy samples taken later from this patient did not contain *T. gondii* antigen, and were consistent with immune-complex nephritis in which the offending antigen is only found early in the disease. Unfortunately, *T. gondii* is rarely looked for early in such illnesses, and thus the true incidence of the condition is unknown. Nevertheless, the strong experimental evidence of renal disease (Wickbom & Winberg 1972; Ginsberg et al. 1974) suggests that the condition may not be uncommon.

An interesting association of toxoplasmosis and polyarthritis has been described (Gemou et al. 1983). The patient did not respond to salicylates, but made a good response to antitoxoplasma treatment. This patient had no recurrences for 4 years to follow up. The authors suggest that *T. gondii* infection should be considered in children with chronic polyarthritis who have no evidence of collagen disease and do not respond to salicylates.

Summary

Acquired toxoplasma infection in normal individuals is being recognized as having a large spectrum of clinical presentations. While a number of factors influence the clinical picture, strain virulence and circumstances of the exposure are important considerations. Asymptomatic and nonspecific illness are probably very common. However infection of the reticulo-endothelial system is prominent with significant management problems. Respiratory and haemopoietic infections are probably under-recognized. Central nervous system involvement is increasingly identified and chronic active infection may be a real problem of the future. Clinicians must be aware of the whole spectrum of disease associated with acquired toxoplasmosis.

REFERENCES

Abdul-Fattah, M. M., Sanad, M. M., Darwish, R. A. & Yousef, S. M. (1992). Is immuno-protection against toxoplasma strain specific? *Journal of the Egyptian Society of Parasitology*, 22, 77–82.

Adams, E. M., Hafez, G. R., Carnes, M., Weisner, J. K. & Graziano, F. M. (1984). The development of polymyositis in a patient with toxoplasmosis: clinical and pathologic findings and review of literature. *Clinical and Experimental Rheumatology*, 2, 207–8.

Armstrong, C. & MacMurray, F. G. (1953). Toxoplasmosis found by recovery of *Toxoplasma gondii* from excised axillary gland. *Journal of the American Medical Association*, 151, 1103–4.

Bach, M. C. & Armstrong, R. H. (1983). Acute toxoplasmic encephalitis in a normal adult. *Archives of Neurology*, 40, 596–7.

Behan, W. M. H., Behan, P. O., Draper, I. T. & Williams, H. (1983). Does toxoplasma cause polymyositis? *Acta Neuropathologica*, 61, 246–52.

Benenson, M. W., Takafuji, E. T., Lemon, S. M., Greenup, R. L. & Sulzer, A. J. (1982). Oocyst-transmitted toxoplasmosis associated with ingestion of contaminated drinking water. *New England Journal of Medicine*, 307, 666–9.

Beverley, J. K. A. & Beattie, C. P. (1958). Glandular toxoplasmosis. A Survey of 30 cases. *Lancet*, ii, 379–84.

Beverley, J. K. A., Fleck, D. G., Kwantes, N. & Ludlam, G. B. (1976). Age–sex distribution of various diseases with particular reference to toxoplasmic lymphadenopathy. *Journal of Hygiene*, 76, 215–18.

Binazzi, M. (1986). Profile of cutaneous toxoplasmosis. *International Journal of Dermatology*, 25, 357–63.

Candolfi, E., de Blay, F., Rey, D., Christmann, D., Treisser, A., Pauli, G. & Kien, T. A. (1993). Parasitologically proven case of *Toxoplasma* pneumonia in an immunocompetent pregnant woman. *Journal of Infection*, 26, 79–81.

Catterall, J. R., Hofflin, J. M. & Remington, J. S. (1986). Pulmonary toxoplasmosis. *American Reviews of Respiratory Diseases*, 133, 704–5.

Cunningham, T. (1982). Pancarditis in acute toxoplasmosis. *American Journal of Clinical Pathology*, 78, 403–5.

Derouin, F. & Garin, Y. J. F. (1991). *Toxoplasma gondii* blood and tissue kinetics during acute and chronic infections in mice. *Experimental Parasitology*, 73, 46–8.

Feldman, H. A. (1974). Toxoplasmosis: an overview. *Bulletin New York Academy of Medicine*, 50, 110–27.

Frenkel, J. K. (1973). Toxoplasmosis: parasite life cycle, pathology and immunology. In *The Coccidia, Eimeria, Isospora, Toxoplasma and Related Genera*, ed. D. M. Hammond, P. L. Long, pp. 343–410. Baltimore, MD: University Park Press.

Frenkel, J. K., Ruiz, A. & Chinchilla, M. (1975). Soil survival of toxoplasma oocysts in Kansas and Costa Rica. *American Journal of Tropical Medicine and Hygiene*, 24, 439–43.

Gemou, V., Messaritakis, J., Karpathios, T. & Kingo, A. (1983). Chronic polyarthritis of toxoplasmic etiology. *Helvinica Paediatrica Acta*, 38, 295–6.

Ghatak, N. R., Poon, T. P. & Zimmerman, H. M. (1970). Toxoplasmosis of the central nervous system in the adult. *Archives of Pathology*, 89, 337–48.

Ginsburg, B. E., Wasserman, J., Hudlt, G. & Bergstrand, A. (1974). Case of glomerulonephritis associated with acute toxoplasmosis. *British Medical Journal*, 3, 664–5.

Guy, E. C. & Joynson, D. H. M. (1995). Potential of the polymerase chain reaction in the diagnosis of active toxoplasma infection by detection of parasite in blood. *Journal of Infectious Diseases*, 172, 319–22.

Harland, C. C., Marsden, J. R., Vernon, S. A. & Allen, B. R. (1991). Dermatomyositis responding to treatment of associated toxoplasmosis. *British Journal of Dermatology*, 125, 76–8.

Ho-Yen, D. O. (1992). Clinical features. In *Human Toxoplasmosis*, ed. D. O. Ho-Yen & A. W. L. Joss, pp. 56–78. Oxford: Oxford University Press.

Ho-Yen, D. O. (1999). *Better Recovery from Viral Illnesses*. Inverness: Dodona Books.

Ho-Yen, D. O. & Martin, K. W. (1981). The relationship between atypical lymphocytosis and serological tests for infectious mononucleosis. *Journal of Infection*, 3, 324–31.

Ho-Yen, D. O., Joss, A. W. L., Balfour, A. H., Smyth, E. T. M., Baird, D. & Chatterton, J. M. W. (1992). Use of the polymerase chain reaction to detect *Toxoplasma gondii* in human blood samples. *Journal of Clinical Pathology*, 45, 910–13.

Joss, A. W. L. (1992). Treatment. In *Human Toxoplasmosis*, ed. D. O. Ho-Yen & A. W. L. Joss, pp. 119–43. Oxford: Oxford University Press.

Kalderon, A. E., Kikkawa, Y. & Bernstein, J. (1964). Chronic toxoplasmosis associated with severe hemolytic anemia. *Archives of Internal Medicine*, 114, 95–102.

Kaufman, H. E., Remington, J. S. & Jacobs, L. (1958). Toxoplasmosis: the nature of virulence. *American Journal of Ophthalmology*, 46, 255–61.

Ludlam, G. B. & Beattie, C. P. (1963). Pulmonary toxoplasmosis? *Lancet*, ii, 1136–8.

Luft, B. J. & Remington, J. S. (1985). Toxoplasmosis of the central nervous system. In *Current Clinical Topics in Infectious Diseases*, ed. J. S. Remington, M. N. Swartz, pp. 315–58. New York: McGraw-Hill.

Magaldi, C., Elkis, H., Pattoli, D. & Coscina, A. L. (1969). Epidemic of toxoplasmosis at a University in Sao-Jose-dos-Campos, S. P., Brazil. *Reviews Latin-American Microbiology*, 11, 5–13.

Miettinen, M. & Franssila, K. (1982). Malignant lymphoma simulating lymph node toxoplasmosis. *Histopathology*, 6, 129–40.

Miettinen, M., Saxen, L. & Saxen, E. (1980). Lymph node toxoplasmosis. *Acta Medica Scandinavica*, 208, 431–6.

O'Connell, S., Guy, E. C., Dawson, S., Francis, J. M. & Joynson, D. H. M. (1993). Chronic active toxoplasmosis in an immunocompetent patient. *Journal of Infection*, 27, 305–10.

Prosmanne, O., Chaloni, J., Sylvestre, J. & Lefebrue, R. (1984). Small nodular patterns in the lungs due to opportunistic toxoplasmosis. *Journal of Canadian Association of Radiologists*, 35, 186–8.

Sagrista-Sauleda, J., Permanyer-Miralda, G., Juste-Sanchez, C., de Buen-Sanchez, M. L., Capmany-Pujadas, R., Arcalis-Arce, L. & Soler-Soler, J. (1982). Huge chronic pericardial effusion caused by *Toxoplasma gondii*. *Circulation*, 4, 895–7.

Sexton, R. C., Eyles, D. E. & Dillman, R. E. (1953). Adult toxoplasmosis. *American Journal of Medicine*, 14, 366–77.

Sharpe, M. C., Archard, L. C., Banatvala, J. E., Borysiewicz, L. K., Clare, A. W., David. A., Edwards, R., Hawton KEH., et al. (1991) Chronic fatigue syndrome: Guidelines for research. *Journal of the Royal Society Medicine*, 84, 115–21.

Tan, D. S. K., Zaman, V. & Lopes, M. (1978). Infectious mononucleosis or toxoplasmosis? *Medical Journal of Malaysia*, 33, 23–5.

Tenhunen, A. (1964). Glandular toxoplasmosis: occurrence of the disease in Finland. *Acta Pathological et Microbiologica Scandinavica Supplementum*, 172, 172.

Theologides, A. & Kennedy, B. J. (1969). Toxoplasmic myocarditis and pericarditis. *American Journal of Medicine*, 47, 169–74.

Thomaidis, T., Anastassea-Vlachou, C., Mandalenaki-Lambrou, C., Theodoridis, C. & Vrahnou, E. (1977). Chronic lymphoglandular enlargement and toxoplasmosis in children. *Archives of Diseases in Childhood*, 52, 403–7.

Townsend, J. J., Wolinsky, J. S., Baringer, J. R. & Johnson, P. C. (1975). Acquired toxoplasmosis. A neglected cause of treatable nervous system disease. *Archives of Neurology*, 32, 335–43.

Weitberg, A. B., Alper, D. C., Diamond, I. & Fligiel, Z. (1979). Acute granulomatous hepatitis in the course of acquired toxoplasmosis. *New England Journal of Medicine*, 300, 1093–6.

Wickbom, B. & Winberg, J. (1972). Coincidence of syndrome. *Acta Paediatrica Scandinavica*, 61, 470–2.

Wright, W. H. (1957). A summary of the newer knowledge of toxoplasmosis. *American Journal of Clinical Pathology*, 28, 1–17.

Yermakov, V., Rashid, R. K., Vuletin, J. C., Pertschuk, L. P. & Isaksson, H. (1982). Disseminated toxoplasmosis. *Archives of Pathological Laboratory Medicine*, 106, 524–8.

5

Toxoplasma infection in HIV-infected patients

P. Mariuz[1] and R. T. Steigbigel[2]

[1] Infectious Disease Unit, University of Rochester, School of Medicine and Dentistry, Rochester, USA
[2] Division of Infectious Diseases, Health Science Centre, SUNY Stony Brook, Stony Brook, New York, USA

Introduction

In patients infected with human immunodeficiency virus (HIV) the most frequent manifestation of toxoplasmosis is encephalitis. Toxoplasmic encephalitis is, in fact, the most common cause of focal central nervous system infections in people with acquired immunodeficiency syndrome (AIDS). In addition, toxoplasma infection and disease may occur in other organ systems. The mechanism of disease in the overwhelming majority of patients is reactivation of latent toxoplasma infection subsequent to severe immune suppression. This chapter will consider the epidemiology, clinical presentation, diagnosis, treatment and prognosis of toxoplasma infection in the setting of HIV infection.

Epidemiology

Human infection with *Toxoplasma gondii* occurs primarily from consumption of undercooked meats, particularly lamb and pork (containing tissue cysts) (Weinman & Chandler 1956; Masur et al. 1978; Dubey 1986) or ingestion of food, water or inadvertently of soil or sand contaminated with oocysts (Teutsch et al. 1979; Benenson et al. 1983). The overwhelming majority (>95%) of cases of toxoplasmosis in patients with AIDS occur as a consequence of reactivation of a dormant (latent) infection (Luft & Remington 1988). Latent infection can easily be identified by serological testing. The incidence of toxoplasmic encephalitis is directly proportional to the prevalence of latent toxoplasma infection in any given population. Serological surveys in humans demonstrate that the prevalence of antibodies to *T. gondii* increases with increasing age (Feldman & Miller 1965). There is no significant difference between the sexes. Geographically the prevalence is lower in cold regions, in areas with hot, arid climates and at higher altitudes. Additional factors, which affect the incidence of toxoplasma infection, include: methods of animal husbandry, cultural and hygienic practices regarding the handling, preparation and consumption of food, and oocyst excretion by cats (Weinman & Chandler 1956; Wallace 1973; Dubey & Beattie 1988; Remington & Desmonts 1990).

A serological survey done in 1962 among US military recruits aged 17–26 years revealed that the prevalence of toxoplasma infection varied from 3% to 20% depending upon the geographical area (Feldman 1965). In another study done in 1989, *T. gondii* antibody prevalence among US military recruits varied from 3.2% to 13.3% (Smith et al. 1996). Rates were higher in the eastern and southeastern states and lowest in the mountain region. Another study has confirmed the lower *T. gondii*-antibody-positive rates in the west and southwestern USA (Richards et al. 1994; Wilson et al. 1994). Growing up in a small town and rural environment was also associated with higher *T. gondii*-antibody-positive rates (Smith et al. 1996).

Among adults with AIDS in the US 3–40% are latently infected with *T. gondii*. It is estimated that up to 30% of these patients will develop toxoplasmic encephalitis (Luft & Remington 1988). Toxoplasmic encephalitis was the AIDS-defining illness of 5% of all AIDS patients reported to the Centers for Disease Control in 1989 (Luft & Castro 1991). It was most frequent (7.5%) when the risk factor for HIV infection was heterosexual transmission followed by injecting drug use (5.2%). Amongst male heterosexual noninjecting drug-users, toxoplasmic encephalitis was much more frequent in blacks (12%) compared to whites (4%) (Ambrose *et al.* 1987). Significant differences in the incidence of toxoplasmic encephalitis in different geographical locations and among different ethnic groups have also been noted. The incidence of toxoplasmic encephalitis amongst AIDS patients of Haitian origin in Florida, for example, at 12–40% is three times higher than in other states (Post et al. 1983; Luft & Castro 1991; Glatt 1992). Significantly higher *T. gondii*-antibody-positive rates ranging from 50% to >80% have been observed in Europe (Clumeck 1991) (mainly France, Belgium, Germany, Italy and Spain), Haiti, Africa and Latin America. Toxoplasmic encephalitis is the AIDS-defining illness in 23% of HIV-infected patients in France (Oksenhendler et al. 1994). A study from Austria reported that 47% of *T. gondii*-antibody-positive AIDS patients developed toxoplasmic encephalitis (Zangerle et al. 1991). In Africa and Europe 25–50% of *T. gondii*-antibody-positive patients will develop toxoplasmic encephalitis (Pohl & Eichenlaub 1987). The reasons for the different propensity to develop reactivation of latent toxoplasma infection according to geographical origin remain unknown. It also remains unclear why some (30–50%) AIDS patients latently infected with *T. gondii* develop toxoplasmic encephalitis while others do not. Host factors (e.g. genetic predisposition) (Suzuki et al. 1996) or variations in the virulence among different strains of *T. gondii*, and especially the use of trimethoprim–sulphamethoxazole which decreases the incidence of toxoplasmic encephalitis in *T. gondii*-

antibody-positive patients, are probably important in this regard (Darde et al. 1988; McLeod et al. 1989; Remington & Desmonts 1995; Jones et al. 1996). Adherence or failure to adhere to preventative medication is also another factor (Jones et al. 1998).

The overwhelming majority of HIV-infected patients develop toxoplasmic encephalitis when the CD4 lymphocyte count is less than $100/mm^3$ (Levy et al. 1988; Dannemann et al. 1992; Girard et al. 1993; Jones et al. 1996). In a prospective study of *T. gondii*-antibody-positive, HIV-infected patients, 7.3% and 21.2% of those with CD4 counts between 100 and $200/mm^3$ developed toxoplasmic encephalitis by 12 and 18 months, respectively. Over the same period of time 22% and 40%, respectively, of patients developed toxoplasmic encephalitis when their CD4 cell counts were below $100/mm^3$ (Girard *et al.* 1993).

Asymptomatic primary *T. gondii* infection in HIV-infected patients does occur (Reiter-Owana et al. 1998). A prospective study in France reported a 5.5% *T. gondii* seroconversion rate during a median observation period of 28 months (Partisani et al. 1991). *Toxoplasma gondii*-antibody-negative individuals should be instructed about methods to prevent infection (see 'Prevention of toxoplasma infection in *T. gondii*-antibody-negative patients'). Primary *T. gondii* infection in patients with AIDS may present as disseminated disease (Strittmatter et al. 1992).

Pathology and clinical manifestations

Toxoplasmic encephalitis without other organ involvement is the most frequent manifestation of toxoplasmosis in patients with AIDS. Occasionally toxoplasmic encephalitis will be part of a multisystem infection while isolated extracerebral toxoplasmosis is rare. Most often toxoplasmic encephalitis presents with multiple lesions in the brain which vary in size from microscopic (Hooper 1957; Strittmatter et al. 1992) to involvement of a large portion of a cerebral hemisphere (Navia et al. 1989). Location in the cerebral hemispheres (particularly of the corticomedullary junction) is most frequent. Involvement of the cerebellum and brainstem is also common. However, white matter as well as any other part of the central nervous system may be involved (Post et al. 1983; Luft et al. 1984; Milligan et al. 1984; Wanke et al. 1987) though the meninges are usually not affected. Cerebral oedema, vasculitis and haemorrhage contribute to the disease process (Casado-Naranjo et al. 1989; Chaudhari et al. 1989; Engstrom et al. 1989; Berlit et al. 1996). Typically three histopathological zones are identified in untreated patients: the central zone, which contains necrotic amorphous material with few if any organisms, an intermediate zone comprised of engorged blood vessels, spotty necrosis, numerous extra- and intracellular tachyzoites, rare cysts, and endothelial cell hyperplasia with vasculitis, and the outer zone in which tissue cysts predominate, necrosis is rare and vascular lesions are minimal (Post et al. 1983). Widespread poorly demarcated confluent

Table 5.1. Neurological manifestations of toxoplasmic encephalitis

Focal neurological defects	Generalized/global cerebral dysfunction	Neuropsychiatric abnormalities
Hemiparesis, hemiplegia, dysphasia	Lethargy	Dementia
Aphasia, dysarthria	Altered level of consciousness	Anxiety
Visual impairment	Confusion	Psychosis
Movement disorders (hemichorea, hemiballismus)	Coma	Personality changes
Cranial nerve deficits	Mood abnormalities and memory	
Deficits		
Hemisensory loss and hemisensory deficits	Global cognitive impairment (similar to AIDS dementia)	
Singultus (hiccups)		

areas of necrosis (necrotizing toxoplasmic encephalitis) have been noted, particularly in patients who had not received chemotherapy (Strittmatter et al. 1992).

In treated patients chronic abscesses are the predominant finding. These consist of small cystic spaces, which contain lipid-laden and haemosiderin-containing macrophages with surrounding gliosis. A diffuse form of toxoplasmic encephalitis in which abscess formation is absent has been described where the brain tissue appears normal (Gray et al. 1989; Khuong et al. 1990; Strittmatter et al. 1992; Caramello et al. 1993). However, histopathological analysis demonstrates the presence of microglial nodules containing cysts and free tachyzoites mostly involving cerebral grey matter (Gray et al. 1989; Khuong et al. 1990).

The clinical manifestations of toxoplasmic encephalitis depend upon the location, number and size of the lesions. Toxoplasmic encephalitis may present with focal or generalized signs and symptoms of central nervous system dysfunction (Table 5.1). Most frequently, patients present with a combination of focal neurological defects and generalized cerebral dysfunction (Levy et al. 1985; McArthur 1987; Navia et al. 1989; Luft & Remington 1992; Porter & Sande 1992; Renold et al. 1992). The onset of illness is usually subacute with focal defects developing over a period of days to weeks (up to 4–6 weeks) during which nonfocal symptoms (headache, lethargy, cognitive impairment) become evident. Acute fulminant presentations rarely occur. Seizures accompany the initial manifestations of toxoplasmic encephalitis in 15–29% of cases (Levy et al. 1985; Porter & Sande 1992; Renold et al. 1992). Headache is present in as many as 55% of patients (Porter & Sande 1992). Fever is variably present (7% to 56%) (McArthur 1987; Navia et al. 1989; Renold et al. 1992). Occasionally neuropsychiatric abnormalities dominate the clinical picture (Navia et al. 1989; Arendt et al. 1991) (Table 5.1). In two large studies (Porter & Sande 1992; Renold et al. 1992) the most frequent focal neurological deficits were hemiparesis or hemiplegia, ataxia and cranial nerve palsies. Of the nonfocal manifestations of toxoplasmic encephalitis, confusion, psychomotor retardation, lethargy, headache and fever predominated. Other abnormalities include diabetes insipidus, panhypopituitarism, inappropriate antidiuretic hormone secretion (SIADH) and hydrocephalus (Luft et al. 1984; Milligan et al. 1984; Helweg-Larsen et al. 1986; Nolla-Sallas et al. 1987; Navia et al. 1989; Bourgonin et al. 1992). Meningeal involvement is rare so that signs and symptoms of meningeal irritation are unusual and examination of cerebrospinal fluid is not helpful except to exclude other diseases. Ventriculo-meningo-encephalomyelitis has been described (Artigas et al. 1994).

The diffuse form of toxoplasmic encephalitis appears to be unique to AIDS patients (Gray et al. 1989; Caramello et al. 1993). Clinical manifestations are a rapidly progressive, generalized cerebral dysfunction, without focal neurological deficits, which is usually fatal. Neuroradiological studies have been unable to demonstrate focal lesions. Macroscopic examination was normal in three of four cases. Histopathological examination revealed numerous scattered (hence the term diffuse) microglial nodules most of which contained *T. gondii* tachyzoites and cysts. An autopsy series of 55 cases of toxoplasmic encephalitis revealed diffuse encephalitis in seven patients (Khuong et al. 1990). In one case the diagnosis was made by tissue culture of the cerebrospinal fluid (CSF) (Caramello et al. 1993). Computerized tomography scans of the brain (even with contrast) are frequently negative in these cases.

Toxoplasmosis of the spinal cord is a rare manifestation of central nervous system toxoplasma infection (Vyas & Ebright 1996). Sites of involvement include the cervical, thoracic and lumbar spine (Mehren et al. 1988; Herskovitz et al. 1989; Harris et al. 1990; Poon et al. 1992). Concomitant toxoplasmic encephalitis is not always present (Mehren et al. 1988; Herskovitz et al. 1989; Harris et al. 1990; Poon et al. 1992; Vyas & Ebright 1996). Most patients present with acute or subacute myelopathy manifested by paraparesis and a sensory level. Neuroradiology reveals contrast-enhancing intramedullary lesions (Vyas & Ebright 1996). Antitoxoplasma therapy appears to be effective particularly when started within a few weeks of the onset of disease (Vyas & Ebright 1996). Conus medullaris syndrome has also been described (Kayser et al. 1990; Overhage et al. 1990).

Extracerebral toxoplasmosis in HIV-infected patients occurs infrequently (May et al. 1993). In a French national survey of this condition, the estimated prevalence was 1.5% to 2% (Rabaud et al. 1994); the lungs were the most common sites. In a 33-month French national survey, 64 cases of HIV-associated pulmonary toxoplasmosis were identified. A total of 39 patients (61%) had isolated pulmonary infection, while 12 had concomitant toxoplasmic encephalitis. Pulmonary toxoplasmosis was part of a widely disseminated infection in nine patients (Rabaud et al. 1996). Extrapulmonary organs involved include bone marrow, muscle, liver and eyes. Serological data were available in 60 cases. Of these, only two patients were *T. gondii*-antibody-negative. Postmortem evidence of extracerebral toxoplasmosis is more frequent and has been reported in 2.7–16.2% of autopsy surveys (Klatt 1988; Tschirhardt & Klatt 1988; Hofman et al. 1993*b*; Jautzke et al. 1993). Although the exact prevalence of pulmonary toxoplasmosis is not known, a 1990 French prospective study of bronchoalveolar lavage fluid in HIV-infected patients reported a prevalence rate of 4.1% (Derouin et al. 1990), while another study from France reported a prevalence of 6.4% in bronchoalveolor lavage fluid (Oksenhendler et al. 1990). This is in contrast to a 1984 US study of pulmonary pathology in 441 HIV-infected patients in which pulmonary toxoplasmosis accounted for less than 1% of cases (Murray et al. 1984). Pulmonary toxoplasmosis is associated with very low CD4 cell counts ($40 \pm 75/mm^3$) with 70% of the patients having CD4 counts below $50/mm^3$. The mortality of patients with pulmonary toxoplasmosis is high (35–50%) (Pomeroy & Felice 1992). The clinical manifestations of pulmonary toxoplasmosis are nonspecific and similar to those of pneumonia due to *Pneumocystis carinii* (Tourani et al. 1985; Catterall et al. 1986; Mendelson et al. 1987; Oksenhendler et al. 1990; Pomeroy & Felice 1992; Schnapp et al. 1992; Rabaud et al. 1996). Most present with fever, cough (productive or nonproductive), dyspnoea, and, occasionally, haemoptysis. Rales may be present (Mendelson et al. 1987; Oksenhendler et al. 1990; Pomeroy & Felice 1992; Schnapp et al. 1992; Rabaud et al. 1996). Chest roentgenograms typically reveal bilateral basal interstitial infiltrates (Pomeroy & Felice 1992; Rabaud et al. 1996). Multiple nodular infiltrates, single nodules, isolated cavitary disease, lobar infiltrates, pleural effusion and hilar lymphadenopathy have been described (Tourani et al. 1985; Pomeroy & Felice 1992; Schnapp et al. 1992; Rabaud et al. 1996). Pneumothorax complicating pulmonary toxoplasmosis has been noted (Libanore et al. 1991; Rabaud et al. 1996). Septic shock with thrombocytopaenia and elevated plasma lactase dehydrogenase levels (>1000 units/l) has been reported to occur in 15.6% of patients with pulmonary toxoplasmosis (Rabaud et al. 1996). Histopathological examination usually reveals areas of coagulative necrosis, mixed inflammatory cell interstitial infiltrates and marked alveolar capillary congestion. Organisms may be found within alveolar macrophages, alveolar lining cells and free-floating within alveoli and the areas of necrosis (Hofman et al. 1993*a*; Jautzke et al. 1993).

Ocular toxoplasmosis is infrequently reported in patients with AIDS (Weiss et al. 1986). Ocular toxoplasmosis may be the sole manifestation of infection or present with concomitant toxoplasmic encephalitis or disseminated disease (De Smet 1992;

May et al. 1993). Patients presenting with ocular toxoplasmosis should therefore be evaluated for concomitant toxoplasmic encephalitis (Weiss et al. 1986; Friedman et al. 1990). Rarely, ocular toxoplasmosis is the initial manifestation of AIDS (Fabricius et al. 1993). The most common clinical manifestation is decreased visual acuity and less frequently ocular pain. Involvement may be unilateral (70%) or bilateral (30%) (De Smet 1992). Fundoscopic examination reveals single or multiple yellow–white areas of necrotizing retinochoroiditis with ill-defined fluffy margins. The lesions can be difficult to distinguish from those of cytomegalovirus retinitis. However, toxoplasmic retinochoroiditis tends to occur at the posterior pole, be nonhaemorrhagic and may be associated with a moderate to severe inflammatory response in the vitreous and anterior chamber (Friedman 1984; Parke & Font 1986; Holland et al. 1988; Smith 1988; Friedman et al. 1990; Cochereau-Massin et al. 1992; De Smet 1992). Fluorescein angiography may also be helpful in this regard. Unilateral toxoplasmic iridocyclitis has been reported (Rehder et al. 1988). Decreased visual acuity with or without ocular pain in a *T. gondii*-antibody-positive patient with AIDS should raise the suspicion of ocular toxoplasmosis. A prompt response to specific antitoxoplasma therapy is helpful diagnostically. A definitive diagnosis can be made by demonstrating organisms in retinal biopsy specimens isolating *T. gondii* from vitreal fluid, by the detection of *T. gondii* DNA or by determining serum and ocular fluid *T. gondii* antibody concentrations (Smith 1988; Friedman et al. 1990; Cochereau-Massin et al. 1992).

Toxoplasmic myocarditis in patients with AIDS is usually asymptomatic and found only at autopsy, frequently in the setting of widely disseminated infection (Roldan et al. 1987; Tschirhardt & Klatt 1988; Hofman et al. 1991; Jautzke et al. 1993; Sell et al. 1993; Rabaud et al. 1996). The clinical manifestations of symptomatic myocarditis include cardiac tamponade or biventricular heart failure (Roldan et al. 1987; Adair et al. 1989; Grange et al. 1990; Machler et al. 1993). The definitive diagnosis requires an endomyocardial biopsy. The diagnostic yield of this procedure can be hampered by the small size of the specimens obtained and the patchy nature of the infection. A sepsis syndrome in the setting of disseminated toxoplasmosis with prominent cardiopulmonary disease has been reported (Albrecht et al. 1993). As with the other manifestations of toxoplasmosis in patients with AIDS, reactivation of latent toxoplasmosis is the pathogenic mechanism in the majority of cases.

Clinical manifestations attributable to isolated involvement of other organs occur infrequently. Testicular (Nistral et al. 1986; Crider et al. 1988), gastrointestinal (Isrealski et al. 1988; Marche et al. 1989; Smart et al. 1990; Garcia et al. 1991; Pauwels et al. 1992;), pancreatic (Brivet et al. 1987; Dowell et al. 1990; Ahuja et al. 1993), renal (Patrick et al. 1986), hepatic (Brion et al. 1992), adrenal (Groll et al. 1990), skeletal muscle (Gherardi et al. 1992) and bladder (Hofman et al. 1993b) involvement have been reported to occur in HIV-infected patients.

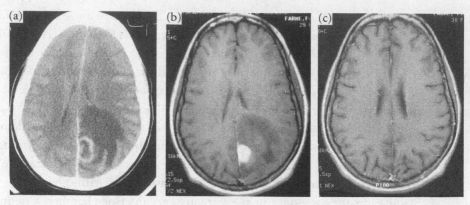

Figure 5.1   Computerized tomography (CT) (a) and magnetic resonance imaging (MRI) (b) showing a single contrast-enhancing lesion involving the left posterior occipital region. MRI shows complete resolution after 6 weeks of therapy (c).

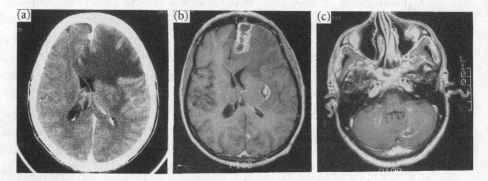

Figure 5.2   Contrast-enhanced CT showing multiple lesions involving the left frontal lobe and basal ganglia (a). MRI scan demonstrating additional lesions in the left occipital lobe (b) and posterior fossa (c).

Diagnosis

The definitive diagnosis of toxoplasmic encephalitis requires a brain biopsy. However, given the difficulty of biopsy, the morbidity associated with this procedure and the reluctance of many neurosurgeons to perform biopsies, the clinical practice of empirical therapy based on a presumptive diagnosis is widely accepted.

An initial presumptive diagnosis of toxoplasmic encephalitis can be made based upon clinical manifestations, neuroimaging studies (Figures 5.1 and 5.2), *T. gondii* antibody positivity and with subsequent clinical and radiological response to therapy. Computerized tomography scanning with contrast typically shows multiple lesions of various sizes located in the basal ganglia and corticomedullary junctions of the cerebral hemispheres (Whelan et al. 1983; Post et al. 1985; Levy et al. 1986). Surrounding oedema and mass effect are variably present. Concomitant cerebral haemorrhage is a rare complication (Levy et al. 1986; Casado-Naranjo et al. 1989; Chaudhari et al. 1989; Engstrom et al. 1989). Computerized tomography with contrast most commonly demonstrates ring-enhancement with central hypo-density (Post et al. 1983). This neuroradiographic appearance correlates with the pathological findings discussed above (Post et al. 1986). The region of avascular necrosis corresponds to the central hypodensity on computerized tomography while the surrounding inflammation accounts for the contrast enhancement. Solid or nodular enhancement is very common. Magnetic resonance imaging demon-strates similar enhancement patterns. In addition, because of its greater sensitivity compared to computerized tomography, magnetic resonance imaging can detect a larger number of lesions and may show lesions not seen with computerized tomog-raphy (Levy et al. 1986; McArthur 1987; Porter & Sande 1992).

Serological tests for the diagnosis of toxoplasma infection, as discussed in Chapter 12, are useful for identifying individuals at risk of developing toxoplasmic encephal-itis and for supporting this diagnosis in patients with focal brain lesions on neuro-radiographic imaging studies. The determination of baseline toxoplasma antibody levels in sera collected when the initial diagnosis of HIV infection is made can be helpful in this context. Nearly 100% of patients with AIDS with toxoplasmic enceph-alitis are *T. gondii*-antibody-positive by dye test or indirect immunofluorescence assay (Levy et al. 1985; Grant et al. 1990; Luft & Hafner 1990; Luft & Remington 1992; Renold et al. 1992). A recent study showed that high anti- *T. gondii* IgG antibody titres ($\geq$ 150 international units/ml IgG by enzyme-linked immunosorbent assay) are a prognostic indicator of toxoplasmic encephalitis (Derouin et al. 1996). In one study the presence of characteristic computerized tomography or magnetic resonance imaging abnormalities and *T. gondii* antibody had a predictive value of 80% (Cohn et al. 1989). The predictive value of *T. gondii*-positive serology may be decreased, however, in patient populations in whom other central nervous system pathologies are more prevalent (e.g. injecting drug users) (Bishburg et al. 1989), in those who have been receiving prophylactic trimethoprim-sulfamethoxazole and when single lesions are found on neuroimaging studies, particularly magnetic resonance imaging (Luft & Remington 1992).

A clinical response to empirical treatment (i.e. a therapeutic trial) should be expected within 10–14 days (Luft & Remington 1988, 1992). In a recent study which used quantified neurological assessment to prospectively evaluate clinical outcome, 50% and 86% of patients had a clinical response after 5 and 7 days of therapy, respectively (Luft et al. 1993). Over 90% of patients who respond to therapy will have an improvement in relevant signs and symptoms by day 14 of therapy (Luft et al. 1993). Patients who did not respond to empirical therapy had either progression of relevant signs and symptoms or developed new abnormalities within the first 10 days of treatment. Neither headache nor seizures were reliable indicators of therapeutic efficacy. Among patients with a clinical response 91% also had improvement on serial neuroradiographic studies within 2–6 weeks of starting therapy. Therefore, follow-up scans should be obtained 10–14 days after starting therapy and all lesions should be assessed for response as some patients may have more than one condition (Chang et al. 1995). Brain biopsy should be considered in patients with any of the following:

1 no improvement of baseline clinical abnormalities (except headache and sei-zures) within 10–14 days of starting therapy;

2 clinical deterioration early in the course of therapy;

3 single lesions on neuroimaging studies, particularly magnetic resonance imaging (in one large retrospective study of toxoplasmic encephalitis in patients with AIDS, single lesions were noted in 28% of computerized tomography scans and 14% of magnetic resonance imaging, respectively) (Porter & Sande 1992);

4 *T. gondii* antibody negativity;

5 use of trimethoprim-sulphamethoxazole for *Pneumocystis carinii* pneumonia and toxoplasmic encephalitis prophylaxis. The lack of a response to empiric treatment does not exclude toxoplasmic encephalitis as a diagnosis since, despite optimal therapy, therapeutic failure and death do occur (Dannemann et al. 1992; Renold et al. 1992; Luft et al. 1993).

Primary central nervous system lymphoma is the major entity in the differential diagnosis of toxoplasmic encephalitis. Other infectious or neoplastic lesions are much less common; neither clinical manifestations nor neuroradiographic findings can reliably distinguish between these diseases (Remick et al. 1990; Goldstein et al. 1991; Luft & Remington 1992; Walot et al. 1996). The probability of central nervous system lymphoma is higher than toxoplasmic encephalitis when there is a solitary lesion on magnetic resonance imaging (Ciricillo & Rosenblum 1990). Other radiological findings suggestive of lymphoma include location within the corpus callosum or periventricular white matter, subependymal spread or ven-tricular encasement (Ciricillo & Rosenblum 1990; Dina 1991). Thallium-201 brain single-photon emission computerized tomography imaging has been employed to make this distinction (Ruiz et al. 1994; Chang et al. 1995). Lymphomas and other metabolically active tissue take up more thallium-201 relative to surrounding parenchyma whereas inflammatory lesions do not (O'Malley et al. 1994). However, the exact specificity and sensitivity of this technique in the setting of AIDS remains unknown (Walot et al. 1996). The sensitivity of thallium-201 brain single-photon emission computerized tomography is limited when the tumour size is small (<6–8 mm) in the subependymal region (Hansman Whiteman et al. 1997). A report comparing thallium-201 chloride and 99Tc(m)-sestamibi SPET concluded that the latter was the better technique for differentiating lymphoma from cerebral toxoplasmosis (Naddaf et al. 1998).

The diagnosis of pulmonary toxoplasmosis should be suspected in a *T. gondii*-antibody-positive patient with a CD4 count of <200 cells/ml and clinical presentation suggestive of *Pneumocystis carinii* pneumonia. A definitive diagnosis can be made by identifying tachyzoites in bronchoalveolar lavage fluid using Giemsa staining, whole animal or tissue culture (Derouin et al. 1989*a*, *b*; Bottone 1991; Pomeroy & Felice 1992). Detection of *T. gondii* DNA in bronchoalveolar lavage fluid and induced sputum by polymerase chain reaction may become a useful diagnostic tool (Lavrard et al. 1992; Pomeroy & Felice 1992; Roth et al. 1992).

Definitive diagnosis is made from specimens stained with haematoxylin and eosin or Giemsa stains, and demonstration of the tachyzoite form of *T. gondii* in tissue sections, smears or body fluids. *Toxoplasma gondii* or its antigens can be identified in specimens using direct or indirect immunofluorescence antibody methods or detection with peroxidase-antiperoxidase (Conley et al. 1981; Moskowitz et al. 1984). Inoculation of clinical specimens into mice or tissue culture may yield the diagnosis (Derouin et al. 1989*a*). Polymerase chain reaction can be used to detect *T. gondii* nucleic acid in tissue specimens and body fluids (Holliman et al. 1990; Roth et al. 1992; Cingolani et al. 1996; Antinori et al. 1997; d'Arminio Monforte et al. 1997). The efficacy of polymerase chain reaction for the detection of *T. gondii* DNA in CSF from patients with central nervous system mass lesions has been variable (Novati et al. 1994; Eggers et al. 1995; Cingolani et al. 1996; Antinori et al. 1997; d'Arminio Monforte et al. 1997).

Therapy

It is currently standard practice to initiate empirical treatment of toxoplasmic encephalitis based upon clinical and neurological findings. This has evolved because a definitive diagnosis requires a brain biopsy and in the setting of a toxoplasma antibody-positive patient with a compatible clinical syndrome and multiple contrast-enhancing lesions on neuroradiographic studies the predictive value for toxoplasmic encephalitis is approximately 80% (Cohn et al. 1989). The efficacy of this approach has been confirmed in both prospective and retrospective studies (Wanke et al. 1987; Leport *et al.* 1988; Dannemann et al. 1992; Porter & Sande 1992; Renold et al. 1992; Luft et al. 1993; Katlama 1992; Katlama et al. 1996). The combination of pyrimethamine and sulphadiazine with folinic acid (leucovorin) remains the treatment of choice for toxoplasmic encephalitis and extraneural forms of toxoplasmosis (Table 5.2). Unfortunately, up to 40–50% of patients develop adverse effects, which require discontinuation of therapy (Dannemann et al. 1992; Katlama et al. 1996). Oral folinic acid is used for preventing the haematological

Table 5.2. Drugs of choice for acute treatment of toxoplasmic encephalitis and extracerebral toxoplasmosis

Drug	Dosing	Adverse effects
Pyrimethamine oral use only	100 mg orally twice daily for 1 day, (loading dose) – then 50–75 mg orally daily for 3–6 weeks; with folinic acid(leucovorin) 10–20 mg orally daily	Gastrointestinal upset Rash Cytopaenias
Pyrimethamine oral use with sulphadiazine or trisulphapyrimidines oral use only	100 mg/kg (4–8 g in four divided doses) orally daily for 3–6 weeks	Gastrointestinal upset Rash (including Stevens–Johnson Syndrome) Cytopaenias Interstitial nephritis Crystalluria Encephalopathy
or Clindamycin	600 mg every 6 hours for 3–6 weeks, orally or IV use	Gastrointestinal upset Rash Pseudomembranous colitis

toxicity associated with antifolate drugs. In the sulpha-intolerant patient the combination of pyrimethamine and clindamycin is the regimen of choice (Table 5.2). This combination seems equal in efficacy to pyrimethamine/sulphadiazine during the acute phase of therapy (Dannemann et al. 1992; Katlama et al. 1996) but also has comparable rates of toxicity (Dannemann et al. 1992; Katlama et al. 1996). Overall a response to therapy with these combinations has been reported in 68–95% of patients (Luft et al. 1983; Dannemann et al. 1988, 1992; Luft & Remington 1992; Porter & Sande 1992; Renold et al. 1992; Katlama et al. 1996). In a prospective study of 49 patients with toxoplasmic encephalitis a quantifiable neurological response was seen in 71% of patients by day 7 and in 91% of patients by day 14 of therapy, respectively (Luft et al. 1993). Patients not responding to therapy had progressive or new neurological abnormalities within the first 12 days of therapy. Seizures and headaches could not be used to assess the clinical response to therapy. A complete response to therapy (i.e. absence of neurological sequelae), however, was noted in only 18–55% of patients in three prospective studies (Dannemann et al. 1992; Luft et al. 1993; Katlama et al. 1996). Mortality rates of 6–16% during the first 3 weeks of therapy have been reported (Pedrol et al. 1990; Dannemann et al. 1992). Treatment failure resulting in progressive toxoplasmic encephalitis has been noted in 5–12% of patients (Porter & Sande 1992; Renold et al. 1992; Luft et al. 1993). A complete radiological response (i. e. disappearance of all initial lesions in the absence of any new lesions) was seen in 25% and 32% of patients treated with pyrimethamine/clindamycin and pyrimethamine/sulphadiazine respectively (Katlama et al. 1996). Overall, 52% of patients will have a quantifiable response on neuroradiological studies within 6 weeks of initiating therapy (Luft & Remington 1988; Katlama et al. 1996). Acute therapy is given for 3 weeks while 6 weeks or more may be indicated for severely ill patients. Brain biopsy (see section entitled 'Diagnosis') should be considered in patients who have evidence of progressive disease after 3 days of empirical therapy or no clinical improvement after 10–14 days of treatment. In one study of patients with no clinical improvement after 7 days of empirical therapy for toxoplasmic encephalitis, 36% had primary central nervous system lymphoma, 24% had progressive multifocal leukoencephalopathy and only 8% had toxoplasmic encephalitis on brain biopsy (Chappell et al. 1992). The prophylactic use of anticonvulsants is not recommended. Steroids are not routinely recommended unless there is evidence of increased intracranial pressure, as there is no difference in the overall response rate or rate of response to therapy in patients who receive corticosteroids versus those who do not (Luft et al. 1993).

Despite the reported efficacy of pyrimethamine/sulphadiazine and pyrimethamine/clindamycin numerous problems exist with these regimens. The early mortality rate (within the first 3 weeks of treatment) approaches 20% (Luft &

Remington 1988; Pedrol et al. 1990). Many patients have significant neurological dysfunction despite therapy (Luft & Hafner 1990). Adverse effects may preclude the use of these regimens in almost 40% of patients. These regimens are inactive against the tissue cyst, making chronic suppressive (maintenance) therapy necessary. Multiple daily doses of sulphadiazine and clindamycin are necessary because of their short serum half-life. There is concern about the possible emergence of drug-resistant strains of *T. gondii*. Thus there is great interest in finding new drugs for treating toxoplasmic encephalitis (Table 5.3). Trimethoprim-sulphamethoxazole by intravenous infusion has been used for acute therapy of toxoplasmic encephalitis (Menichetti et al. 1991; Herrera et al. 1991; Canessa et al. 1992; Solbreux et al. 1992; Torre et al. 1998*b*). The results of a large multicentre - randomized prospective study of trimethoprim-sulphamethoxazole versus pyrimethamine-sulphadiazine for acute therapy of toxoplasmic encephalitis suggest that trimethoprim-sulphamethoxazole is an acceptable alternative to pyrimethamine-sulphadiazine, particularly in patients unable to take oral medications (Torre et al. 1998*a*). However, adverse reactions associated with the use of trimethoprim-sulphamethoxazole have been reported in 25–50% of patients (Canessa et al. 1992; Klein et al. 1992).

Azithromycin, a macrolide antibiotic, has activity against *T. gondii in vitro* and in animal models (Derouin & Chastang 1990; Derouin et al. 1992). Used alone, azithromycin is ineffective (Lane et al. 1994) while there is anecdotal evidence of its efficacy in combination with pyrimethamine (Saba et al. 1993; Godofsky 1994). The combination of azithromycin and pyrimethamine has been evaluated in a dose-escalating study sponsored by the AIDS Clinical Trials Group and may have some role as an alternative therapy (Mariuz et al. 1996). The results of this trial have not been published. Clarithromycin, another macrolide antibiotic, has been evaluated in combination with pyrimethamine in a small pilot study of 13 patients with toxoplasmic encephalitis (Fernandez-Martin et al. 1991). A total of 62% of patients had a complete response. However, adverse events occurred in 38% of patients and clarithromycin had to be discontinued in 27% of surviving patients. Further studies are necessary to confirm these results and determine the efficacy of a lower dose of clarithromycin.

Atovaquone, a hydroxynaphthoquinone, has excellent activity against *T. gondii in vitro* and in animal studies (Araujo et al. 1991; Huskinson-Mark et al. 1991). In studies of atovaquone monotherapy most patients had a partial clinical and radiographic response to therapy (Kovacs 1992; Behbahani et al. 1995; Torres et al. 1997). Response rates appear to correlate with atovaquone serum levels (Torres et al. 1997). There is concern about the high relapse rate when atovaquone is used alone for maintenance therapy (Wong & Remington 1994). There is little published data on the use of atovaquone in combination with pyrimethamine (Kovacs 1992). A

Table 5.3. Alternative/experimental drugs for the acute treatment of toxoplasma encephalitis

Drug	Dosing	Adverse effects
Trimethoprim-sulphamethoxazole oral/IV use	Trimethoprim 5–10 mg/kg, sulphamethoxazole 25–50 mg/kg orally/IV, four times daily for 3–6 weeks	Rash Gastrointestinal upset Cytopaenias
	Folinic acid 10–20 mg orally once daily for 3–6 weeks, added by some authors (Canessa et al. 1992)	
Azithromycin oral	1250–1500 mg orally once daily for 3–6 weeks with pyrimethamine; maintenance: same	Gastrointestinal upset
Clarithromycin oral	1000 mg orally twice daily for 3–6 weeks with pyrimethamine; maintenance: same	Gastrointestinal upset Hearing loss Elevated liver function tests
Atovaquone oral	1500 mg orally twice daily for 3–6 weeks with pyrimethamine; maintenance: same	Gastrointestinal upset Elevated liver function tests Rash

Table 5.4. Maintenance/suppressive therapy for toxoplasmic encephalitis

Drug	Dose
Pyrimethamine oral and	25–50 mg orally once daily with folinic acid 10–20 mg orally once daily
Sulphadiazine oral or	500 mg to 1 gram orally four times daily
Clindamycin oral	300 mg orally four times daily

large, international, multi-centred AIDS Clinical Trials Group study started in July 1994 to evaluate a new, better absorbed liquid formulation of atovaquone in combination with pyrimethamine or sulphadiazine or clarithromycin. Whenever possible atovaquone should be used in combination with pyrimethamine. Atovaquone is well tolerated; the most common adverse effects are rash, nausea, diarrhoea and elevated liver function tests.

Maintenance therapy

Chronic suppressive (maintenance) therapy for toxoplasmic encephalitis is necessary because the available chemotherapeutic agents are ineffective against the tissue cyst form of *T. gondii* and an adequate cell-mediated immune response is not re-established. The combination of pyrimethamine/sulphadiazine or pyrimethamine/clindamycin in the sulpha-drug intolerant patient is recommended for maintenance therapy (Table 5.4). However, pyrimethamine/sulphadiazine is superior to pyrimethamine/clindamycin given the higher relapse rate when pyrimethamine/clindamycin is used in this setting compared with pyrimethamine/sulphadiazine (22% versus 11%) (Pedrol et al. 1990; Maslo et al. 1992; Katlama et al. 1996).

Another advantage of pyrimethamine/sulphadiazine is that it offers adequate prophylaxis against *Pneumocytis carinii* pneumonia (Heald et al. 1991). Relapse rates of 10–26% have been reported in patients receiving some form of maintenance therapy (Pedrol et al. 1990; Ragnaud et al. 1991; Porter & Sande 1992; Renold et al. 1992; Katlama et al. 1996). It is likely that some of these relapses are the result of patient noncompliance or intolerance to the prescribed medication.

The use of bi-weekly or tri-weekly pyrimethamine/sulphadiazine or pyrimethamine/clindamycin for maintenance therapy (at doses noted in Table 5.5) has been reported (Pedrol et al. 1990; Fong et al. 1992). However, because of the small number of patients studied and the retrospective nature of one of these trials (Fong et al. 1992), an unqualified recommendation cannot be given for these regimens at the present time. Monotherapy with pyrimethamine (50–100 mg daily by mouth)

Table 5.5. Maintenance therapy for toxoplasmic encephalitis

Drug	Dose
Bi-weekly maintenance therapy for toxoplasmic encephalitis (Pedrol et al. 1990)	
Pyrimethamine (oral) and	25 mg orally for one day twice week
Sulphadiazine (oral) or	75 mg/kg orally for one day twice week
Clindamycin (oral)	600 mg orally four times for one day twice weekly
Folinic acid (oral)	10 mg orally once daily
Tri-weekly maintenance therapy for toxoplasmic encephalitis (Fong et al. 1992)	
Pyrimethamine (oral) and	25 mg orally for one day thrice weekly
Sulfadiazine (oral) or	1 g orally twice for one day thrice weekly
Clindamycin (oral)	300 mg orally four times for one day thrice weekly

has also been reported (deGans et al. 1992; Maslo et al. 1992). Relapse rates ranged from 10–28% with 50 mg to 5% with the 100 mg dosing. When an alternative regimen (Table 5.3) is used for acute therapy of toxoplasmic encephalitis, the same drugs have been continued for maintenance therapy.

Primary prophylaxis

The prophylaxis of toxoplasmic encephalitis is indicated in the AIDS patients with a CD4 count <200/mm^3 and who are *T. gondii*-antibody-positive. Several drug regimens have been reported to be efficacious in this regard (Table 5.6) (Richards et al. 1994). Trimethoprim-sulphamethoxazole has been shown to be highly effective in preventing toxoplasmic encephalitis in studies of its use for prophylaxis against *Pneumocystis carinii* pneumonia (Carr et al. 1992; Hardy et al. 1992; Michelet et al. 1992; Podzamczer et al. 1993, 1995; May et al. 1994; Bozette et al. 1995). The incidence of toxoplasmic encephalitis in these studies varies from 0% to 9%.

Clinical data also suggest that a combination of dapsone and pyrimethamine is effective for the primary prophylaxis of toxoplasmic encephalitis (Clotet et al. 1991, 1992; Girard et al. 1993; Podzamczer et al. 1993; Opravil et al. 1995). The incidence of toxoplasmic encephalitis in these studies varies from 0% to 15%, compared with 25% in patients not receiving this drug regimen.

Pyrimethamine with folinic acid has been evaluated for the primary prophylaxis of toxoplasmic encephalitis (Bachmeyer et al. 1994; Leport et al. 1996;

Table 5.6. Drugs used for primary prophylaxis of toxoplasmic encephalitis

Trimethoprim-sulphamethoxazole oral	One DS* tablet orally daily or two DS tablets orally twice weekly
Pyrimethamine/dapsone oral	Pyrimethamine 50 mg orally once weekly with 50 mg orally dapsone once daily
Folinic acid (leucovorin)	Folinic acid 10–15 mg orally is given with pyrimethamine or
	Pyrimethamine 25mg orally twice weekly with dapsone 100mg orally twice weekly
Folinic acid 10–15 mg orally is given with pyrimethamine or Pyrimethamine 75 mg orally once weekly with Dapsone 200 mg orally once weekly Folinic acid 10–15 mg orally is given with pyrimethamine	
Pyrimethamine oral	Pyrimethamine 50 mg orally once daily with folinic acid 50 mg orally twice weekly or
Folinic acid (leucovorin)	Pyrimethamine 100mg loading dose, then 50 mg orally thrice weekly with folinic acid 15 mg orally thrice weekly

*One DS (Double Strength) tablet contains 160 mg trimethoprim/800 mg sulphamethoxazole.

Rousseau et al. 1997). In an open study of 44 patients (Bachmeyer et al. 1994), only 59% tolerated a full dose of pyrimethamine. None of these patients developed toxoplasmic encephalitis compared with 44% of patients not receiving pyrimethamine. In a double-blind, randomized trial (Leport et al. 1996) the incidence of toxoplasmic encephalitis and survival rate was similar in the pyrimethamine-treated (12%) and placebo (13%) groups on an intent-to-treat analysis. In the on-treatment analysis, however, the incidence of toxoplasmic encephalitis was 4% in the pyrimethamine arm and 12% in the placebo arm. The most common side-effect was rash which occurred in 7% of patients on pyrimethamine. The authors conclude that pyrimethamine should be considered for patients who are intolerant of trimethoprim-sulphamethoxazole.

Prevention of toxoplasma infection in *T. gondii*-antibody-negative patients

The following measures can significantly reduce the risk of infection with *T. gondii* in susceptible patients:

1 Limiting exposure to cats, their litter, and soil contaminated with cat faeces; cat litter should be disposed of daily before the oocysts become infectious. Thorough handwashing after handling cats, their litter, faeces or soil. When possible, cats should be kept indoors and fed only commercial cat food or well-cooked food. Gloves should be used when gardening (see Appendices).

2 Eating only well-cooked meats. Meat should be cooked to an internal temperature of over 60 °C (until the meat is no longer pink inside). Microwave ovens may not provide even cooking temperatures throughout the meat and are therefore unreliable. Frozen meats (−20 °C for at least 24 hours) which have been thawed or *correctly* smoked or cured in brine are also safe (Remington & Desmont 1990) though home freezers may not reach such temperatures (see Chapter 3).

Summary

Toxoplasmic encephalitis is the most common cause of focal central nervous system infections in people with AIDS. Serological tests are useful for identifying individuals at risk of developing toxoplasmic encephalitis and therefore appropriate for primary prophylaxis. A presumptive diagnosis of toxoplasmic encephalitis may be made based upon clinical manifestations, neuroimaging studies, *T. gondii* antibody positivity and subsequent clinical and radiological response to therapy. A definitive diagnosis can be made by brain biopsy. Despite the reported efficacy of currently available drug regimens, morbidity, mortality and adverse drug effects continue to be a problem. In addition, the lack of activity against the tissue cyst form of *T. gondii* makes chronic maintenance therapy necessary to avoid relapses of toxoplasma encephalitis. Patients who are *T. gondii* antibody negative should be instructed on how to prevent toxoplasma infection.

REFERENCES

Adair, O. V., Randive, N. & Krasnow, N. (1989). Isolated toxoplasma myocarditis in acquired immunodeficiency syndrome. *American Heart Journal*, 118, 856–7.

Ahuja, S. K., Ahuja, S. S., Thelma, W. *et al.* (1993). Necrotizing pancreatitis and multiorgan failure associated with toxoplasmosis in a patient with AIDS. *Clinical Infectious Diseases*, 16, 432–4.

Albrecht, H., Skorde, J., Arasteh *et al.* (1993). Disseminated toxoplasmosis (DT) causing a sepsis like illness – report of 16 cases. In *Programs and Abstracts of the XI International Conference on AIDS*. Berlin, Germany, June 6–11 [Abstract].

Ambrose, R. A., Lee, E. Y. & Sharer, L. R. (1987). The acquired immunodeficiency syndrome in intravenous drug abusers and patients with a sexual risk: clinical and postmortem comparisons. *Human Pathology*, **18**, 1109–14.

Antinori, A., Ammassari, A., DeLuca, A. *et al.* (1997). Diagnosis of AIDS-related focal brain lesions – a decision-making analysis based on clinical and neuroradiologic characteristics combined with polymerase chain reaction assays in CSF. *Neurology*, **48**, 687–694.

Araujo, F. G., Huskinson-Mark, J. & Remington, J. S. (1991). Remarkable *in vitro* and *in vivo* activities of the hydroxynaphthoquinone 566C80 against tachyzoites and tissue cysts of *Toxoplasma gondii*. *Antimicrobial Agents and Chemotherapy*, **35**, 293–9.

Arendt, G., Hefter, H., Figge, C. *et al.* (1991). Two cases of cerebral toxoplasmosis in AIDS patients mimicking HIV-related dementia. *Journal of Neurology*, **238**, 439–42.

Artigas, J., Gross, G., Niedobitek, F. *et al.* (1994). Severe toxoplasmic ventriculo- meningoencephalomyelitis in two AIDS patients following treatment of cerebral toxoplasmic granuloma. *Clinical Neuropathology*, **13**, 120–6.

Bachmeyer, C., Gorin, I., Deleuze, J. *et al.* (1994). Pyrimethamine as primary prophylaxis for toxoplamosis in patients infected with human immunodeficiency virus. Open study [Letter]. *Clinical Infectious Diseases*, **18**, 479–80.

Behbahani, R., Mersedeh, M. & Baxter, J. D. (1995). Therapeutic approaches for AIDS-related toxoplasmosis. *Annals of Pharmacotherapy*, **29**, 760–8.

Benenson, M. W., Takafugi, E. T., Lemon, S. M. *et al.* (1983). Oocyst-transmitted toxoplasmosis associated with ingestion of contaminated water. *The New England Journal of Medicine*, **307**, 666–9.

Berlit, P., Popescu, O., Weng, Y. & Málessa, R. (1996). Disseminated cerebral hemorrhages as unusual manifestations of toxoplasmic encephalitis in AIDS. *Journal of Neurological Science*, **143**, 187–9.

Bishburg, E., Engh, R. H., Slim, J. *et al.* (1989). Brain lesions in patients with the acquired immunodeficiency syndrome. *Archives of Internal Medicine*, **149**, 941–3.

Bottone, J. (1991). Diagnosis of acute pulmonary toxoplasmosis by visualization of invasive and intracellular tachyzoites in Giemsa-stained smear of bronchoalveolar lavage fluid. *Clinical Microbiology*, **29**, 2626–7.

Bourgonin, P. M., Melancon, D., Carpenter, S. *et al.* (1992). Hydrocephalus and prominence of the choroid plexus: an unusual computed tomographic presentation of cerebral toxoplasmosis. *Canadian Association of Radiology Journal*, **43**, 55–9.

Bozzette, S. A., Finkelstein, D. M., Spector, S. A. *et al.* (1995). A randomized trial of three antipneumocystis agents in patients with advanced human immunodeficiency virus infection. *The New England Journal of Medicine*, **332**, 693–9.

Brion, J. P., Pelloux, H., Le Marc'hadour, F. *et al.* (1992). Acute toxoplasmic hepatitis in a patient with AIDS. *Clinical Infectious Diseases*, **15**, 183–4.

Brivet, F., Coffin, B., Bedossa, P. et al. (1987). Pancreatic lesions in AIDS [Letter]. *Lancet*, **2**, 570–1.

Canessa, A., DelBono, V., Deleo, P. et al. (1992). Cotrimoxazole therapy of *Toxoplasma gondii* encephalitis in AIDS patients. *European Journal of Clinical Microbiology and Infectious Diseases*, **11**, 125–30.

Caramello, P., Forno, B., Lucchini, A. et al. (1993). Toxoplasmosis diffuse encephalitis diagnosed by isolation of *Toxoplasma gondii* in cell culture. In *Programs and Abstracts of the XI International Conference on AIDS*. Berlin, Germany, June 6–11. [Abstract].

Carr, A., Tindall, B., Brew, B. J. et al. (1992). Low-dose trimethoprim-sulfamethoxazole prophylaxis for toxoplasmic encephalitis in patients with AIDS. *Annals of Internal Medicine*, 117, 106–11.

Casado-Naranjo, I., Lopez-Trigo, J., Ferrandiz, A. et al. (1989). Hemorrhagic abscess in a patient with acquired immunodeficiency syndrome. *Neuroradiology*, 31, 289.

Catterall, J. R., Hofflin, J. M. & Remington, J. S. (1986). Pulmonary toxoplasmosis. *American Review of Respiratory Diseases*, 133, 704–5.

Chang, L., Cornford, M. E., Chiang, F. L. et al. (1995). Radiologic–pathologic correlation: cerebral toxoplasmosis and lymphoma in AIDS. *American Journal of Neuroradiology*, 16, 1653–63.

Chappell, E. T., Guthrie, B. L. & Orenstein, J. (1992). The role of stereotactic biopsy in the management of HIV related focal brain lesions. *Neurosurgery*, 30, 825–9.

Chaudhari, A. B., Singh, A., Jindal, S. et al. (1989). Hemorrhage in cerebral toxoplasmosis: a report on a patient with acquired immunodeficiency syndrome. *South African Medical Journal*, 76, 272–4.

Cingolani, A., DeLuca, A., Ammassari, A. et al. (1996). PCR detection of *Toxoplasma gondii* DNA in CSF for the differential diagnosis of AIDS-related focal brain lesions. *Journal of Medical Microbiology*, 45, 472–6.

Ciricillo, S. F. & Rosenblum, M. L. (1990). Use of CT and MR imaging to distinguish intracranial lesions and to define the need for biopsy in AIDS patients. *Journal of Neurosurgery*, 73, 720–4.

Ciricillo, S. F. & Rosenblum, M. L. (1991). Imaging of solitary lesions in AIDS [Letter]. *Journal of Neurosurgery*, 74, 1029.

Clotet, B., Sirena, G., Romeu, J. et al. (1991). Twice-weekly dapsone-pyrimethamine for presenting PCP and cerebral toxoplasmosis. *Acquired Immunodeficiency Syndrome*, 5, 601–2.

Clotet, B., Romeu, J. & Sirena, G. (1992). Cerebral toxoplasmosis and prophylaxis for *Pneumocystis carinii* pneumonia [Letter]. *Annals of Internal Medicine*, 117, 169.

Clumeck, N. (1991). Some aspects of the epidemiology of toxoplasmosis and pneumocystosis in AIDS in Europe. *European Journal of Clinical Microbiology and Infectious Diseases*, 10, 177–8.

Cochereau-Massin, I., LeHoang, P., Lautier-Frau, M. et al. (1992). Ocular toxoplasmosis in human immunodeficiency virus-infected patients. *American Journal of Ophthalmology*, 114, 130–5.

Cohn, J., McMeeking, A., Cohen, W. et al. (1989). Evaluation of the policy of empirical treatment of suspected toxoplasmic encephalitis in patients with the acquired immunodeficiency syndrome. *American Journal of Medicine*, 86, 521–7.

Conley, F. K., Jenkins, K. A. & Remington, J. S. (1981). *Toxoplasma gondii* infection of the central nervous system: use of the peroxidase-antiperoxidase method to demonstrate toxoplasma in formalin-fixed paraffin embedded tissue sections. *Human Pathology*, 12, 690–8.

Crider, S. R., Horstman, W. G. & Massay, G. S. (1988). Toxoplasma orchitis: report of a case and review of the literature. *American Journal of Medicine*, 85, 421.

Dannemann, B., Israelski, D. M. & Remington, J. S. (1988). Treatment of toxoplasmic encephalitis with intravenous clindamycin. *Archives of Internal Medicine*, **148**, 2477–82.

Dannemann, B., McCutchan, J. A., Israelski, D. et al. (1992). Treatment of toxoplasmic encephalitis in patients with AIDS, a randomized trial comparing pyrimethamine plus clindamycin to pyrimethamine plus sulfadiazine. *Annals of Internal Medicine*, **116**, 33–43.

Darde, M. L., Bouteille, B. & Pestre-Alexandre, M. (1988). Isoenzymatic characterization of seven strains of *Toxoplasma gondii* by isoelectrofocusing in polyacrylamide gels. *American Journal of Tropical Medicine and Hygiene*, **39**, 551–8.

d'Arminio Monforte, A., Cinque, P., Vago, I. et al. (1997). A comparison of brain biopsy and CSF-PCR in the diagnosis of CNS lesions in AIDS patients. *Journal of Neurology*, **244**, 35–9.

deGans, J., Portegies, P., Reiss, P. et al. (1992). Pyrimethamine alone as maintenance therapy for central nervous system toxoplasmosis. *Journal of Acquired Immune Deficiency Syndrome*, **5**, 137–42.

Derouin, F. & Chastang, C. (1990). Activity *in vitro* against *Toxoplasma gondii* of azithromycin and clarithromycin alone and with pyrimethamine. *Journal of Antimicrobial Agents and Chemotherapy*, **25**, 708–11.

Derouin, F., Mazeron, M. C., Grin, Y. J. F. (1989*a*). Comparative study of tissue culture and mouse inoculation methods for demonstration of *Toxoplasma gondii. Journal of Clinical Microbiology*, **25**, 1597–600.

Derouin, F., Sarfati, C., Beauvais, B. et al. (1989*b*). Laboratory diagnosis of pulmonary toxoplasmosis in patients with acquired immunodeficiency syndrome. *Journal of Clinical Microbiology*, **27**, 1661–3.

Derouin, F., Sarfati, C., Beauvais, B. et al. (1990). Prevalence of pulmonary toxoplasmosis in HIV-infected patients. *Acquired Immunodeficiency Syndrome*, **4**, 1036.

Derouin, F., Almadany, R., Chua, F. et al. (1992). Synergistic activity of azithromycin and pyrimethamine or sulfadiazine in acute experimental toxoplasmosis. *Antimicrobial Agents and Chemotherapy*, **36**, 997–1001.

Derouin, F., LePort, C., Pueyo, S. et al. (1996). Predictive value of *Toxoplasma gondii* titers on the occurrence of toxoplasma encephalitis in HIV infected patients. *Acquired Immunodeficiency Syndrome*, **10**, 1521–7.

De Smet, M. D. (1992). Differential diagnosis of retinitis and choroiditis in patients with acquired immunodeficiency syndrome. *American Journal of Medicine*, **92** [Suppl. 2A], 17–21.

Dina, T. S. (1991). Primary central nervous system lymphoma versus tomoplasmosis in AIDS. *Radiology*, **179**, 823–8.

Dowell, S. F., Moore, G. W. & Hutchins, G. M. (1990). The spectrum of pancreatic pathology in patients with AIDS. *Modern Pathology*, **3**, 49–53.

Dubey, J. P. (1986). A review of toxoplasmosis in pigs. *Veterinary Parasitology*, **19**, 181–23.

Dubey, J. P. & Beattie, C. P. (1988). *Toxoplasmosis of Animals and Man*. Boca Raton, FL: CRC Press.

Eggers, C., Gross, U., Klinker, H. et al. (1995). Limited value of cerebrospinal fluid for detection of *Toxoplasma gondii* in toxoplasmic encephalitis associated with AIDS. *Journal of Neurology*, **242**, 644–9.

Engstrom, J. W., Lowenstein, D. H. & Bredesen, D. E. (1989). Cerebral infarctions and transient neurological deficits with the acquired immunodeficiency syndrome. *American Journal of Medicine*, **86**, 528–32.

Fabricius, E. M., Patzak, A., Horwick, H. et al. (1993). Ocular diseases as the initial manifestation of AIDS. In *Programs and Abstracts of the IX International Conference on AIDS*. Berlin, Germany, June 6–11. [Abstract].

Feldman, H. A. (1965). Nationwide serum survey of United States military recruits, 1962 VI. Toxoplasma antibodies. *American Journal of Epidemiology*, **81**, 385–91.

Feldman, H. A. & Miller, L. T. (1965). Serological study of toxoplasmosis prevalence. *American Journal of Hygiene*, **64**, 320–35.

Fernandez-Martin, J., Leport, C., Morlat, P. et al. (1991). Pyrimethamine-clarithromycin combination for therapy of acute toxoplasmic encephalitis in patients with AIDS. *Antimicrobial Agents and Chemotherapy*, **35**, 2049–52.

Fong, I. W., Glazer, S., Fletcher, D. et al. (1992). Recurrence of CNS toxoplasmosis in AIDS patients on chronic suppressive treatment. In *VIII International Conference on AIDS*. Amsterdam, The Netherlands, July 19–24. [Abstract POB3171].

Friedman, A. H. (1984). The retinal lesions of the acquired immunodeficiency syndrome. *Transactions of the American Ophthalmological Society*, **82**, 447–91.

Friedman, A. H., Orellana, J., Gaggiuso, D. J. et al. (1990). Ocular toxoplasmosis in AIDS patients. *Transactions of the American Ophthalmological Society*, **88**, 63–88.

Garcia, L. W., Hemphill, R. B., Marasco, W. A. et al. (1991). Acquired immunodeficiency syndrome with disseminated toxoplasmosis presenting as an acute pulmonary and gastrointestinal illness. *Archives of Pathology Laboratory Medicine*, **115**, 459–63.

Gherardi, R., Baudrimont, M., Lionnet, T. et al. (1992). Skeletal muscle toxoplasmosis in patients with acquired immunodeficiency syndrome: a clinical and pathological study. *Annals of Neurology*, **32**, 535–42.

Girard, P. M., Landman, R., Gaudebout, C. et al. (1993). Dapsone-pyrimethamine compared with aerosolized pentamidine as primary prophylaxis against *Pneumocystis carinii* pneumonia and toxoplasmosis in HIV infection. *The New England Journal of Medicine*, **328**, 1514–20.

Glatt, A. E. (1992). *Toxoplasma gondii* serologies in patients with human immunodeficiency virus infection. *Infectious Diseases in Clinical Practice*, **1**, 237.

Godofsky, E. W. (1994). Treatment of presumed cerebral toxoplasmosis with azithromycin. *The New England Journal of Medicine*, **330**, 575–6.

Goldstein, J. D., Zeifer, B., Chao, C. et al. (1991). CT appearance of primary CNS lymphoma in patients with acquired immunodeficiency syndrome. *Journal of Computer Assisted Tomography*, **15**, 39–44.

Grange, F., Kinney, E. L., Monseux et al. (1990). Successful therapy for *Toxoplasma gondii* myocarditis in acquired immunodeficiency syndrome. *American Heart Journal*, **120**, 443–4.

Grant, I. H., Gold, J. W. M., Rosenblum, M. et al. (1990). *Toxoplasma gondii* serology in HIV-infected patients: the development of central nervous toxoplasmosis. *Acquired Immunodeficiency Syndrome*, **4**, 319–521.

Gray, F., Gherardi, R., Wingate, E. et al. (1989). Diffuse encephalitic cerebral toxoplasmosis in AIDS. Report of four cases. *Journal of Neurology*, **236**, 273–7.

Groll, A., Schneider, M., Althoft, P. H. et al. (1990). Morphologic and clinical significance of

AIDS-related lesions in the adrenals and pituitary. *Deutsch Medicine Wochenschrift*, **115**, 483–8.

Hansman Whiteman, M. L., Post, J. D. & Sklar, E. (1997). Neuroimaging of acquired immunodeficiency syndrome. In *AIDS and the Nervous System*, 2nd edn., ed. J. R. Berger & R. M. Levy, pp. 297–381. Philadelphia: Lippincott–Raven Publishers.

Hardy, W. D., Feinber, J., Finkelstein, D. M. et al. (1992). Trimethoprim-sulfamethoxazole versus aerosolized pentamidine for secondary prophylaxis of *Pneumocystis carinii* pneumonia in AIDS patients receiving zidovudine. *The New England Journal of Medicine*, **327**, 1842–8.

Harris, T. M., Smith, R., Bognanno, J. R. et al. (1990). Toxoplasmic myelitis in AIDS gadolinium-enhanced MR. *Journal of Computer Assisted Tomography*, **14**, 809–11.

Heald, A., Flepp, M. & Chave, J.-P. (1991). Treatment for cerebral toxoplasmosis protects against *Pneumocystis carinii* pneumonia in patients with AIDS. *Annals of Internal Medicine*, **115**, 760–3.

Helweg-Larsen, S., Jakobsen, J., Boeser, F. & Artier-Siberg, P. (1986). Neurological complications and concomitants of AIDS. *Acta Neurologica Scandanavica*, **74**, 467–74.

Herrera, G., Villala, O. & Visona, K. (1991). Trimethoprim-sulfamethoxazole treatment of toxoplasma encephalitis in AIDS patients. In *VII International Conference on AIDS*. Florence, Italy, June 16–21. [Abstract WB2321].

Herskovitz, S., Siegel, S. E., Schneider, A. T. et al. (1989). Spinal cord toxoplasmosis in AIDS. *Neurology*, **39**, 1552–3.

Hofman, P., Michiels, J.-F., Maingnene, C. et al. (1991). Cardiac toxoplasmosis in acquired immunodeficiency syndrome (AIDS). A post mortem study of 15 cases. In *Programs and Abstracts of the VII International Conference on AIDS*. Florence, Italy, June 16–21. [Abstract].

Hofman, P., Bernard, E. & Michiels, J.-F. (1993a). Extracerebral toxoplasmosis in the acquired immunodeficiency syndrome (AIDS). *Pathology Research Practices*, **189**, 894–901.

Hofman, P., Quintens, H., Michiels, J.-F et al. (1993b). Toxoplasma cystitis associated with acquired immunodeficiency syndrome. *Urology*, **42**, 589–92.

Holland, G. N., Engstrom, R. E., Jr., Glasgow, B. J. et al. (1988). Ocular toxoplasmosis in patients with the acquired immunodeficiency syndrome. *American Journal of Ophthalmology*, **106**, 653–67.

Holliman, R. E., Johnson, J. D. & Savva, D. (1990). Diagnosis of cerebral toxoplasmosis in association with AIDS using the polymerase chain reaction. *Scandinavian Journal of Infectious Diseases*, **22**, 243–4.

Hooper, A. D. (1957). Acquired toxoplasmosis: report of a case with autopsy findings. *American Archives of Pathology*, **64**, 1–6.

Huskinson-Mark, J., Araujo, F. G. & Remington, J. S. (1991). Evaluation of the effect of drugs on the cyst form of *Toxoplasma gondii*. *Journal of Infectious Diseases*, **164**, 170–7.

Isrealski, D. M., Skowron, G., Leventhal, J. P. et al. (1988). Toxoplasma peritonitis in a patient with acquired immunodeficiency syndrome. *Archives of Internal Medicine*, **148**, 1655–7.

Jautzke, G., Sell, M. & Thalman, U. (1993). Extracerebral toxoplasmosis in AIDS: histological and immunohistological findings based on 80 autopsy cases. *Pathology Research Practices*, **189**, 428–36.

Jones, J. L., Hanson, D. L. & Chu, C. A. (1996). Toxoplasmic encephalitis in HIV infected persons: risk factors and trends. *Acquired Immunodeficiency Syndrome*, 10, 1393–9.

Jones, J. L., Hanson, D. L., Dworkin, M. S. et al. (1998). Trends in AIDS-related opportunistic infections among men who have sex with men and among injecting drug users, 1991–1996. *Journal of Infectious Diseases*, 178, 114–20.

Katlama, C. (1992). New perspectives on the treatment and prophylaxis of *Toxoplasma gondii* infection. *Current Opinion in Infectious Diseases*, 5, 833–9.

Katlama, C., DeWit, S., O'Doherty, E. et al. (1996). Pyrimethamine-clindamycin vs. pyrimethamine sulfadiazine as acute and long-term therapy for toxoplasmic encephalitis in patients with AIDS. *Clinical Infectious Diseases*, 22, 268–75.

Kayser, C., Campbell, R., Sartorius, C. et al. (1990). Toxoplasmosis of the conus medularis in a patient with hemophilia A-associated AIDS. *Journal of Neurosurgery*, 73, 951–3.

Khuong M. A., Matherson, S., Marche, C. et al. (1990). Diffuse toxoplasmic encephalitis without abscess in AIDS patients. In *Program and Abstracts of the Interscience Congress of Antimicrobial Agents and Chemotherapy*. Atlanta, Georgia, October 21–24. [Abstract 1157].

Klatt, E. C. (1988). Diagnostic findings in patients with acquired immunodeficiency syndrome (AIDS). *Journal of Acquired Immunodeficiency Syndrome*, 1, 454–65.

Klein, N. C., Duncanson, F. P., Lenox, T. H. et al. (1992). Trimethoprim-sulfamethoxazole for *Pneumocystis carinii* in AIDS patients: results of a large prospective randomized treatment trial. *Acquired Immunodeficiency Syndrome*, 6, 301–5.

Kovacs, J. A. (1992). Efficacy of atovaquone in treatment of toxoplasmosis in patients with AIDS. *Lancet*, 340, 637–8.

Lane, H. C., Laughon, B. E., Falloon, J., Kovacs, J., Davey, R. T., Polis, M. A. & Masur, H. (1994). Recent advances in the management of AIDS-related opportunistic infections. *Annals of Internal Medicine*, 120, 945–55.

Lavrard, I., Roux, P., Poirot, J. et al. (1992). Pulmonary toxoplasmosis. Detection of *Toxoplasma gondii* DNA by polymerase chain reaction in bronchoalveolar lavage fluid and induced sputum. In *VIII International Conference on AIDS*. Amsterdam, The Netherlands, July 19–24 1992. [Abstract P0B3204].

Leport, C., Raffi, F., Matheron, S. et al. (1988). Treatment of central nervous system toxoplasmosis with pyrimethamine/sulfadiazine combination in 35 patients with the acquired immunodeficiency syndrome: efficacy of long-term continuous therapy. *American Journal of Medicine*, 84, 94–100.

Leport, C., Morlat, P., Chene, G et al. (1996). Pyrimethamine for primary prophylaxis of toxoplasmosis in HIV patients. A double blind randomized trial. *Journal of Infectious Diseases*, 173, 91–7.

Levy, R. M., Bredesen, D. E. & Rosenblum, M. L. (1985). Neurological manifestations of the acquired immunodeficiency syndrome (AIDS): experience at UCSF and review of the literature. *Journal of Neurosurgery*, 62, 475–95.

Levy, R. M., Rosenbloom, S. & Perett, L. V. (1986). Neuroradiological findings in the acquired immunodeficiency syndrome (AIDS): a review of 200 cases. *American Journal of Neuroradiology*, 7, 833–9.

Levy, R. M., Janssen, R. S., Bush, T. J. & Rosenblum, M. L. (1988). Neuroepidemiology of acquired immunodeficiency syndrome. *Journal of Acquired Immune Deficiency Syndrome*, 1, 31–40.

Libanore, M., Biccochi, R., Sighonolfi, L. et al. (1991). Pneumothorax during pulmonary toxoplasmosis in the AIDS patient. *Chest*, 100, 1184.

Luft, B. J. & Castro, K. G. (1991). An overview of the problem of toxoplasmosis and pneumocystosis in AIDS in the USA: implications for future therapeutic trials. *European Journal of Clinical Microbiology and Infectious Diseases*, 10, 178–81.

Luft, B. J. & Hafner, R. (1990). Toxoplasmic encephalitis [Editorial]. *Acquired Immunodeficiency Syndrome*, 4, 593–5.

Luft, B. J. & Remington, J. S. (1988). AIDS commentary: toxoplasmic encephalitis. *Journal of Infectious Diseases*, 157, 1–6.

Luft, B. J., & Remington, J. S. (1992). Toxoplasmic encephalitis in AIDS. *Clinical Infectious Diseases*, 15, 211–22.

Luft, B. J., Conley, T. K., Remington, J. S. et al. (1983). Outbreak of CNS toxoplasmosis in Western Europe and North America. *Lancet*, 1, 781–4.

Luft, B. J., Brooks, R. G., Conley, F. K. et al. (1984). Toxoplasmic encephalitis in patients with the acquired immunodeficiency syndrome (AIDS) and other immunocompromising diseases. *Journal of the American Medical Association*, 252, 913–17.

Luft, B. J., Hafner, R., Korzun, A. H. et al. (1993). Toxoplasmic encephalitis in patients with the acquired immunodeficiency syndrome. *The New England Journal of Medicine*, 329, 995–1000.

Lunden, A. & Uggla, A. (1992). Infectivity of *Toxoplasma gondii* in mutton following curing, smoking, freezing or microwave cooking. *International Journal of Food Microbiology*, 15, 357–63.

Machler, G., Meyer, E. & Emminger, C. (1993). *Toxoplasma gondii* infection in seven HIV patients with mycocarditis. In *Programs and Abstracts of the IX International Conference on AIDS*. Berlin, Germany, June 6–11. [Abstract].

Marche, C., Mayorga, R., Clair, B. et al. (1989). Localisations de la Toxoplasmose dans le Tube Digestif au Cours du Sida. Etude Anatomoclinique. In *Programs and Abstracts of the V International Conference on AIDS*. Montreal, June 19–23. [Abstract].

Mariuz, P., Bosler, E. & Luft, B. J. (1996). Toxoplasmosis. In *AIDS and the Central Nervous System*, 2nd edn., ed. J. R. Berger & R. M. Levy, pp. 641–59. Philadelphia: Lippincottt–Raven Publishers.

Maslo, C., Matheron, S. & Saimot, A. G. (1992). Cerebral toxoplasmosis: assessment of maintenance therapy. In *VIII International Conference on AIDS*. Amsterdam, The Netherlands, July 19–24. [Abstract POB3218].

Masur, H., Jones, T. C., Lempert, J. A. & Cherubini, T. D. (1978). Outbreak of toxoplasmosis in a family and documentation of acquired retinochoroiditis. *American Journal of Medicine*, 64, 396–402.

May, T. H., Rabaud, C., Amiel, C. et al. (1993). Extracerebral toxoplasmosis in HIV infected patients: a French national survey. In *Programs and Abstracts of the IX International Conference on AIDS*. Berlin, Germany, June 6–11. [Abstract].

May, T. H., Beuscart, C., Reynew, J. et al. (1994). Trimethoprim-sulfamethoxazole versus aerosolized pentamidine for primary prophylaxis of *Pneumocystis carinii* pneumonia: a prospective, randomized controlled clinical trial. *Journal of Acquired Immune Deficiency Syndrome,* **7**, 457–62.

McArthur, J. C. (1987). Neurological manifestations of AIDS. *Medicine, Baltimore,* **66**, 407–37.

McLeod, R., Skamenae, E., Brown, C. R. et al. (1989). Genetic regulation of early survival and cyst number after perioral *Toxoplasma gondii* infection of AxB/BxA recombinant inbred and B/O congenic mice. *Journal of Immunology,* **143**, 3031–4.

Mehren, M., Burns, P. J., Mamani, F. et al. (1988). Toxoplasmic myelitis mimicking intramedullary spinal cord tumor. *Neurology,* **38**, 1648–50.

Mendelson, M. H., Finkel, L. J., Meyers, B. R. et al. (1987). Pulmonary toxoplasmosis in AIDS. *Scandanavian Journal of Infectious Diseases,* **19**, 703–6.

Menichetti, F., Marroni, M., diCandilo, F. et al. (1991). Cotrimoxazole (T/S) for cerebral toxoplasmosis (CT) in AIDS. In *VII International Conference on AIDS.* Florence, Italy, June 16–21. [Abstract WB2311].

Michelet, C. H., Raffi, F., Besnier, J. et al. (1992). Cotrimoxazole (CMX) versus aerosolized pentamidine (AP) for primary prophylaxis of *Pneumocystis carinii* pneumonia (PCP). In *VIII International Conference on AIDS.* Amsterdam, The Netherlands, July 19–24. [Abstract POB3312].

Milligan, S. A., Katz, M. S., Craven, P. C. et al. (1984). Toxoplasmosis presenting as panhypopituitarism in a patient with the acquired immunodeficiency syndrome. *American Journal of Medicine,* **77**, 760–4.

Moskowitz, L. B., Hensley, G. T. & Chan, J. C. (1984). The neuropathology of acquired immunodeficiency syndrome. *Archives of Pathology and Laboratory Medicine,* **108**, 867–72.

Murray, J. F., Folton, C. P., Garay, S. M. et al. (1984). Pulmonary complications of the acquired immunodeficiency syndrome. *The New England Journal of Medicine,* **310**, 1682–8.

Naddaf, S. Y., Akisik, M. F., Aziz, A. et al. (1998). Comparison between 201 TI-chloride and 99 Tc(m)-sestamibi SPET brain imaging for differentiating intracranial lymphoma from non-malignant lesions in AIDS patients. *Nuclear Medicine Communication,* **19**, 47–53.

Navia, B. A., Petito, C. K., Gold, J. W. M. *et al.* (1989). Cerebral toxoplasmosis complicating the acquired immunodeficiency syndrome. Clinical and neuropathological findings in 27 patients. *Annals of Neurology,* **19**, 224–8.

Nistral, M., Samtana, A., Pamiagua, R. et al. (1986). Testicular toxoplasmosis in two men with the acquired immunodeficiency syndrome (AIDS). *Archives of Pathology Laboratory Medicine,* **110**, 744–6.

Nolla-Sallas, J., Ricart, D., Ohlaberringue, F. et al. (1987). Hydrocephalus: an unusual CT presentation of cerebral toxoplasmosis in a patient with the acquired immunodeficiency syndrome. *European Neurology,* **27**, 130–2.

Novati, R., Castagna, A., Morsica, G. et al. (1994). Polymerase chain reaction for *Toxoplasma gondii* DNA in the cerebrospinal fluids of AIDS patients with focal brain lesions. *AIDS,* **8**, 1691–4.

Oksenhendler, E., Cadranel, J., Sarafati, C. et al. (1990). *Toxoplasma gondii* pneumonia in patients with the acquired immunodeficiency syndrome. *American Journal of Medicine,* **88**, 18–21.

Oksenhendler, E., Charreau, I., Tournerie, C. et al. (1994). *Toxoplasma gondii* infection in advanced HIV infection. *Acquired Immunodeficiency Syndrome*, 8, 483–7.

O'Malley, J. P., Ziessman, H. A., Kumar, P. N. et al. (1994). Diagnosis of intracranial lymphoma in patients with AIDS: value of 201 TI single-photon emission computed tomography. *American Journal of Roentgenology*, 163, 417–21.

Opravil M, Hirschel B, Lazzarin, A. et al. (1995). Once weekly administration of dapsone/pyrimethamine vs aerosolized pentamidine as combined prophylaxis for *Pneumocystis carinii* pneumonia and toxoplasma encephalitis in human immunodeficiency virus-infected patients. *Clinical Infectious Diseases*, 20, 531–41.

Overhage, J. M., Greist, A., & Brown, D. R. (1990). Conus medullaris syndrome resulting from *Toxoplasma gondii* infection in a patient with the acquired immunodeficiency syndrome. *American Journal of Medicine*, 8, 814–15.

Parke, D. W. & Font, R. L. (1986). Diffuse toxoplasmic retinochoroiditis in a patient with AIDS. *Archives of Ophthalmology*, 104, 571–5.

Partisani, M., Candolfi, H., Demautort et al. (1991). Seroprevalence of latent *T. gondii* infection in HIV infected individuals and long–term follow–up of toxoplasma seronegative subjects. In *Programs and Abstracts of the VII International Conference on AIDS*. Florence, Italy. [Abstract Wb2294].

Patrick, A. L., Roberts, L. A., Burton, E. N. et al. (1986). Focal sequential glomerulosclerosis in the acquired immunodeficiency syndrome patient. *Wisconsin Medical Journal*, 15, 200–3.

Pauwels, A., Meyohas, M. C., Eliaszewicz, M. et al. (1992). Toxoplasma colitis in the acquired immunodeficiency syndrome. *American Journal of Gastroenterology*, 87, 518–19.

Pedrol, E., Gonzalez-Clementz, J. M., Gatell, J. M. et al. (1990). Central nervous toxoplasmosis in AIDS patients: efficacy of an intermittent maintenance therapy. *Acquired Immunodeficiency Syndrome*, 4, 511–17.

Podzamczer, D., Satin, M., Jimenez, J. et al. (1993). Thrice weekly cotrimazole is better than weekly dapsone-pyrimethamine for primary prevention of *Pneumocystis carinii* pneumonia in HIV-infected patients. *Acquired Immunodeficiency Syndrome*, 7, 501–6.

Podzamczer, D., Miro, J., Bolao, F. et al. (1995). Twice-weekly maintenance therapy with sulfadiazine-pyrimethamine to prevent recurrent toxoplasmic encephalitis in patients with AIDS. *Annals of Internal Medicine*, 123, 175–80.

Pohl, H. D. & Eichenlaub, D. (1987). Toxoplasmosis of the CNS in AIDS Patients. In *Program of Berlin Symposium: HIV and the Nervous System*. Berlin, Germany.

Pomeroy, C. & Felice, G. A. (1992). Pulmonary toxoplasmosis. A review. *Clinical Infectious Diseases*, 14, 863–70.

Poon, T. P., Tchertkoff, V., Pares, G. F. et al. (1992). Spinal cord toxoplasma lesion in AIDS: MRI findings. *Journal of Computer Assisted Tomography*, 16, 817–19.

Porter, S. B. & Sande, M. (1992). Toxoplasmosis of the central nervous system in the acquired immunodeficiency syndrome. *The New England Journal of Medicine*, 327, 1643–8.

Post, M. J. D., Chan, J. C. & Hensley, G. T. (1983). Toxoplasma encephalitis in Haitian adults with acquired immunodeficiency syndrome: a clinical–pathologic–CT correlation. *American Journal of Roentgenology*, 140, 861–8.

Post, M. J. D., Kursunoglu, S. J., Hensley, G. T. et al. (1985). Cranial CT in acquired immunodeficiency syndrome: spectrum of diseases and optimal contrast enhancement technique. *American Journal of Neuroradiology*, 6, 743–54.

Post, M. J. D., Sheldon, J. J., Hensley, G. T. et al. (1986). Central nervous system disease in acquired immunodeficiency syndrome: prospective correlation using CT, MR imaging and pathological studies. *Radiology*, 158, 141–8.

Rabaud, C., May, T. H, Amiel, C. et al. (1994). Extracerebral toxoplasmosis in patients infected with HIV: a French national survey. *Medicine (Baltimore)*, 73, 306–14.

Rabaud, C., Thierry, M., Lucet, J. C. et al. (1996). Pulmonary toxoplasmosis in patients infected with human immunodeficiency virus: a French national survey. *Clinical Infectious Diseases*, 23, 1249–54.

Ragnaud, J.-M., Beylot, J. & Lacut, J. Y. (1991). Toxoplasmic encephalitis in 73 AIDS patients. In *VII International Conference on AIDS*. Florence, Italy, June 16–21. [Abstract MB2090].

Rehder, J. R., Burnier, M., Pavesio, C. E. et al. (1988). Unilateral toxoplasmic iridocyclitis. *American Journal of Ophthalmology*, 106, 740–1.

Reiter-Owana, L., Bialek, R., Rockstroh, J. K. & Seitz, H. M. (1998). The probability of acquiring primary toxoplasma infection in HIV-infected patients: results of a 8-year retrospective study. *Infection*, 26, 20–5.

Remick, S. C., Diamond, C., Migliozzi, J. A. et al. (1990). Primary central nervous system lymphoma in patients with and without acquired immunodeficiency syndrome: a retrospective analysis and review of the literature. *Medicine, (Baltimore)* 69, 345–60.

Remington, J. S. & Desmonts, G. (1990). Toxoplasmosis. In *Infectious Diseases of the Fetus and Newborn Infants*, 3rd. edn. ed. J. S. Remington & J. D. Klein, p. 89. Philadelphia: Saunders.

Remington, J. S. & Desmonts, G. (1995). Toxoplasmosis. In *Infectious Diseases of the Fetus and Newborn Infants*, 4th edn. ed. J. S. Remington & J. D. Klein, pp. 1–140. Philadelphia: Saunders.

Renold, C., Sugar, A., Chave, J.-D. et al. (1992). Toxoplasma encephalitis in patients with the acquired immunodeficiency syndrome. *Medicine*, 71, 224–39.

Richards, T. O., Jr., Kovacs, J. A. & Luft, B. J. (1994). Preventing toxoplasmic encephalitis in persons infected with human immunodeficiency virus. *Clinical Infectious Diseases*, 21 [Suppl. 1], S49–56.

Roldan, E. D., Moskowitz, L. & Hensley, G. T. (1987). Pathology of the heart in acquired immunodeficiency syndrome. *Archives of Pathology Laboratory Medicine*, 111, 943–6.

Roth, A., Roth, A., Hoffken, G. et al. (1992). Applications of the polymerase chain reaction in the diagnosis of pulmonary toxoplasmosis in immunocompromised patients. *European Journal of Clinical Microbiology and Infectious Diseases*, 11, 1177–81.

Rousseau, F., Pueyo, S., Morlat, P. et al. (1997). Increased risk of toxoplasmic encephalitis in human immunodeficiency virus-infected patients with pyrimethamine related rash. ANRS 005– ACTG 154 Trial Group Agence Nationale Recherche sur le sida (ANRS–INSERM) and the NIAID-AIDS Clinical Trials Group. *Clinical Infectious Diseases*, 3, 396–402.

Ruiz, A., Ganz, W. I., Post, J. D. et al. (1994). Use of thallium-201 brain SPECT to differentiate cerebral lymphoma from toxoplasma encephalitis in AIDS patients. *American Journal of Neuroradiology*, 15, 1885–94.

Saba, J., Morlat, P., Raffi, F. et al. (1993). Pyrimethamine plus azithromycin for treatment of acute toxoplasmic encephalitis in patients with AIDS. *European Journal of Clinical Microbiology and Infectious Diseases*, 12, 853–6.

Schnapp, L., Geaghan, S., Campagna, A. et al. (1992). *Toxoplasma gondii* pneumonitis in patients infected with the human immunodeficiency virus. *Archives of Internal Medicine*, 152, 1073–7.

Sell, M., Grunewald, T. H., Koppens, S. et al. (1993). Extracerebral toxoplasmsosis in AIDS: results of a histopathological study in autopsied cases. In *Programs and Abstracts of the IX International Conference on AIDS*. Berlin, Germany, June 6–11. [Abstract].

Smart, P. E., Weinfeld, A., Thompson, M. E. et al. (1990). Toxoplasmosis of the stomach: a cause of antral narrowing. *Radiology*, 174, 369–70.

Smith, K. L., Wilson, M., Hightower, A. W. et al. (1996). Prevalence of *Toxoplasma gondii* antibodies in US military recruits in 1989: comparison with data published in 1965. *Clinical Infectious Diseases*, 23, 1182–3.

Smith, R. E. (1988). Toxoplasmic retinochoroiditis as an emerging problem in AIDS patients. [Editorial]. *American Journal of Ophthalmology*, 106, 738–9.

Solbreux, P., Sonnet, J. & Zech, F. (1992). A retrospective study about the use of cotrimoxazole as diagnostic support and treatment of suspected cerebral toxoplasmosis in AIDS. *ACTA Clinica Belgica*, 45, 85–96.

Strittmatter, C., Lang, W., Wiestler, O. D. & Kleihues, P. (1992). The changing pattern of human immunodeficiency virus associated cerebral toxoplasmosis: a study of 46 postmortem cases. *ACTA Neuropathology*, 83, 475–81.

Suzuki, Y., Wong, S. & Grumet, F. (1996). Evidence for genetic regulation of the susceptibility to toxoplasmic encephalitis in AIDS patients. *Journal of Infectious Diseases*, 173, 265–8.

Teutsch, S. M., Juranek, D. D. & Sulzer, A. (1979). Epidemic toxoplasmosis associated with infected cats. *The New England Journal of Medicine*, 300, 695–9.

Torre, D., Casari, S., Speranza, F. et al. (1998a). Randomized trial of trimethoprim-sulfamethaxazole vs. pyrimethamine-sulfadiazine for therapy of toxoplasmic encephalitis in patients with AIDS. *Antimicrobial Agents and Chemotherapy*, 42, 1346–9.

Torre, D., Speranza, F., Martegani, R. et al. (1998b). A retrospective study of treatment of cerebral toxoplasmosis in AIDS patients with trimethoprim-sulfamethaxazole. *Journal of Infection*, 37, 15–18.

Torres, R., Weinberg, J., Stansell, G. et al. (1997). Atovaquone for salvage treatment and suppression of toxoplasmic encephalitis in patients with AIDS. Atovaquone/toxoplasmic encephalitis study group. *Clinical Infectious Diseases*, 24, 422–9.

Tourani, J. M., Isreal-Biet, D., Vemet, A. et al. (1985). Unusual pulmonary infection in a puzzling presentation of AIDS. *Lancet*, 1, 989.

Tschirhardt, D. & Klatt, E. C. (1988). Disseminated toxoplasmosis in the acquired immunodeficiency syndrome. *Archives of Pathology and Laboratory Medicine*, 112, 1237–41.

Vyas, R. & Ebright, J. R. (1996). Toxoplasmosis of the spinal cord in a patient with AIDS: case report and review. *Clinical Infectious Diseases*, 23, 1061–5.

Wallace, G. D. (1973). The role of the cat in the natural history of *Toxoplasma gondii*. *American Journal of Tropical Medicine and Hygiene*, 22, 313–22.

Walot, I., Miller, B. L., Chang, L. & Mehringer, C. M. (1996). Neuroimaging findings in patients with AIDS. *Clinical Infectious Diseases*, 22, 906–19.

Wanke, C., Tuazon, C. V., Kovacs, C. et al. (1987). Toxoplasmic encephalitis in patients with the acquired immunodeficiency syndrome. Diagnosis and response to therapy. *American Journal of Tropical Medicine Hygiene*, 36, 509–16.

Weiss, A., Margo, E. C., Ledford, D. K. et al. (1986). Toxoplasmic retinochoroiditis as an initial manifestation of the acquired immunodeficiency syndrome. *American Journal of Ophthalmology*, 101, 248–9.

Whelan, M. A., Kricheff, I. I., Handler, M. et al. (1983). Acquired immunodeficiency syndrome: cerebral computed tomographic manifestations. *Radiology*, 149, 477–84.

Wienman, D. & Chandler, A. H. (1956). Toxoplasmosis in man and swine – an investigation of the possible relationship. *Journal of the American Medical Association*, 161, 229–32.

Wilson, M., Lewis, B. & Fried, J. (1994). Seroepidemiology of toxoplasmosis in the US. In *9th General Meeting of the American Society of Microbiology*, Las Vegas, May 1994. [Abstract C545].

Wong, S. Y. & Remington, J. S. (1994). Toxoplasmosis in the Setting of AIDS. In *Textbook of AIDS Medicine*, ed. S. Broder, T. Merigan & D. Bolognesi. Baltimore, MD: Williams and Wilkinson.

Zangerle, R., Allerberger, F., Pohl, P., Fritsch, P. & Dierich, M. P. (1991). High risk of developing toxoplasmic encephalitis in AIDS patients seropositive to *Toxoplasma gondii*. *Medical Microbiology & Immunology*, 180, 59–66.

6

Toxoplasma infection in immunosuppressed (HIV-negative) patients

T. G. Wreghitt[1] and D. H. M. Joynson[2]

[1] Public Health Laboratory, Addenbrooke's Hospital, Cambridge, UK
[2] Toxoplasma Reference Unit, Public Health Laboratory, Singleton Hospital, Swansea, Wales

Introduction

Toxoplasma gondii is a classic example of an organism that has re-emerged as a threat to human health due in main to two external factors – the advent of HIV infection (discussed in Chapter 5) and advances in medical techniques and treatment such as transplantation and chemotherapy for malignancy – and the intrinsic ability of the protozoan to produce a persistent but latent infection via tissue cysts.

Toxoplasma gondii infection in an immunocompetent person is usually a trivial event which is normally asymptomatic; severe life-threatening disease is very rare. However, this is not the case in immunosuppressed patients (Table 6.1), in whom toxoplasma infection can result in significant morbidity and mortality. Clinically the situation can be complicated since the symptoms and signs of toxoplasma infection can mimic, confound or compound the presentation of the underlying disease and the possibility of infection may not even be considered. Diagnosis of infection is not always straightforward since the immune response in these patients may be atypical; clinical awareness of the possibility of infection must, therefore, be paramount.

Toxoplasma infection can be acute, chronic, latent or reactivated. Though naturally acquired acute infection can and does occur in immunosuppressed patients, it is not a common occurrence and reactivation of a previously latent infection is the usual scenario. The risk of infection in the individual patient depends on two factors – the prevalence of toxoplasma infection in that particular patient's community and the degree and nature of immunosuppression. It is important to note that *T. gondii* antibody prevalence rates can vary greatly even within the same continent; for example, within Europe *T. gondii* antibody prevalence in the UK is about 20–40% whilst in France it is 70–80%.

As in HIV-infected patients, the deficiency in the immune system probably resides primarily within the cell-mediated arm. Reactivation of toxoplasma infection in animal models has been induced by steroids, cyclophosphamide and

Table 6.1. Patient groups at particular risk of life-threatening toxoplasma infection due to immunosuppression

Organ and bone marrow transplant recipients
Patients with malignancy
Patients receiving anticancer chemotherapy
Patients receiving corticosteroid treatment
Patients with connective tissue/collagen vascular disease

Table 6.2. *Toxoplasma gondii* infections in transplant recipients

Type of transplant	Risk of donor-acquired toxoplasmosis in *T. gondii*-antibody-negative recipients of organs from *T. gondii*-antibody-positive recipients	Risk of *T. gondii* reactivation in *T. gondii*-antibody-positive recipients	Symptoms
Heart	50–60%	1–2%[*]	Fever
Liver	20%	1–2%[*]	Pneumonia
Kidney	<1%	1–2%[*]	Encephalitis
Bone marrow		0.5–2%[*+]	Myocarditis leukopaenia

[*]The incidence of *T. gondii* reactivation will be greater in those patients receiving increased immunosuppression.
[+]The incidence and severity of *T. gondii* reactivation is greater in those bone marrow transplant recipients with graft-versus-host disease.

whole-body irradiation. However, this chapter will not consider the biology and immunology of toxoplasma infection, as they are discussed in Chapters 1 and 2 respectively.

Transplant patients

Toxoplasma gondii infections arise in all transplant recipient groups, but at varying frequencies (Table 6.2). Heart and heart-lung recipients are more likely to have symptomatic infection than liver or kidney patients. Primary infections are almost always acquired from the donor organ(s). Speirs et al. (1988) reported that 57% heart, 20% liver and 0% kidney transplant recipients who were *T. gondii* antibody-negative before transplantation and who received organs from *T. gondii*-antibody-positive donors acquired primary *T. gondii* infection. *Toxoplasma gondii* is occasionally transmitted by donated kidneys, but this is an infrequent occurrence (Mason et al. 1987).

Reactivation of latent *T. gondii* infection in transplant patients is uncommon, but does occur. The incidence of reactivation is greater in patient groups receiving more aggressive immunosuppression. In the early period of the Papworth Hospital series of heart, heart-lung and lung transplant recipients, only five of 250 (2%) *T. gondii*-antibody-positive patients had serological evidence of *T. gondii* reactivation and only one was symptomatic (Wreghitt et al. 1989). One study has reported a high incidence of *T. gondii* reactivation after heart transplantation, but there were technical problems with the conduct of this study and most of the reported cases were false positive, a result of cross-reactions in the IgM serological assay employed to make the diagnosis (Luft et al. 1983). In the early years of transplantation, when high doses of immunosuppressive drugs were used, the rate of *T. gondii* reactivation was higher than that in patients who currently receive less aggressive triple therapy (low-dose cyclosporin A, steroids and azathioprine). Also the more recent use of co-trimoxazole prophylaxis for *Pneumocystis carinii* has virtually eliminated *T. gondii* reactivation in transplant recipients.

Toxoplasma gondii has much in common with cytomegalovirus (CMV) in transplant patients. Both produce the most serious symptoms in solid-organ recipients when infection is transmitted by the donor organ, and in both infections symptoms usually present 1–2 months after transplantation (Wreghitt et al. 1986). All symptomatic solid-organ transplant recipients with primary *T. gondii* infection have fever. Some also have one or more of the following symptoms: pneumonia, encephalitis and myocarditis (Luft et al. 1983; Sluiters et al. 1989; Wreghitt et al. 1989).

Heart/lung transplants

Several studies have documented *T. gondii* infections in heart, heart-lung and lung transplant recipients (Luft et al. 1983; Wreghitt et al. 1986; Sluiters et al. 1989; Andersson et al. 1992; Orr et al. 1994; Gallino et al. 1996). In our study of 250 patients transplanted at Papworth Hospital, Cambridge, of seven *T. gondii*-antibody-negative recipients of organs from *T. gondii*-antibody-positive donors, four (57%) acquired primary infection and two died (Wreghitt et al. 1986) (Table 6.3). Other series of transplant patients have reported a similar percentage of *T. gondii*-mismatched patients acquiring primary infection (Sluiters et al. 1989 – 50%; Gallino et al. 1996 – 61%). Primary infections are almost always symptomatic with symptoms occurring in the fourth week after transplantation.

Reactivation of *T. gondii* after transplantation in *T. gondii*-antibody-positive

Table 6.3. Effect of pyrimethamine prophylaxis on the development of *T. gondii* infection and symptoms in *T. gondii* antibody-negative patients who received hearts from *T. gondii* antibody-positive donors

No anti-*T. gondii* prophylaxis			Pyrimethamine anti-*T. gondii* prophylaxis		
No. of patients *T. gondii* antibody donor positive, recipient negative	No. (%) of patients with primary *T. gondii* infection	No. (%) of patients with symptoms	No. of patients *T. gondii* antibody donor positive, recipient negative	No. (%) of patients with primary *T. gondii* infection	No (%) patients with symptoms
7	4 (57%)	4 (100%)	83	8 (10%)	1 (1.2%)

recipients is relatively rare and is almost certainly more frequent if severe immuno-suppressive regimes are employed. In this latest period of our Papworth series, 1.2% *T. gondii*-antibody-positive recipients studied over a period of at least a year after transplantation had a significant rise in *T. gondii* IgG, consistent with *T. gondii* reactivation. Reactivation was noted on days 30, 75 and 270 after transplantation. This compared with 2% in the earlier period when more aggressive immuno-suppression was used (Wreghitt et al. 1989). Two patients were symptomatic; both had fever, one also had enlarged cervical nodes, rash and malaise, the second had a lower lobe pneumonia. Additionally the two patients in the earlier period who survived primary *T. gondii* infection after appropriate treatment had a series of asymptomatic *T. gondii* reactivations at two-yearly intervals (Wreghitt et al. 1989).

Kidney transplants

The risk of donor-acquired *T. gondii* infection in kidney recipients is much lower than in heart and liver recipients and is probably around 1%. However, some donors have transmitted *T. gondii* infection to both recipients of kidneys (Mason et al. 1987; Renoult et al. 1997), probably because the donor had recently acquired the *T. gondii* infection. Renoult et al. (1997) reported five primary *T. gondii* infections in 373 consecutive kidney transplants performed between 1989 and 1995, including four cases where infection was acquired from two donors. Patients first developed symptoms on days 15–41 after transplantation and symptoms included fever, cough, pneumonia, leukopenia and encephalitis, and two of the five patients died.

Several studies have documented *T. gondii* infection in kidney transplant recipient (Mejia et al. 1983; Mason et al. 1987; Rostaing et al. 1995; Renoult et al. 1997). Many of these cases were first diagnosed post mortem. Most symptoms arose in the first month after transplantation, but one patient first had *T. gondii*-related symptoms at 13 months.

It is difficult to estimate the incidence of *T. gondii* reactivation in kidney transplant recipients, since no prospective studies of patients who are *T. gondii* antibody positive at the time of transplantation have been conducted. However, the incidence is probably low. Renoult et al. (1997), in a review of *T. gondii* infection in kidney transplant recipients, documented several patients with *T. gondii* reactivation. Patients had fever, thrombocytopaenia, pneumonia and encephalitis and some died. These infections were documented because they were symptomatic and there are no data on the incidence of asymptomatic *T. gondii* reactivations. The overall mortality of primary and reactivated *T. gondii* infections reported by Renoult et al. (1997) was 64.5%.

Liver transplants

There are fewer reports of *T. gondii* infection in liver transplant recipients (Anthony 1972; Wreghitt 1987; Lappalainen et al. 1988; Mayes et al. 1995; Blanc-Jouvan et al. 1996) and most are single case reports. We reviewed *T. gondii* infections in 54 liver transplant recipients in Cambridge (Wreghitt 1987). Two cases of *T. gondii* infection were identified: one was a donor-acquired primary infection who developed grand mal fits one month after transplantation and subsequently died. The second case experienced *T. gondii* reactivation one month after transplantation and died one month later with reactivated CMV disease.

Both primary and reactivated *T. gondii* infections have been reported in liver transplant recipients, with an overall mortality of 80%. Patients usually develop symptoms a month after transplantation, which include fever, pneumonia, encephalitis, chorioretinitis and multi-organ failure.

Extensive prospective studies to establish the incidence of *T. gondii* infection in liver transplant recipients have not been reported, but Speirs et al. (1988) reported that 20% of *T. gondii*-antibody-negative recipients of livers from *T. gondii*-antibody-positive donors acquired primary *T. gondii* infection. Asymptomatic *T. gondii* reactivation infection probably occurs, but with unknown frequency. *Toxoplasma gondii* infection should be considered in liver transplant patients with fever, pneumonia, retinochoroiditis or encephalitis, especially in the first few months after transplantation.

Bone marrow transplants

Bone marrow transplant recipients are at high risk of acquiring opportunistic infections, including toxoplasmosis. There are many reports of *T. gondii* infections in bone marrow transplant recipients (Lowenberg et al. 1983; Hirsch et al. 1984; Derouin et al. 1992; Israelski & Remington 1993*a*; McCabe & Chirurgi 1993; Slavin et al. 1994; Bretagne et al. 1995; Chandrasekar & Momin 1997). Most infections are reactivations occurring in *T. gondii*-antibody-positive recipients; however, some primary infections in *T. gondii*-antibody-negative recipients have been reported (Chandrasekar & Momin 1997).

Shepp et al. (1985) reported an incidence of 0.5% (10 in 2000) cases of toxoplasmosis in bone marrow transplant recipients at the Fred Hutchinson Cancer Research Centre. Later, Slavin et al. (1994) reported an incidence of 0.31% (12 in 3803) cases of toxoplasmosis over a 20-year period in bone marrow recipients. The median day of clinical presentation of symptoms (encephalitis, fever, pneumonitis, myocarditis) was 59 days after transplantation (range 35–97 days). Eleven patients had graft versus host disease (GVHD) and all died. An increased incidence of toxoplasmosis after treatment for GVHD has also been reported by Beclen et al. (1986), Derouin et al. (1986) and Martino et al. (2000). Derouin et al. (1992) reported an incidence of 2.3% (7 in 296) of toxoplasmosis in bone marrow recipients. Enhanced immunosuppression exposes patients to an increased risk of toxoplasmosis after bone marrow transplantation.

Malignancy

Symptomatic reactivation of toxoplasma infection in patients with malignancies is relatively rare, despite *T. gondii* antibody prevalences worldwide ranging from 30% to 80%. Vietzke et al. (1968) reported six cases in a 5-year period and a further 39 cases identified at another centre over an 11-year period have been reported (Carey et al. 1973; Hawkes & Armstrong 1983). In the latter group, Hodgkin's disease was the most commonly occurring malignancy and the incidence of toxoplasmosis was estimated to be about 3% compared with rates in chronic lymphatic leukaemia and breast cancer of 366 and 2 per 10,000 patients respectively (Hawkes & Armstrong 1983).

Extensive reviews of toxoplasmosis in immunocompromised (nonAIDS) patients (Ruskin & Remington 1976; Israelski & Remington 1993b) have confirmed the predominance of Hodgkin's disease as the underlying condition in some 40% of the cases reviewed by the authors. Toxoplasmosis has also been reported in association with non-Hodgkin's lymphoma and acute and chronic lymphatic and myeloid leukaemia (Wertlake & Winter 1965; Strannegard et al. 1971; Carey et al. 1973; Re et al. 1999). Hairy-cell leukaemia (leukaemic reticuloendotheliosis) has been reported as being associated with a high incidence (21%) of reactivated toxoplasma infection (Knecht et al. 1986). Other malignancies that have occasionally been reported include multiple myeloma (Theologides et al. 1966) and angioimmunoblastic lymphadenopathy (Narasimham et al. 1979). Reports of *T. gondii* reactivation with solid tumours are very uncommon. However, in patients who have received chemotherapy, *T. gondii* reactivation occurs more frequently (Hawkes & Armstrong 1983).

Virtually any system in the body can be involved as a result of toxoplasma reactivation but the commonest sites are the central nervous system (CNS) and eye followed by the heart and lungs (Israelski & Remington 1993a). Myositis has been noted in patients with hairy-cell leukamia (Knecht et al. 1986). However, widely disseminated toxoplasma infection has also been described (Cohen 1970). The presenting signs and symptoms (Table 6.4), e.g. altered mental state, focal neurological signs, impaired visual acuity, congestive heart failure, bundle branch block,

Table 6.4. *Toxoplasma gondii* infection in patients with malignancies

Type of malignancy	Symptoms	Suggested treatment regimen
Lymphoma	Encephalitis Pyrexia Lymphadenopathy Hepatosplenomegaly Retinochoroiditis Pneumonitis	Pyrimethamine 100 mg orally twice daily for 1 day then 25–50 mg orally daily for 3–4 weeks or until symptoms resolve
Leukaemia	Fever Encephalitis Rash Myocarditis Pneumonitis Hepatosplenomegaly	Plus Sulphadiazine 50–100 mg/kg (up to 8g) orally daily (divided doses) for 3–4 weeks or until symptoms resolve
Other malignancies including: • angioimmunoblastic lymphadenopathy • breast cancer • melanoma • myeloma	Pyrexia Lymphadenopathy Encephalitis Myocarditis	Plus Folinic acid (leucovorin) 5–10 mg orally daily for 3–4 weeks or until symptoms resolve N.B. Haematological monitoring due to risk of bone marrow suppression

dyspnoea and cough, will, of course, depend upon the organ(s) involved. Fever is frequently present (Israelski & Remington 1993*b*).

It has been postulated that toxoplasma infection is a risk factor for gliomas (Schuman et al. 1967) but a later study found no link between toxoplasma infection and glioma but a possible association with meningioma (Ryan et al. 1993).

Co-infections with CMV have been frequently demonstrated in patients with cancer who have developed toxoplasmosis (McCabe 1990). It has been suggested that CMV infection may predispose the patient to toxoplasmosis as CMV is immunosuppressive and has been shown to produce reactivation of toxoplasma in animal models (Pomeroy et al. 1989).

Corticosteroids and anti-cancer chemotherapy

The immunosuppressive effects of large doses and extended courses of corticosteroids are well known and thus it is not surprising that reactivation of toxoplasma infection has been reported in patients treated with these drugs (Townsend et al.

1975). Corticosteroids are, of course, often given in combination with cytotoxic drugs to patients with malignancies or other potentially immunosuppressive disease, and it is therefore difficult to ascertain which drugs cause the reactivation to occur. The treatment of toxoplasmic retinochoroditis with corticosteroids alone (i.e. without concomitant antitoxoplasma therapy) has been reported to result in the worsening of the eye disease, leading to blindness or deterioration of the eye (O'Connor & Frenkel 1976).

Reactivation of latent infection has been reported in patients receiving anticancer chemotherapy (Hawkes & Armstrong 1983) but it is uncertain whether the immunosuppression resulting in reactivation was due to the therapy or the underlying disease.

Connective tissue disease

An association between toxoplasmosis and systemic lupus erythematosus (SLE) has been mooted in the past but reactivation of infection is invariably linked to concurrent treatment with corticosteroids. Recurrent congenital toxoplasmosis in two consecutive pregnancies has been reported in a woman with SLE treated with corticosteroids (D'Ercole et al. 1995).

Treatment and prophylaxis

Although the morbidity and mortality of untreated, reactivated *T. gondii* infection in patients with malignancy have been reported as being very high (98%) (Israelski & Remington 1993*a*), antitoxoplasma chemotherapy resulted in an improvement in 68%. (Similar results have been shown in organ transplant recipients.) At the present time, the treatment of choice is still a combination of pyrimethamine, sulphadiazine and folinic acid, which should be given until the signs and symptoms of the toxoplasma infection have resolved (Table 6.4). It is, however, important to be alert to the potential toxic effect of these antibiotics on the bone marrow which may possibly be exacerbated by concomitant anticancer chemotherapy.

The need for suppressive or maintenance antitoxoplasma therapy in *T. gondii*-antibody-positive patients with malignancies is uncertain but this may well be required while the patient remains immunosuppressed whether due to the underlying disease or as a result of treatment for that particular disease.

The benefit of prophylaxis against *T. gondii* in *T. gondii*-antibody-negative heart transplant recipients who receive organs from *T. gondii*-antibody-positive donors has been demonstrated. In our Papworth series of heart and heart-lung transplant recipients, a 6-week prophylactic course of pyrimethamine (25 mg/day) significantly reduced the incidence of donor-acquired primary *T. gondii* infection from 57% to 14% (Wreghitt et al. 1989, 1992). Subsequently, in an enlarged series of patients, transmission has been reduced to 10% (Table 6.3). Sluiters et al. (1989) showed that spiramycin prophylaxis was ineffective in preventing donor-acquired *T. gondii* infection in heart transplant recipients. Orr et al. (1994) showed that Trimethoprim–sulphamethoxazole (co-trimoxazole) prophylaxis to prevent *Pneumocystis carinii* infection after a heart transplant also effectively reduced the incidence of donor-acquired *T. gondii* infection. Of nine patients studied, three received 480 mg co-trimoxazole twice daily orally for 3 months and one acquired *T. gondii* infection with symptoms of fever, malaise, nausea and abdominal pain. Six patients received 960 mg co-trimoxazole twice daily orally three times a week for 3 months; none acquired *T. gondii* infection. Following this report, we investigated the incidence of *T. gondii* infection in Papworth heart transplant recipients who had been given co-trimoxazole prophylaxis (for *Pneumocystis carinii*) (480 mg daily for 1 year). None of the 28 *T. gondii* mismatched patients who received co-trimoxazole prophylaxis acquired *T. gondii* infection as judged by serology (Wreghitt et al. 1995).

Because of the significant risk of donor-acquired *T. gondii* infection in heart and liver transplant recipients, we feel that patients should be investigated for donor and recipient *T. gondii* antibody status and given prophylaxis for at least 3 months if the recipient is *T. gondii* antibody-negative and the donor *T. gondii* antibody-positive.

The identification of 'toxoplasma mismatches', i. e. an organ from a toxoplasma antibody-positive donor being transplanted into a toxoplasma antibody-negative recipient, together with the administration of prophylaxis markedly reduces the risk of an acute toxoplasma infection. However, if it does occur antitoxoplasma chemotherapy must be instituted. The suggested treatment of choice is a combination of pyrimethamine, sulphadiazine and folinic acid (leucovorin), which should be continued for 4–6 weeks after resolution of the infection. If the use of sulphamonamide is contraindicated because of side-effects clindamycin can be substituted.

However, as this regimen has a potentially toxic effect on bone marrow, its use may be inappropriate when toxoplasma reactivation occurs in bone marrow transplants. Atovaquone and azithromycin are suggested alternative treatments in this circumstance (Table 6.5).

Diagnosis

The clinical diagnosis of toxoplasmosis in immunosuppressed patients can be difficult and the signs and symptoms of the infection such as lymphadenopathy, fever and focal lesion in the brain can also be caused by malignancies. Clinical awareness and acumen are the key to the appropriate management of such patients.

Table 6.5. Suggested treatment regimens in transplant patients for acute toxoplasma infection

Patient group	Treatment
Heart liver and kidney transplant recipients	
Adults	Pyrimethamine 100 mg orally twice daily for 1 day then 25–50 mg daily for 4–6 weeks after resolution of infection; plus sulphadiazine 50–100 mg/kg (up to 8g) orally daily – duration as for pyrimethamine; plus folinic acid (leucovorin) 5–10 mg orally – duration as for pyrimethamine.
Children	Pyrimethamine 2 mg/kg orally daily for 3–4 days then 1 mg/kg orally daily for 4–6 weeks after resolution of infection; plus sulphadiazine 100 mg/kg orally daily – duration as for pyrimethamine; plus folinic acid (leucovorin) 5–10 mg orally daily – duration as for pyrimethamine.
Bone marrow transplant recipients	
Possible alternative treatments to be considered:	Atovaquone 750 mg (liquid form) orally three times daily; or azithromycin 500 mg orally daily.
Prophylaxis in heart and liver transplant patients (adult)	Trimethoprim-sulphamethoxazole (co-trimoxazole) 480 mg orally twice daily for 6 weeks post transplant.
Alternative treatment	Pyrimethamine 25 mg orally daily for 6 weeks post transplant plus folinic acid (leucovorin) 5–10 mg orally daily – duration as for pyrimethamine.

The laboratory diagnosis of primary *T. gondii* infection or reactivation (Chapter 12) is usually serological with the demonstration of an increase in IgG titres when serum samples taken at different times are tested in parallel or by the appearance of *T. gondii* IgM. Serology may occasionally be unhelpful and demonstration of the organism by culture or nucleic acid detection (e.g. polymerase chain reaction,

PCR) or histopathological special stains may be required. However, diagnosis in bone marrow recipients is more difficult.

Most cases of toxoplasmosis in bone marrow transplant recipients have been diagnosed post mortem (84% in the series reported by Slavin et al. 1994). Serology is often not useful in these patients, since most are not capable of mounting a good antibody response. The diagnosis, therefore, may require either PCR, culture or histopathology to be done. *Toxoplasma gondii* infection should be considered in antibody-positive bone marrow transplant recipients with compatible symptoms (diffuse encephalitis, myocarditis, fever or pneumonia), and even in apparently *T. gondii*-antibody-negative patients, although the likelihood of infection is much lower.

The determination of baseline *T. gondii* antibody status in serum samples collected when the underlying cause of immunosuppression (especially haematological and lymphoproliferative malignancies) presents, and in organ recipients and donors prior to transplantation cannot be overemphasized.

Summary

Toxoplasmosis should be considered in *T. gondii*-antibody-positive patients with malignancies, on large doses of corticosteroids or in transplant recipients if they experience myocarditis, pneumonia or encephalitis in the first year after disease presentation or immunosuppression. *Toxoplasma gondii*-antibody-negative recipients of organs from *T. gondii*-antibody-positive donors are at increased risk of infection; prophylaxis should be provided for heart and liver recipients. Patients with symptoms compatible with toxoplasma infection should be treated while laboratory diagnosis is being conducted. Determination of the baseline toxoplasma antibody status of immunosuppressed patients is essential. Since many infections are only recognized post mortem clinical suspicion of *T. gondii* infection is paramount.

REFERENCES

Andersson, R., Sandberg, T., Berglin, E. & Jeansson, S. (1992). CMV infections and toxoplasmosis in heart transplant recipients in Sweden. *Scandinavian Journal of Infectious Diseases*, **24**, 411–17.

Anthony, C. W. (1972). Disseminated toxoplasmosis in a liver transplant patient. *Journal of the American Medical Womens Association*, **27**, 601–3.

Beclen, D. W., Mahmoud, H. K., Mlynek, M. I., et al. (1986). Toxoplasmosis after bone marrow transplantations. *Immunitat und infection*, **5**, 183–7.

Blanc-Jouvan, M., Boibieux, J., Fleury, N., Fortel, N., Gandilhon, F., Dupouy-Camet, J., Peyron,

F. & Ducert, C. (1996). Chorioretinitis following liver transplantation: detection of *Toxoplasma gondii* in aqueous humor. *Clinical Infectious Diseases*, 22, 184–5.

Bretagne, S., Costa, J. M., Kuentz, M. et al. (1995). Late toxoplasmosis evidenced by PCR in a marrow transplant recipient. *Bone Marrow Transplantation*, 15, 809–11.

Carey, R. M., Kimball, A. C., Armstrong, D. & Leiberman, P. H. (1973). Toxoplasmosis: clinical experiences in a cancer hospital. *American Journal of Medicine*, 54, 30–8.

Chandrasekar, P. H. & Momin, F. (1997). Disseminated toxoplasmosis in marrow recipients: a report of three cases and a review of the literature. *Bone Marrow Transplantation*, 19, 685–9.

Cohen, S. M. (1970). Toxoplasmosis in patients receiving immunosuppressive therapy. *Journal of American Medical Association*, 211, 657– 60.

D'Ercole, C., Boubli, L., Frank, J., Costa, M., Harle, J. R., Chagnon, C., Cravello, L., Leclaire, M. & Blanc, B. (1995). Recurrent congenital toxoplasmosis in a woman with lupus erythematosis. *Prenatal Diagnosis*, 15, 1171–5.

Derouin, F., Gluckman, E., Beauvais, B., et al. (1986). Toxoplasma infection after human allogeneic bone marrow transplantation: clinical and serological study of 80 patients. *Bone Marrow Transplantation*, 1, 67–73.

Derouin, F., Devergie, A., Auber, P., et al. (1992). Toxoplasmosis in bone marrow-transplant recipients: report of seven cases and review. *Clinical Infectious Diseases*, 15, 267–70.

Gallino, A., Maggiorini, M., Kiowski, W., Martin, X., Wonderli, W., Schneider, J., Turina, M. & Follath, F. (1996). Toxoplasmosis in heart transplant recipients. *European Journal of Clinical Microbiology and Infectious Diseases*, 15, 389–93.

Hawkes, T. B. & Armstrong, D. (1983). Toxoplasmosis: problems in diagnosis and treatment. *Cancer*, 52, 1535–40.

Hirsch, R., Burke, B. A. & Kersey, J. H. (1984). Toxoplasmosis in bone marrow transplant recipients. *Journal of Pediatrics*, 105, 426–8.

Israelski, D. M. & Remington, J. S. (1993a). Toxoplasmosis in patients with cancer. *Clinical Infectious Diseases*, 17 [Suppl. 2], S423–5.

Israelski, D. M. & Remington, J. S. (1993b). Toxoplasmosis in the non-AIDS immunocompromised host. In *Current Clinical Topics in Infectious Diseases*, vol. 13, ed. J. S. Remington & M. N. Swartz, pp. 322–56. Oxford: Blackwell Scientific Publications.

Knecht, H., Rhuner, K. & Struli, R. A. (1986). Toxoplasmosis in hairy-cell leukaemia. *British Journal of Haematology*, 62, 65–73.

Lappalainen, M., Jokiranta, T. S., Halme, L., Tynninen, O., Lautenschlager, I., Hedman, K., Hockerstedt, K. & Meri, S. (1988). Disseminated toxoplasmosis after liver transplantation: case report and review. *Clinical Infectious Diseases*, 27, 1327–8.

Lowenberg, B., van Gijn, J., Prins, E. & Polderman, A. M. (1983). Fatal cerebral toxoplasmosis in a bone marrow transplant recipient with leukaemia. *Transplantation*, 35, 30–4.

Luft, B. J., Naot, Y., Araujo, F. G., Stinson, E. B. & Remington, J. S. (1983). Primary and reactivated Toxoplasma infection in patients with cardiac transplants. Clinical spectrum and problems in diagnosis in a defined population. *Annals of Internal Medicine*, 99, 27–31.

Martino, R., Maertens, J., Bretagne, S., Rovira, M., Deconinck, E., Ullman, A. J. & Held, T. (2000). Toxoplasmosis after hematopoietic stem cell transplantation. *Clinical Infectious Disease*, 31, 1188–94.

Mason, J. C., Ordelheide, K. S., Grames, G. M., Thrasher, T. V., Harris, R. D., Bui, R. H. D. & Mackett, M. C. T. (1987). Toxoplasmosis in two renal transplant recipients from a single donor. *Transplantation*, **44**, 588–91.

Mayes, J. T., O'Connor, B. J., Avery, R., Castellani, W. & Carey, W. (1995). Transmission of *Toxoplasma gondii* infection by liver transplantation. *Clinical Infectious Diseases*, **21**, 511–15.

McCabe, R. E. (1990). Current diagnosis and management of toxoplasmosis in cancer patients. *Oncology*, **4**, 81–90.

McCabe, R. & Chirurgi, V. (1993). Issues in toxoplasmosis. *Infectious Disease Clinics of North America*, **7**, 587–604.

Mejia, G., Leiderman, E., Builes, M. et al. (1983). Transmission of toxoplasmosis by renal transplant. *American Journal of Kidney Diseases*, **2**, 615–17.

Narasimham, P., Ahn, B. H., Levy, R. N. & Glasberg, S. S. (1979). Immunoblastic lymphadenopathy: high serum toxoplasma titres. *New York State Journal of Medicine*, **79**, 241–4.

O'Connor, G. R. & Frenkel, J. K. (1976). Dangers of steroid treatment in toxoplasmosis. *Archives of Ophthalmology*, **94**, 213.

Orr, K. E., Gould, F. K., Short, G., Dark, J. H., Hilton, C. J., Corris, P. A. & Freeman, R. (1994). Outcome of *Toxoplasma gondii* mismatches in heart transplant recipients over a period of 8 years. *Journal of Infection*, **29**, 249–53.

Pomeroy, C., Kline, E., Jordan, M. C. & Felice, G. A. (1989). Reactivation of *Toxoplasma gondii* by cytomegalovirus disease in mice. Antimicrobial activities of macrophages. *Journal of Infectious Diseases*, **160**, 305–11.

Re, D., Reiser, M., Bamborschke, S., Schröder, R., Lehroke, R., Tosch, H., Salzberger, B., Diehe, V. & Fätkenheuer, L. (1999). Two cases of toxoplasmic encephalitis in patients with acute T-cell leukaemia and lymphoma. *Journal of Infection*, **38**, 26–9.

Renoult, E., Georges, E., Biava, M.-F., Hulin, C., Frimat, L., Hestin, D. & Kessler, M. (1997). Toxoplasmosis in kidney transplant recipients: report of six cases and review. *Clinical Infectious Diseases*, **24**, 625–34.

Rostaing, L., Baron, E., Fillola, O. et al. (1995). Toxoplasmosis in two renal transplant recipients: diagnosis by bone marrow aspiration. *Transplantation Proceedings*, **27**, 1733–4.

Ruskin, J. & Remington, J. S. (1976). Toxoplasmosis in the compromised host. *Annals Internal Medicine*, **84**, 193–9.

Ryan, P., Hurley, S., Johnson, A., Saltzberg, M., Lee, M. W., North, J. B., McNeil, J. J. & McMichael, A. J. (1993). Tumours of the brain and presence of antibodies to *Toxoplasma gondii*. *International Journal of Epidemiology*, **22**, 412–19.

Schuman, L. M., Choi, N. W. & Gullen, W. H. (1967). Relationship of central nervous system neoplasms to *Toxoplasma gondii* infection. *American Journal of Public Health*, **57**, 848–56.

Shepp, D. H., Hackman, R. C., Conley, F. K., Anderson, J. B. & Myers, D. J. (1985). Toxoplasma reactivation identified by parasitaemia in tissue culture. *Annals of Internal Medicine*, **103**, 218–21.

Slavin, M. A., Meyers, J. D., Remington, J. S. & Hartsman, R. C. (1994). *Toxoplasma gondii* infection in bone marrow transplant recipients: a 20 year experience. *Bone Marrow Transplantations*, **13**, 549–57.

Sluiters, J. F., Balk, A. H., Essed, C. E., Mochtar, B., Weimar, W., Simoons, M. L. & Ijzerman, E.

P. (1989). Indirect ELISA for IgG and four immunoassays for IgM to *Toxoplasma gondii* in a series of heart transplant recipients. *Journal of Clinical Microbiology*, 27, 529–35.

Speirs, G. E., Hakim, M., Calne, R. Y. & Wreghitt, T. G. (1988). Relative risk of donor-transmitted *Toxoplasma gondii* infection in heart, liver and kidney transplant recipients. *Clinical Transplantation*, 2, 257–60.

Strannegard, O., Holm, S. E., Weinfeld, A. & Westin, J. (1971). Serological studies of infections in patients with haematologic malignancy. *Scandinavian Journal of Infectious Diseases*, 5, 181–6.

Theologides, A., Osterberg, K. & Kennedy, B. J. (1966). Cerebral toxoplasmosis in multiple myeloma. *Annals of Internal Medicine*, 64, 1071–4.

Townsend, J. J., Wolinksy, J. S., Baringer, J. R. & Johnson, P. C. (1975). Acquired toxoplasmosis: a neglected cause of treatable nervous system disease. *Archives Neurology*, 21, 335–43.

Vietzke, W. M., Gelderman, A. H., Grimley, P. M. & Valsamis, M. P. (1968). Toxoplasmosis complicating malignancy: experience at the National Cancer Institute. *Cancer*, 21, 816–27.

Wertlake, P. T. & Winter, T. S. (1965). Fatal toxoplasma myocarditis in an adult patient with acute lymphocytic leukaemia. *New England Journal of Medicine*, 118, 782–7.

Wreghitt, T. G. (1987). Viral and *Toxoplasma gondii* infections. In *Liver Transplantation*, ed. R. Y. Calne, pp. 365–83. Grune and Stratton, New York.

Wreghitt, T. G., Hakim, M., Cory-Pearce, R., English, T. A. H. & Wallwork, J. (1986). The impact of donor-transmitted CMV and *Toxoplasma gondii* disease in cardiac transplantation. *Transplantation Proceedings*, XVIII, 1375–6.

Wreghitt, T. G., Hakim, M., Gray, J. J., Balfour, A. H., Stovin, P. G. I., Stewart, S., Scott, J., English, T. A. H. & Wallwork, J. (1989). Toxoplasmosis in heart and heart and lung transplant recipients. *Journal of Clinical Pathology*, 42, 194–9.

Wreghitt, T. G., Gray, J. J., Pavel, P., et al. (1992). Efficacy of pyrimethamine for the prevention of donor-required *Toxoplasma gondii* infection in heart and heart-lung transplant patients. *Transplant International*, 5, 197–200.

Wreghitt, T. G., McNeil, K., Roth, C., et al. (1995). Antibiotic prophylaxis for the prevention of donor-acquired *Toxoplasma gondii* in transplant patients. *Journal of Infection*, 31, 253–4.

7

Maternal and foetal infection

P. Thulliez

Institute de Puériculture de Paris, ADHMI, Laboratoire de Serologie et de Recherche sur la Toxoplasmose, Paris, France

In recent years, significant progress has been made in the early diagnosis of toxoplasma infection in the mother, the foetus and the newborn. The management of women infected during pregnancy has been greatly improved by the ability to diagnose the infection prenatally; also, the treatment of congenital infection is now initiated before birth. However, the prevention of infection in pregnant women should be reinforced with education about hygiene; in addition, advances in the prevention of late sequellae in infected offsprings should be made by using optimal treatments that have yet to be evaluated.

Maternal infection

Every instance of primary maternal toxoplasmosis occuring during pregnancy exposes the foetus to the risk of infection via the transplacental route, whereas the foetus is protected when maternal infection is prior to pregnancy. However, rare cases of congenital infection as the result of a maternal infection primarily acquired before pregnancy have been reported, either in immunocompromised women or in women infected shortly before conception.

Incidence

The rate of primary infection in pregnant women can be estimated by a serological follow-up of those who are susceptible (seronegative) at the beginning of pregnancy, or by age-specific seroprevalence surveys (Papoz et al. 1986; Ades & Nokes 1993). The prevalence of specific IgG antibodies indicating past exposure to toxoplasma may vary according to the sensitivity of the serological method used, but mainly depends on the epidemiological conditions pertaining to each geographical area. In the UK for instance, the incidence rate is 2 per 1000 pregnancies (Joynson 1992) whereas it is 5 per 1000 in the Paris area (Jeannel et al. 1988). It is thought that primary prevention with specific hygiene measures should reduce the incidence of infection. Foulon et al. (1994) reported a reduction in the number of seroconversions by 63% in seronegative women who had received written recommendations on how to avoid infection.

Clinical aspects

Primary infection acquired during pregnancy is asymptomatic in about 60% of cases (Daffos et al 1988) and the clinical features are the same as in other immunocompetent individuals. When present, signs and symptoms are mild and nonspecific: fatigue, malaise, low-grade fever, myalgia and lymphadenopathy. The latter may be localized or may involve multiple areas but it is more common in the neck; the most characteristic sign is a lymph node enlargement of the posterior cervical region. The lymphadenopathy can be tender for a few days and is unattached to the overlying skin; in some patients it may persist for several months but there is no tendency towards suppuration. Signs of acute infection are commonly unrecognized and symptoms are often so slight that they are not noticed by the patients; however, when the serology of a pregnant woman suggests a recent infection, it is especially important to search for symptoms by retrospective questioning, since the time of their onset may reliably indicate the time of infection with respect to the date of conception.

When enlarged nodes are present, the contemporaneous serological results usually suggest a recent infection: tests for specific IgG and IgM are positive. They seldom happen to be negative; the only time this may happen is when the patient's blood is sampled only a few days after the onset of the lymphadenopathy. The diagnosis of recent toxoplasmosis cannot be definitively excluded and the study of a later sample, 10 or 15 days after the previous one, should confirm the diagnosis.

Finally, because they occur rarely and are not particularly specific, the clinical features of acquired infection are not diagnostic and the identification of all primary infections occurring in a given population of pregnant women requires systematic serological screening.

Diagnosis

Very few countries have implemented a serological screening programme for toxoplasmosis, but some are discussing their introduction. Ideally, every woman should know her serological status before or very early in pregnancy, so that tests are repeatedly performed for those who are nonimmune in order to detect any seroconversion. The frequency of sampling differs in countries with a screening programme: it can be one per trimester, as in Austria (Aspöck & Pollak 1992), or one per month, as in France (Thulliez 1992); the latter allows for more rapid management after the onset of infection. Whatever screening programme is considered, it is particularly important that the last maternal serological test is performed at delivery or within the following 3 weeks so that infections acquired very late in pregnancy are not missed.

The laboratory diagnosis of a seroconversion is generally easy provided that serial sera sampled during pregnancy are examined together in the same series of tests. In these conditions, a high sensitivity to detect low titres of IgG and IgM is necessary for an early diagnosis of the infection. Since some methods for IgM can give false-positive results in the absence of a toxoplasma infection (Remington et al. 1995), seroconversion is definitively proven only if IgG is also demonstrated.

In the absence of seroconversion, the diagnosis of recent infection requires the demonstration of a rise in IgG antibody titre and the presence of IgM in serial serum specimens obtained during pregnancy, preferably 3 weeks apart, that are tested in parallel. To estimate the date of infection with regard to the date of conception, it is necessary to know the relationship between the kinetics of the IgG titre and the serological method used. A stable IgG titre means that infection was acquired at least 2 months before the first specimen was obtained. However, patients are often evaluated late in pregnancy and also IgM antibodies may sometimes be detected for over a year after the infection (Remington et al. 1995). Thus, in certain cases when IgM antibodies are detected it may be unclear whether the infection was acquired during or prior to pregnancy. With this problem in mind, various serological tests have been developed to differentiate between recent and past infection.

Specific IgA antibodies may be detected in acutely infected patients, but IgA production varies greatly across a population (Bessières et al., 1992; Francis & Joynson, 1993) and the results can also differ according to the commercial kits used for assay (Decoster et al. 1995). Furthermore, IgA cannot be demonstrated in some seroconversions occurring during pregnancy (Wong et al. 1993).

Pinon et al. (1990) detected specific IgE antibodies with immunosorbent agglutination assay (ISAGA) in sera from 25 (86%) out of 29 women who either seroconverted or had a rising IgG titre and the presence of IgM during pregnancy. IgE antibodies had been present for less than 4 months in 23 serially tested patients. In another study of eight seroconverters during pregnancy, IgE antibodies were detected with both ISAGA and enzyme-linked immunosorbent assay (ELISA) in the first sample, which was positive in dye-test and IgM-ISAGA (Wong et al. 1993). The antibodies had been present for a varied length of time, i. e. from 7 to 36 weeks. The authors emphasized that variations of IgE titres were also observed in an individual patient and between the two methods evaluated. In their study of patients with lymphadenopathy, Ashburn et al. (1995) reported results indicating that IgE may persist for up to 9 months and suggested that patients with persisting symptoms may produce more IgE than asymptomatic patients.

Other methods for measuring IgG antibodies specific to the acute stage of infection seem to be less susceptible to individual variations. The differential agglu-tination (HS/AC) test compares the IgG titres obtained with formalin-fixed tachy-zoites (HS antigen) with those obtained with methanol-fixed tachyzoites (AC antigen) (Dannemann et al. 1990). Suzuki et al. (1988) reported that the AC prep-aration contains stage-specific antigens that are recognized by IgG antibodies early in infection. This method is helpful in routine testing for pregnant women whose sera contain both IgM and IgG titres of around 100 IU, in order to define whether infection has been recently acquired. In these conditions, the high predictive value of a nonacute pattern excludes an infection acquired during pregnancy. Hedman et al. (1989) developed an ELISA to measure the antigen binding avidity of specific IgG using urea to elute the low avidity IgG associated with recent infection. Several studies using different ELISAs showed that this method could appropriately distin-guish between sera taken at the early stage of infection from those taken 3–6 months after infection (Joynson et al. 1990; Lecolier & Pucheu 1993; Holliman et al. 1994). Under screening conditions, results suggest that measuring IgG avidity is suitable for verifying acute primary infection during pregnancy and serves as a very useful adjunct to currently available tests (Lappalainen et al. 1993).

In conclusion, the demonstration of seroconversion or a rise in IgG titre with the presence of IgM enables the date of infection to be assessed in most cases. The differential agglutination test or the avidity ELISA may clarify the situation in other cases of suspected recent toxoplasmosis infection, while the demonstration of a low IgG avidity can be helpful in determining the risk for the pregnancy.

Infection before pregnancy

Although the development of maternal immunity before conception should prevent the infection from being transmitted to the foetus, a few cases of congeni-tal infection have been reported in infants born to women who had a primary infec-tion before conception. There have been three reports of immunologically normal women who had acquired toxoplasma within 3 months before conception and who then transmitted the infection to their foetus (Desmonts et al. 1990; Marty et al. 1991; Pons et al. 1995). In two cases a rise in IgG titres was observed after a period of stable titres. These data suggest that a recrudescence of recent maternal infection occurred during pregnancy and was associated with a parasitaemia. Although these cases are very uncommon it seems justified to advise women with well-docu-mented recent infection to postpone pregnancy for at least 3 months. If the patient is already pregnant and the infection was acquired a few months before conception, a treatment with spiramycin could be given throughout pregnancy and ultrasound monitoring should be performed. One case report (Fortier et al. 1991) has raised the possibility of parasitaemia occurring in an immune pregnant woman due to toxoplasma reinfection by the ingestion of oocysts.

In the past, many studies have been performed to determine whether latent toxoplasma infection causes abortion. Very few of them report any substantial evidence suggesting that there is an association between past infection and sporadic abortion. This must be considered as exceedingly uncommon. In addition, no study has unequivocally proven that toxoplasmosis can cause recurrent abortion (Remington et al. 1995).

More examples of reactivation of a latent maternal infection and transmission to the foetus have been documented in women with a cell-mediated immunity defect. This has been associated with lupus erythematosus and pancytopaenia (both treated with corticosteroids), as well as in Hodgkin's disease and in human immunodeficiency virus (HIV) infection (Desmonts et al. 1990; Mitchell et al. 1990; Marty et al. 1994; D'Ercole et al. 1995). With the advent of pregnancies among such immunocompromised women, an increase in the prevalence of congenital infection in this population is to be feared. The demonstration of toxoplasma IgG antibodies, even if they are consistent with a past infection, should lead to a careful follow-up of the pregnancies. Women should at least receive spiramycin throughout their pregnancy, but treatment with pyrimethamine and sulphadiazine or trimethoprim and sulphamethoxazole may also be considered, especially in HIV-infected women. Furthermore, infants should be clinically and biologically followed-up as if they were born to mothers who were infected during their pregnancy.

Foetal infection

Infection of the placenta is a prerequisite for congenital transmission. The placenta is infected during the maternal parasitaemic phase, which results almost exclusively from a primary infection acquired after conception or extremely rarely from the reactivation of an infection prior to pregnancy. The placenta then acts as a source of parasites which are transmitted to the foetus almost immediately after maternal infection but possibly with a delay of several weeks or longer (Remington et al. 1995). Modifying factors may be the virulence of the *T. gondii* strain and the inoculum size, but the most important factor is the development of the placental blood flow. This is probably the reason why the later in pregnancy the maternal infection is acquired, the more frequently the infection is transmitted to the foetus.

Incidence

In the 1970s the rate of transmission of infection from mother to foetus was estimated to increase from about 14% in the first trimester to 29% in the second and 59% in the third (Desmonts & Couvreur 1984). More recent data obtained from French studies on the reliability of prenatal diagnosis reveal lower transmission rates (see Table 7.1). This may be attributed to early treatment with spiramycin which is given as soon as the maternal infection is proven or highly suspected on the basis of a monthly screening programme. Nevertheless, several drawbacks make it difficult to make comparisons between studies. For instance, in past surveys, rates of transmission could have been overestimated if they included mothers whose diagnosis of congenital infection had been made from their offspring. Other factors may contribute to the tendency to underestimate the risk of transmission:

- no recording of spontaneous abortions occurring before women are referred to centres for prenatal diagnosis;
- no examination of foetuses dead *in utero*;
- serological screening not continued until delivery – thus missing late maternal infections;
- infants apparently normal at birth but not followed-up until one year old.

One inevitable bias concerns the diagnosis of infection early in pregnancy, which is most often based on the demonstration of a high IgG titre or on other results rather than seroconversion. This can result in preconceptional infections being mistakenly thought of as having been acquired during pregnancy and, as a consequence, reducing the calculated rate of transmission. The use of a classification system and case definitions as proposed by Lebech et al. (1996) would help improve the data collected.

Clinical aspects

The severity of infection in the foetus depends upon the gestational age at the time of transmission of parasites and this, in turn, determines the manifestations of the infection.

If transplacental transmission occurs early, that is if the mother has acquired infection early and if there has only been a short delay before the parasites spread from the placenta to the foetus, a progressive disease will occur. This may result in foetal death *in utero* and spontaneous abortion, or in the delivery of a live child with signs of central nervous system involvement including hydrocephalus, meningoencephalitis, intracranial calcifications and chorioretinitis. Signs of generalized infection may also be present including hepatosplenomegaly, jaundice, rash, anaemia and thrombocytopaenia.

If transmission to the foetus occurs late, either because of late acquisition of infection by the mother or because of delayed spreading of parasites from the placenta to the foetus, the congenital infection will be subclinical at birth and may only present months or years after birth, usually as eye lesions.

Maternal infection early in pregnancy is rarely transmitted, but if it is it results in severe foetal infection. Conversely, late maternal infection is frequently transmitted but generally results in mild or subclinical foetal infection; as a consequence,

Table 7.1. Risk of congenital infection according to gestational age at the time of maternal infection

	Risk of congenital infection							
	Desmonts & Couvreur (1984)*			Pratlong et al. (1994)**			Hohlfeld et al. (1994)***		
	Before 1977			Period of survey					
				1985–1991			1983–1992		
Weeks of gestation	0–15	16–28	29–40	7–15	16–28	>28	3–14	15–26	27–34
Maternal infection	120	241	128	102	70	15	1398	745	38
Congenital infection	11	68	76	4	12	8	52	123	11
Transmission rate (%)	9.1	28.2	59.3	3.9	17.1	53.1	3.7	16.5	28.9

*Almost two-thirds of mothers were given spiramycin, 2–3 g daily for 1 month at least. Eleven foetal and neonatal deaths are not included.

**Mothers were given spiramycin, 3 g daily throughout pregnancy. Thirty-two children with a negative prenatal diagnosis were not followed-up.

***Mothers were given spiramycin, 3 g daily throughout pregnancy. The number of children lost to follow-up is not specified.

approximately 85% of live infants with congenital infection appear normal at birth (Remington et al. 1995).

In pregnancies in which dizygotic twins are involved, both placentas can be infected or one only can be infected so that one twin escapes infection. When both twins are infected, discrepancies in clinical findings are frequent; for example, one may have a subclinical infection while the other may be severely damaged. Thus, prenatal or postnatal diagnosis of infection in one twin should prompt investigation of the other (Couvreur et al 1976). Conversely, in monozygotic twins the risk of congenital infection is the same and the clinical pattern is usually very similar.

Prospective studies monitoring women infected during pregnancy can provide estimates of the incidence of severe consequences for the foetus. However, the rate of spontaneous abortion or stillbirth is poorly documented and is probably underestimated since women who acquire infection very early in pregnancy may be excluded from some studies (Berrebi et al. 1994) or not examined for evidence of toxoplasma infection before they miscarry. Desmonts and Couvreur (1984) reported 12 cases of foetal death and stillbirth out of 542 pregnancies; six with a maternal infection of the first trimester, five of the second trimester; and the date of maternal infection was unknown in the last case. *T. gondii* was isolated in five of seven foetuses examined. Another study of 206 maternal infections reported three intra-uterine deaths due to severe toxoplasmosis at 23, 24, and 30 weeks (Berrebi et al. 1994).

The consequences of foetal infection can also be evaluated by ultrasound examinations repeatedly performed during pregnancy. Of 20 infected foetuses from 190 maternal infections acquired after 7 weeks of gestation, Pratlong et al. (1994) reported abnormalities in four cases: one with hydrocephalus and three with hepatomegaly. Berrebi et al. (1994) reported one cerebral ventricular dilatation, one bilateral hydronephrosis and one growth retardation among 24 infected foetuses excluding three deaths *in utero*, from 163 mothers infected from 8 to 26 weeks of gestation. In a larger series of 148 foetal infections diagnosed among 2030 infected mothers, Daffos et al. (1994) reported the following frequencies of abnormal ultrasound findings according to the time of maternal infection:

- before 16 weeks: 31/52 foetuses (60%) of whom 48% had cerebral ventricular dilatation;
- between 17 and 23 weeks: 16/63 foetuses (25%) of whom 12% had cerebral ventricular dilatation but no case was identified among mothers with seroconversion after the 22nd week;
- after 24 weeks: 1/33 (3%) foetuses had abnormal ultrasound without ventricular dilatation.

Table 7.2. Signs in 27 infected foetuses with an abnormal ultrasound examination* (adapted from Hohlfeld *et al.* 1991)

Signs	n	(%)
Brain lesions		
• Ventricular dilatation	25	(93)
• Intracranial densities	6	(22)
Placental inflammation		
• Increased thickness	11	(41)
• Hyperdensity	2	(7)
Liver lesions		
• Intrahepatic densities	4	(15)
• Hepatomegaly	2	(7)
Ascites	5	(19)
• Pericardial effusion	2	(7)
• Pleural effusion	1	(4)

*One sign was observed in 13 cases and two or more in 14 cases.

Cerebral ventricular dilatation, usually bilateral and symmetrical, is the most common and characteristic sign (see Table 7.2); it occurs first in the occipital region before involving the entire lateral ventricles. Its evolution may be very rapid over a period of a few days and it is associated with a poor prognosis. Intracranial densities correspond to intracranical calcifications observed after birth; they are often poorly calcified at the time of prenatal diagnosis and less frequently demonstrated than ventricular dilatation (Hohlfeld et al. 1991). Other ultrasonographic signs correspond to placental inflammation, hepatic involvement and effusions, showing that foetal toxoplasmosis is a multisystemic disease. Some of the signs may be transient.

Ultrasound monitoring alone is not adequate for a definitive diagnosis of foetal infection because the above findings are not specific to toxoplasma infection. Additionally, their demonstration can be delayed since their appearance depends on the date of transmission and, above all, most infected foetuses are not severely damaged. Thus, study of foetal blood and/or amniotic fluid is required.

Laboratory diagnosis

Cordocentesis and amniocentesis are designed to detect the parasite in the foetal blood and/or amniotic fluid, to detect a specific foetal immune response and infection-related abnormalities which may be indicative of foetal infection.

Nonspecific laboratory abnormalities

Nonspecific biological tests of foetal blood sampled from 20 weeks of gestation include the determination of total IgM levels, glutamyltransferase and lactic dehydrogenase activities, and leucocyte, eosinophil and platelet counts. None of these tests is 100% reliable but, when grouped together, the results of the various tests have high predictive values (Daffos et al. 1988). Although these findings are not specific to foetal toxoplasma infection, abnormal results have been used to justify the start of treatment with pyrimethamine and sulphadiazine while awaiting the results of other tests. None of these abnormalities has been recognized as being predictive of the severity of foetal lesions.

Detection of a specific antibody response

Overall, specific IgM antibodies are detected in only 30% of infected foetuses when using ISAGA. The frequency of positive results increases with the gestational age at the time of sampling: 12% in foetuses from 22 to 24 weeks, 39% from 25 to 30 weeks and 59% from 30 to 34 weeks (Hohlfeld et al. 1994). No positive result has been reported before 22 weeks of gestation.

The suitability of serological examination of the foetus might be improved by the detection of specific IgA but few data are available. Decoster et al. (1992) detected IgA antibodies with ELISA in five of ten infected foetuses of which two had no IgM. With ISAGA, Bessières et al. (1992) reported four positive results for IgA and four for IgM among ten infected foetuses. With the same technique Pratlong et al. (1994) detected eight out of ten infected foetuses, which, in combination with IgM detection, gave an overall sensitivity of 65% in 20 infected foetuses.

However, a positive result for IgM or IgA must only be considered when contamination of the foetal blood sample by maternal blood has been ruled out by several tests: haematological indices, Betke–Kleihauer staining procedure and human chorionic gonadotropin measurement (Forestier et al. 1988). However, even when these tests seem to confirm the purity of the foetal blood, positive serological results must be interpreted with caution.

Demonstration of *Toxoplasma gondii*

Isolation of the parasite from foetal blood or amniotic fluid provides unequivocal proof of foetal infection (Desmonts et al. 1985). More recently the use of polymerase chain reaction (PCR) on amniotic fluid samples has proved a reliable diagnostic tool and significantly changed the diagnostic approach.

Isolation of *Toxoplasma gondii*

From 20 weeks of gestation, samples of 1.5–4 ml foetal blood and 10–30 ml amniotic fluid can be sampled for analysis. A pellet of amniotic fluid or whole-blood clot is injected intraperitoneally or subcutaneously into mice. Approximately 5–10 days after intraperitoneal injection, the peritoneal fluid can be examined either fresh or in stained smears for the presence of intracellular and extracellular tachyzoites. Mice that die before 6 weeks are examined for the presence of the organism. With rare exceptions, isolates from infected foetuses are relatively avirulent for mice, and a period of 3–6 weeks is usually required for definitive demonstration of the parasite. Surviving mice are bled for serological testing 3 and 6 weeks after inoculation. If murine *T. gondii* antibodies are present, proof of infection must be obtained by examining wet preparations or stained smears of brain tissue for the demonstration of cysts.

Because the main drawback of mouse inoculation is a 3- to 6-week delay before a result is definitive, inoculation into cell culture combined with fluorescent antibody staining offers an opportunity for more rapid detection of *T. gondii* (Derouin et al. 1988). Amniotic fluid sediment is inoculated into a culture of human embryonic fibroblasts. After 4 days of incubation, parasites are identified in monolayers by an indirect immunofluorescence assay. The buffy coat layer of foetal blood samples may be examined in the same way but the sensitivity is low.

Parasites are isolated from the foetal blood as frequently as from the amniotic fluid (Thulliez et al. 1992). Concerning the amniotic fluid, data obtained from studying more than 100 infected foetuses found tissue culture to be as sensitive as mouse inoculation, although the former appeared less sensitive when the parasite burden was small (Hohlfeld et al. 1994).

Detection of *Toxoplasma gondii* DNA in amniotic fluid

Grover et al. (1990) first reported on the usefulness of PCR-targeting the B1 gene in the testing of amniotic fluid for the rapid prenatal diagnosis of congenital toxoplasma infection. Although sporadic false-positive reactions occurred, PCR was more sensitive than mouse inoculation or tissue culture and correctly identified *T. gondii* in eight of ten samples of amniotic fluid from proven cases of congenital infection. Other promising results were obtained with PCR on amniotic fluid with use of a segment of the 18S ribosomal DNA (Cazenave et al. 1992) or gene of surface protein P30 (Dupouy-Camet et al. 1992).

Further data were reported by Hohlfeld et al. (1994) on 339 consecutive amniotic fluid samples from women infected during pregnancy. The PCR targeted the

B1 gene and used specific decontamination to prevent carryover contamination, together with an internal competitive control to monitor the sensitivity for each sample. Each amniotic fluid sample was studied with this PCR and inoculated into mouse and tissue culture; additionally, foetal blood taken at the same time was tested for specific IgM and inoculated into mice. Congenital infection was demonstrated in 34 foetuses by conventional methods and the PCR was positive in all 34 cases. In three additional cases, the PCR was the only positive test: congenital infection was ultimately confirmed by autopsy findings in two cases and by serological follow-up testing of the infant in the remaining case. There was no false-positive result for the PCR. In one case, all tests including PCR were negative at 22 weeks but they were positive at 34 weeks when detection of ultrasound abnormalities led to further sampling; there was no evidence that the foetus was already infected at the time of the first prenatal diagnosis.

From our experience since 1991 with this PCR test on more than 2000 consecutive amniotic fluid samples, the following conclusions can be drawn:

1 All positive PCR results have been confirmed by autopsy findings or by the clinical and serological follow-up of the infants. Thus, demonstration of *T. gondii* DNA in amniotic fluid provides definitive proof of congenital infection. However, since technical aspects may vary from one laboratory to another, it is clear that, before a given PCR procedure can be considered as a confirmatory diagnostic test, it must be carefully evaluated so that false-positive results are avoided.

2 The PCR assay on amniotic fluid is definitely more sensitive than the other specific tests (tissue culture of amniotic fluid, inoculation of mice with foetal blood and amniotic fluid, determination of specific IgM in foetal blood) considered alone or grouped together. Moreover, since nonspecific biological tests performed on the foetal blood have no prognostic value, foetal blood sampling is not necessary. Sampling the amniotic fluid only makes the prenatal diagnosis safer since it carries a lower risk of foetal loss than foetal blood sampling. Therefore, amniocentesis is the procedure of choice. Our group have ceased using tissue culture except when the amniotic fluid sample contains a lot of blood, which may inhibit the amplification. It is advisable to continue using mouse inoculation because semiquantitative PCR testing has shown that when the parasite burden is low, inoculation could be positive (Hohlfeld et al. 1994). Indeed, on a specimen sampled at 31 weeks, after a maternal infection acquired between 22 and 26 weeks of gestation a false-negative result of the PCR was observed although mouse inoculation was positive. This discrepancy might be explained by both a small parasite burden and the difference of processed volumes: a 10-ml aliquot of amniotic fluid was inoculated into mice whereas 1.5 ml was used for DNA amplification.

Another case of negative PCR result was recorded in a woman who acquired infection in the first month of pregnancy. She had a normal ultrasound at 18 weeks but the following examination at 32 weeks showed a severe cerebral damage; at 36 weeks, tests on the amniotic fluid were negative but specific IgM were demonstrated in the foetal blood. Autopsy of the stillbirth confirmed congenital infection. The failure to detect parasites suggested that, in some cases perhaps, they are not present in the amniotic fluid at some time after the development of the foetal disease and that exceptionally foetal blood examination may provide the answer.

3 The rapidity of the PCR test (the result can be obtained within 1 day of sampling) together with its high specificity allow the very early commencement of a specific treatment with pyrimethamine and sulphadiazine when compared with conventional diagnostic methods. Furthermore, it allows intervention in maternal infections occurring very late in pregnancy since amniocentesis is still feasible at this stage. However, the reliability of the PCR has not been evaluated on specimens sampled before the 18th week of pregnancy. It is probably prudent that prenatal diagnosis should not be attempted until at least 4 weeks after the suspected date of maternal infection, so as not to increase the risk of a negative result due to the delay of transmission of T. gondii from the placenta to the foetus.

4 Since the study by Hohlfeld et al. (1994) was published, our group has recorded several cases of negative prenatal diagnoses including the PCR test on amniotic fluid with evidence of congenital infection as shown by clinical and serological follow-up after birth. Before using the PCR it was known that not all cases of congenital infection are detected prenatally. Of 89 congenital infections, Hohlfeld et al. (1989) reported nine cases (10%) with a negative prenatal diagnosis; among these nine cases one had a severe form. In other series, the rate of congenital infections with no prenatally identified abnormal sign was found to vary from 8% (Berrebi et al. 1994) to 16% (Pratlong et al. 1994). It is probable that the number of infections not recognized by the whole prenatal diagnostic procedure is underestimated in each study, as a significant number of offspring are lost to follow-up after birth. Before using the PCR it was not possible to verify whether these discrepancies were due to a lack of diagnostic procedure sensitivity or to a transmission of parasites after the time of sampling. Evidence of a higher sensitivity of PCR in comparison with conventional methods suggests that in the past congenital infections have been missed prenatally because the conventional methods were not sensitive enough. However, even with PCR some cases are not identified probably because of delayed transmission. This raises the fact that a negative prenatal diagnosis does not necessarily exclude the possibility of congenital infection and consequently emphasizes the absolute necessity of following-up the infants. Failure to do so would deny treatment to infected babies.

Management of maternal–foetal infection

Since the circumstances of diagnosis of maternal infection depend greatly on screening policies in different countries, general guidelines only can be given. The policies in use at the Institut de Puériculture, Paris, concerning treatment, ultrasound monitoring and biological prenatal diagnosis are shown in Figure 7.1.

Desmonts and Couvreur (1984) reported a reduced frequency of congenital infection in infants born to spiramycin-treated (23%) versus untreated (61%) mothers; but among those who were infected, the number of infants with clinical signs was unchanged. In a later study Couvreur et al. (1988) investigated the presence of *T. gondii* in placentae from cases of proven congenital infection. Parasites were detected in 89% (41/46) of the placentae of untreated or inadequately treated women and in 75% (89/118) of women treated with spiramycin for 2 weeks at least. This suggested that treatment decreases the duration of placental infection and/or the parasite burden, and thus the risk of transmission to the foetus. This hypothesis is also supported by results of experimental studies of an animal model which revealed high concentrations of the drug in placental tissues and a reduction in the number of infected foetuses after spiramycin treatment (Schoondermark-Van de Ven et al. 1994). Since the placenta may remain infected for the duration of the pregnancy and the transmission of parasites is often a delayed process, it gives time to start spiramycin treatment (1 g three times daily, i.e. 9×10^6 IU/day) as soon as maternal infection is confirmed or highly suspected. Therapy should be continued without interruption throughout the pregnancy unless foetal infection is demonstrated when therapy is modified. Spiramycin does not modify the pattern of infection in an already infected foetus as it most probably does not enter the foetal brain, so its role should be regarded as reducing the risk of transmission rather than treating congenital infection. Other drugs have proved effective *in vitro* and in animal models, but none has been evaluated in pregnant women infected with *T. gondii*. A recent study (Wallon et al. 1999) has suggested that prenatal antibiotic therapy has no impact on foeto–maternal transmission. Clearly further studies are required to clarify the situation.

Once maternal infection is diagnosed, clinical monitoring of the foetus is achieved by a monthly ultrasound examination in order to detect possible effects of the transmission of infection. If the foetal infection is confirmed or highly suspected by the study of amniotic fluid or foetal blood and if the pregnancy is continued, it is recommended that the examination is performed fortnightly because cerebral ventricular dilatation evolves so rapidly (Daffos et al. 1988).

Prenatal diagnosis should be offered to all women infected during pregnancy. For some authors, cordocentesis is not considered suitable for maternal infections acquired before the seventh or the eighth week. This is either because the procedure

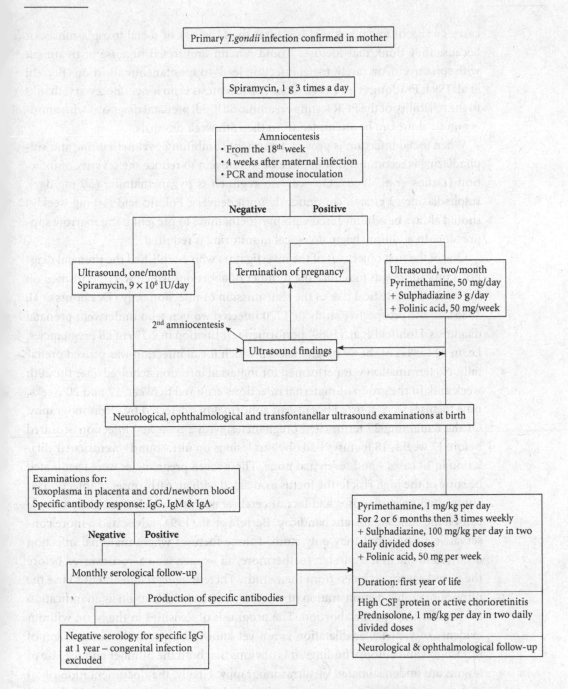

Figure 7.1   Management of primary *T. gondii* maternal infection acquired during pregnancy and management after birth (algorithm in use at Institut de Puériculture)

carries a risk of foetal loss that is greater than the risk of foetal toxoplasmosis, or because they think that foetuses would remain uninfected because of treatment with spiramycin, or, rarely, foetal infection leads to spontaneous abortion (Berrebi et al. 1994; Pratlong et al. 1994). Since cordocentesis is no longer necessary, thanks to the reliability of the PCR testing on amniotic fluid, prenatal diagnosis with amniocentesis alone can be attempted from the 18th week onwards.

When foetal infection is proven, treatment combining pyrimethamine and sulphadiazine is recommended in place of spiramycin to reduce the severity of infection (Daffos et al. 1988). Our current regimen is pyrimethamine (50 mg/day), sulphadiazine (3 g/day), continuously until delivery. Folinic acid (50 mg weekly) should always be administered with pyrimethamine to prevent bone marrow suppression. In addition, haematological monitoring is required.

One of the first objectives of the investigators who established the prenatal diagnosis procedure was to reduce the number of abortions which were performed on the basis of a statistical risk of the transmission of infection only (Desmonts et al. 1985). In the prospective study of 1270 infected women who underwent prenatal diagnosis, Hohlfeld et al. (1989) performed termination in 2.7% of all pregnancies, i.e. in 34 (38%) of the 89 pregnancies in which foetal infection was proved prenatally. No termination was performed for maternal infection acquired after the 20th week and, in the group of maternal infections acquired between 17 and 20 weeks, nine foetuses were aborted because of abnormalities detected by ultrasonography. Of the remaining 25 terminated pregnancies, with a maternal infection acquired before 17 weeks, 18 foetuses had obvious lesions on ultrasound – ventricular dilatation in 14 cases – and seven had none. These seven pregnancies were terminated because of the high risk to the foetus associated with an early onset of infection; at autopsy, all seven foetuses had foci of cerebral necrosis which were likely to have caused the child significant handicap. Berrebi et al. (1994) advocated a more conservative attitude but they only studied three foetuses where maternal infection occurred in the first trimester; furthermore, all women who seroconverted before the 8 weeks were excluded from their study. There is general agreement to use the ultrasonographic demonstration of cerebral ventricular dilatation as an indication to consider therapeutic abortion. The prognosis of densities in the brain without evidence of ventricular dilatation is not yet known, but from the comparison of ultrasound and autopsy findings, it is obvious that both the number and the size of lesions are underestimated by ultrasonography. Finally, the documentation of an early maternal infection combined with an early demonstration of foetal infection without ultrasound abnormalities poses a difficult dilemma since, despite prolonged treatment of the mother with pyrimethamine and sulphadiazine, the offspring may be severely damaged (Pratlong et al. 1994). Parents should be informed of this risk.

Treatment with pyrimethamine and sulphadiazine initiated during pregnancy for a mother whose foetus was identified as infected should be continued in the infant from birth until 1 year of life (Remington et al. 1995). Clinical evaluation includes complete general and neurological examinations as well as ophthalmological and ultrasonographic examinations.

The same evaluation should be performed in infants in whom the prenatal diagnosis was negative or was not attempted. Furthermore, demonstration of *T. gondii* from the placenta or the blood by culture or PCR and detection of a specific humoral response should be attempted (Figure 7.1). If these tests are negative, a monthly serological follow-up must be continued until toxoplasma IgG antibodies become negative, which constitutes definitive proof of the absence of congenital infection. Conversely, the demonstration of specific IgG and IgM or IgA proves congenital infection, but in some cases the only marker is production of specific IgG which may be delayed for several months

Summary

Since most cases of acquired toxoplasma infection are subclinical, their identification in a given population of pregnant women requires repeated testing of those who are seronegative. Vertical transmission occurs by transplacental transfer of the organism from mother to foetus at an average rate of 30% but the rate varies directly with the gestational age at which the mother is infected. In a minority of cases this may result in spontaneous abortion, foetal death or the birth of a severely damaged infant but most infants have a subclinical infection with no overt disease at birth. Following the diagnosis of acute infection in the mother, treatment with spiramycin is begun to try to reduce the risk of transmission of infection to the foetus. Ultrasound follow-up of the foetus is also instituted. Prenatal diagnosis using the PCR method on amniotic fluid should be offered. When foetal infection is proven, treatment with spiramycin is replaced by the combination of pyrimethamine and sulphonamides for the rest of the pregnancy, with the aim of reducing the severity of infection and the incidence of late sequellae.

However, all congenital infections cannot be prenatally identified since delayed transmission of *T. gondii* may occur after the date of amniocentesis. This emphasizes the absolute necessity of following-up the infants in order to exclude congenital infection.

REFERENCES

Ades, A. E. & Nokes, D. J. (1993). Modelling age- and time-specific incidence from seroprevalence: toxoplasmosis. *American Journal of Epidemiology*, 137, 1022–34.

Ashburn, D., Joss, A. W. L., Pennington, T. H. & Ho Yen, D. O. (1995). Specificity and usefulness of an IgE immunosorbent agglutination assay for toxoplasmosis. *Journal of Clinical Pathology*, 48, 64–9.

Aspöck, H. & Pollak, A. (1992). Prevention of prenatal toxoplasmosis by serological screening of pregnant women in Austria. *Scandinavian Journal of Infectious Diseases Supplement*, 84, 32–7.

Berrebi, A., Kobuch, W. E., Bessieres, M. H., Bloom, M. C., Rolland, M., Sarramon, M. F., Roques, C. & Fournie, A. (1994). Termination of pregnancy for maternal toxoplasmosis. *The Lancet*, 344, 36–9.

Bessières, M. H., Roques, C., Berrebi, A., Barre, V., Cazaux, M. & Seguela, J. P. (1992). IgA antibody response during acquired and congenital toxoplasmosis. *Journal of Clinical Pathology*, 45, 605–8.

Cazenave, J., Forestier, F., Bessieres, M. H., Broussin, B. & Begueret, J. (1992). Contribution of a new PCR assay to the prenatal diagnosis of congenital toxoplasmosis. *Prenatal Diagnosis*, 12, 119–27.

Couvreur, J., Desmonts, G. & Gire, J. Y. (1976). Congenital toxoplasmosis in twins. *The Journal of Pediatrics*, 89, 235–40.

Couvreur, J., Desmonts, G. & Thulliez, P. (1988). Prophylaxis of congenital toxoplasmosis. Effects of spiramycin on placental infection. *Journal of Antimicrobial Chemotherapy*, 22, [Suppl. B], 193–200.

Daffos, F., Forestier, F., Capella-Pavlovsky, M., Thulliez, P., Aufrant, C., Valenti, D. & Cox, W. L. (1988). Prenatal management of 746 pregnancies at risk for congenital toxoplasmosis. *The New England Journal of Medicine*, 318, 271–5.

Daffos, F., Mirlesse, V., Hohlfeld, P., Jacquemard, F., Thulliez, P. & Forestier, F. (1994). Toxoplasmosis in pregnancy. *The Lancet*, 344, 541.

Dannemann, B. R., Vaughan, W. C., Thulliez, P. & Remington, J. S. (1990). Differential agglutination test for diagnosis of recently acquired infection with *Toxoplasma gondii*. *Journal of Clinical Microbiology*, 28, 1928–33.

Decoster, A., Darcy, F., Caron, A., Vinatier, D., Houze De L'Aulnoit, D., Vittu, G., Niel, G., Heyer, F., Lecolier B., Delcroix, M., Monnier, J. C., Duhamel, M. & Capron, A. (1992). Anti-P30 IgA antibodies as prenatal markers of congenital toxoplasma infection. *Clinical Experimental Immunology*, 87, 310–15.

Decoster, A., Gontier, P., Dehecq, E., Demory, J. L. & Duhamel, M. (1995). Detection of anti-toxoplasma immunoglobulin A antibodies by Platelia-Toxo IgA directed against P30 and by IMx Toxo IgA for diagnosis of acquired and congenital toxoplasmosis. *Journal of Clinical Microbiology*, 33, 2206–8.

D'Ercole, C., Boubli, L., Franck, J., Casta, M., Harle, J. R., Chagnon, C., Cravello, L., Leclaires, M. & Blanc, B. (1995). Recurrent congenital toxoplasmosis in a woman with lupus erythematosus. *Prenatal Diagnosis*, 15, 1171–5.

Derouin, F., Thulliez, P., Candolfi, E., Daffos, F. & Forestier, F. (1988). Early prenatal diagnosis of congenital toxoplasmosis using amniotic fluid samples and tissue culture. *European Journal of Clinical Microbiology and Infectious Diseases*, 7, 423–5.

Desmonts, G. & Couvreur, J. (1984). Toxoplasmose congénitale – Etude prospective de l'issue de la grossesse chez 542 femmes atteintes de toxoplasmose acquise en cours de gestation. *Annales de Pédiatrie*, 31, 805–9.

Desmonts, G., Daffos, F., Forestier, F., Capella-Pavlovsky, M., Thulliez, P. & Chartier, M. (1985). Prenatal diagnosis of congenital toxoplasmosis. *The Lancet*, i, 500–4.

Desmonts, G., Couvreur, J. & Thulliez, P. (1990). Toxoplasmose congénitale: cinq cas de transmission à l'enfant d'une infection maternelle antérieure à la grossesse. *La Presse Médicale*, 19, 1445–9.

Dupouy-Camet, J., Bougnoux, M. E., Lavareda De Souza, S., Thulliez, P., Dommergues, M., Mandelbrot, L., Ancelle, T., Tourte-Schaefer, C. & Benarous, R. (1992). Comparative value of polymerase chain reaction and conventional biological tests for the prenatal diagnosis of congenital toxoplasmosis. *Annales de Biologie Clinique*, 50, 315–19.

Forestier, F., Cox, W. L., Daffos, F. & Rainaut, M. (1988). The assessment of fetal blood samples. *American Journal of Obstetrics and Gynecology*, 158, 1184–8.

Fortier, B., Aissi, E., Ajana, F., Dieusart, P., Denis, P., Martin De Lassale, E., Lecomte-Houcke, M. & Vinatier, D. (1991). Spontaneous abortion and reinfection by *Toxoplasma gondii*. *The Lancet*, 338, 444.

Foulon, W., Naessens, A. & Derde, M. P. (1994). Evaluation of the possibilities for preventing congenital toxoplasmosis. *American Journal of Perinatology*, 11, 57–62.

Francis, J. M. & Joynson, D. H. M. (1993). Duration of specific immunoglobulin A antibody following acute toxoplasmosis as determined by enzyme immunoassay and immunosorbent agglutination assay. *European Journal of Clinical Microbiology and Infectious Diseases*, 12, 556–9.

Grover, C. M., Thulliez, P., Remington, J. S. & Boothroyd, J. C. (1990). Rapid prenatal diagnosis of congenital *Toxoplasma* infection by using polymerase chain reaction and amniotic fluid. *Journal of Clinical Microbiology*, 28, 2297–301.

Hedman, K., Lappalainen, M., Seppala, I. & Makela, O. (1989). Recent primary Toxoplasma infection indicated by a low avidity of specific IgG. *The Journal of Infectious Diseases*, 159, 736–40.

Hohlfeld, P., Daffos, F., Thulliez, P., Aufrant, J., Couvreur, J., Mac Aleese, D., Descombey, D. & Forestier, F. (1989). Fetal toxoplasmosis: outcome of pregnancy and infant follow-up after *in-utero* treatment. *The Journal of Pediatrics*, 115, 765–9.

Hohlfeld, P., Mac Aleese, J., Capella-Pavlovski, M., Giovangrandi, Y., Thulliez P., Forestier, F. & Daffos, F. (1991). Fetal toxoplasmosis: ultrasonographic signs. *Ultrasound in Obstetrics and Gynecology*, 1, 241–4.

Hohlfeld, P., Daffos, F., Costa, J. M., Thulliez, P., Forestier, F. & Vidaud M. (1994). Prenatal diagnosis of congenital toxoplasmosis with a polymerase-chain-reaction test on amniotic fluid. *The New England Journal of Medicine*, 331, 695–9.

Holliman, R. E, Raymond, R., Renton, N. & Johnson, J. D. (1994). The diagnosis of toxoplasmosis using IgG avidity. *Epidemiology and Infection*, 112, 399–408.

Jeannel, D., Niel, G., Costagliola, D., Danis, M., Traore, B. M. & Gentilini, M. (1988). Epidemiology of toxoplasmosis among pregnant women in the Paris area. *International Journal of Epidemiology,* 17, 595–601.

Joynson, D. H. M. (1992). Epidemiology of toxoplasmosis in the U. K. *Scandinavian Journal of Infectious Diseases Supplement,* 84, 65–9.

Joynson, D. H. M., Payne, R. A., Rawal, B. K. (1990). Potential role of IgG avidity for diagnosing toxoplasmosis. *Journal of Clinical Pathology,* 43, 1032–3.

Lappalainen, M., Koskela, P., Koskiniemi, M., Ammala, P., Hiilesmaa, V., Teramo, K., Raivio, K. O., Remington, J. S. & Hedman, K. (1993). Toxoplasmosis acquired during pregnancy: improved serodiagnosis based on avidity of IgG. *The Journal of Infectious Diseases,* 167, 691–7.

Lebech, M., Joynson, D. H. M., Thulliez, P., Gilbert, R. E., Dutton, G. N. et al. (1996). Classification system and case definitions of *Toxoplasma gondii* infection in immunocompetent pregnant women and congenital infections in their offspring. *European Journal of Clinical Microbiology and Infectious Disease,* 15, 799–805.

Lecolier, B. & Pucheu B. (1993). Interêt de l'étude de l'avidité des IgG pour le diagnostic de la toxoplasmose. *Pathologie Biologie,* 41, 155–8.

Marty, P., Le Fichoux Y., Deville, A. & Forest, H. (1991). Toxoplasmose congénitale et toxoplasmose maternelle préconceptionnelle. *La Presse Médicale,* 20, 387.

Marty, P., Bongain, A., Rahal, A., Thulliez, P., Wasfi, D., Lambert, J. C., Le Fichoux, Y. & Gillet, J. Y. (1994). Prenatal diagnosis of severe fetal toxoplasmosis as a result of toxoplasmic reactivation in an HIV-1 seropositive woman. *Prenatal Diagnosis,* 14, 414–15.

Mitchell, C. D., Erlich, S. S., Mastrucci, M. T., Hutto, S. C., Parks, W. P. & Scott, G. B. (1990). Congenital toxoplasmosis occurring in infants perinatally infected with human immunodeficiency virus 1. *The Pediatric Infectious Disease Journal,* 9, 512–18.

Papoz, L., Simondon, F., Saurin, W. & Sarmini, H. (1986). A simple model relevant to toxoplasmosis applied to epidemiologic results in France. *American Journal of Epidemiology,* 123, 154–61.

Pinon, J. M., Toubas, D., Marx, C., Mougeot, G., Bonnin, A., Bonhomme, A., Villaume, M., Foudrinier, F. & Lepan, H. (1990). Detection of specific immunoglobin E in patients with toxoplasmosis. *Journal of Clinical Microbiology,* 28, 1739–43.

Pons, J. C., Sigrand, C., Grangeot-Keros, L., Frydman, R. & Thulliez, P. (1995). Toxoplasmose congénitale: transmission au foetus d'une infection maternelle antéconceptionnelle. *La Presse Médicale,* 24, 179–82.

Pratlong, F., Boulot, P., Issert, E., Msika, M., Dupont, F., Bachelard, B., Sarda, P., Viala, J. L. & Jarry, D. (1994). Fetal diagnosis of toxoplasmosis in 190 women infected during pregnancy. *Prenatal Diagnosis,* 14, 191–8.

Remington, J. S., McLeod R. & Desmonts, G. (1995). Toxoplasmosis. In *Infectious Diseases of the Fetus and Newborn Infant,* 4th edn., ed. J. S. Remington & J. O. Klein, pp. 140–267. Philadelphia: W. B. Saunders.

Schoondermark-Van de Ven, E., Melchers, W., Camps, W., Eskes, T., Meuwissen, J. & Galama, J. (1994). Effectiveness of spiramycin for treatment of congenital *Toxoplasma gondii* infection in rhesus monkeys. *Antimicrobial Agents and Chemotherapy,* 38, 1930–6.

Suzuki, Y., Thulliez, P., Desmonts, G. & Remington, J. S. (1988). Antigen(s) responsible for immunoglobulin G responses specific for the acute stage of *Toxoplasma* infection in humans. *Journal of Clinical Microbiology*, **26**, 901–5.

Thulliez, P. (1992). Screening programme for congenital toxoplasmosis in France. *Scandinavian Journal of Infectious Disease Supplement*, **84**, 43–5.

Thulliez, P., Daffos, F. & Forestier, F. (1992). Diagnosis of Toxoplasma infection in the pregnant woman and the unborn child: current problems. *Scandinavian Journal of Infectious Diseases Supplement*, **84**, 18–22.

Wallon, M., Liou, C., Garner, P. & Peyron, F. (1999). Congenital toxoplasmosis: systematic review of evidence of efficacy of treatment in pregnancy. *British Medical Journal*, **318**, 1511–14.

Wong, S. Y., Hajdu, M. P., Ramirez, R., Thulliez, P., McLeod, R. & Remington J. S. (1993). Role of specific immunoglobulin E in diagnosis of acute toxoplasma infection and toxoplasmosis. *Journal of clinical microbiology*, **31**, 2952–9.

8

Prenatal screening for toxoplasma infection

R. E. Gilbert and C. S. Peckham

Department of Paediatric Epidemiology, Institute of Child Health, University of London, London, UK

Introduction

Prenatal screening to reduce the risks of congenital toxoplasmosis has always been controversial. The debate centres on two questions, first whether prenatal screening can be justified at all and second, if it can, which screening programme is the most effective.

Measures other than prenatal screening include primary prevention, for example by the provision of health information about how to avoid infection (Ho-Yen et al. 1995) and neonatal screening. The latter approach has been adopted by the Massachusetts newborn screening programme as the most cost-effective (Guerina et al. 1994) and has been evaluated in Denmark (Lebech et al. 1999).

Where prenatal screening is advocated there is controversy about which screening programme is most effective. The French approach (Thulliez 1992) involves monthly retesting of *Toxoplasma gondii* antibody-negative pregnant women whereas in Austria (Aspock & Pollak 1992) retesting is carried out every 3 months. The debate is hampered by inadequate information on the risks of maternal infection and mother-to-child transmission, of clinical manifestations in infected children and the efficacy of antiparasitic treatment prenatally or during infancy in preventing congenital infection or reducing the number of affected children. There have been no published reports of controlled studies of prenatal screening or treatment and the comparative studies which have been undertaken are susceptible to bias. Nevertheless, there is a widespread perception that both the birth prevalence and severity of congenital toxoplasmosis have fallen in France and Austria since prenatal screening was introduced two decades ago. The magnitude of this decline and the extent to which it can be attributed to prenatal screening, or to other factors such as the diminishing risk of exposure to toxoplasma infection, are unknown.

The current diversity of preventive strategies for congenital toxoplasmosis across Europe reflects both the uncertainties about the effectiveness of prenatal screening and the marked regional variation in the risk of exposure to toxoplasma infection.

In addition, decisions about screening are affected by national differences in the organization of health-care, and cultural attitudes, among parents and clinicians, to interventions in pregnancy.

In this chapter we discuss what is currently known about the clinical benefit and potential harm associated with prenatal screening for toxoplasmosis. We stress the need for women to be made aware, before consenting to screening, of the implications of a positive test and the risk of foetal damage and the extent to which this may be prevented by prenatal treatment.

How common is symptomatic congenital toxoplasmosis?

Decisions about screening are heavily influenced by the prevalence and severity of the problem which screening and subsequent intervention aim to prevent. However, it is not easy to determine the 'size of the problem' of symptomatic congenital toxoplasmosis, due to difficulties in diagnosis and the need for long-term follow-up to detect symptoms late in childhood. Other factors that affect screening decisions, such as the prevalence of susceptible women, their risk of infection, treatment efficacy and screening and diagnostic test performance, are also important.

Birth prevalence of congenital toxoplasma infection

Congenital toxoplasmosis is rare, and precise estimates of the birth prevalence (number of congenitally infected births/number of births) can only be derived from studies involving a large, geographically representative population with adequate follow-up to determine the outcome of all infected pregnant women. Many studies to date have been based on the caseload of a referral centre which may overestimate the birth prevalence of congenital toxoplasmosis for two reasons. Women with infected foetuses or infants are more likely to be referred and uninfected infants are more likely to be lost to follow-up as there is less incentive for parents and clinicians to maintain follow-up of healthy, uninfected children than children undergoing treatment or who are at risk of developing sequelae.

The most reliable estimates of the birth prevalence of congenital toxoplasmosis are from prospective, population-based cohort studies of pregnant women with high rates of follow-up of mothers and infants at risk of infection (Conyn van Spaendonck 1991; Lappalainen et al. 1995b), and studies based on the testing of cord blood or neonatal blood samples in liveborns (Guerina et al. 1994; Berger et al. 1995; Lebech et al. 1999) (see Table 8.1). However, these studies underestimate the risk of congenital toxoplasmosis. First, they do not include infected foetuses lost during pregnancy, either spontaneously or due to therapeutic termination. Second, some studies are based on the detection of *T. gondii* IgM or IgA in the neonatal or

Table 8.1. Estimates of the birth prevalence of congenital toxoplasmosis from population-based cohort studies

Study and country	Method of detection	Year(s) of study	Number of liveborns in study	Number of liveborns with congenital toxoplasmosis	Birth prevalence per 10,000 liveborns (95% confidence interval)
Retrospective cohort studies					
Kimball et al. (1971) USA	Paired testing of IgG in prenatal and delivery blood	1967–69	4048	2	4.9 (0.6–17.8)
Sever et al. (1988) USA	Paired testing of IgG in prenatal and cord blood	1959–66	22,845	2	0.9 (0.1–3.2)
Prospective cohort studies					
Conyn van Spaendonck (1991) The Netherlands	Repeat testing for IgG in prenatal samples	1987	28,049	12	4.3 (2.2–7.5)
Lappalainen et al. (1992, 1995a) Finland	Repeat testing for IgG, IgM and IgG avidity in prenatal samples	1988–89	16,733	4	2.4 (0.7–6.1)
Guerina et al. (1994)£ USA	IgM detected in neonatal Guthrie card blood spots	1986–92	635,000	54	0.8 (0.6–1.1)
Berger et al. (1995) Switzerland	IgG titre, IgM, IgA in cord blood	1986–94	30,000	5$	1.7 (0.5–3.9)
Lebech et al. $$£ (1999) Denmark	Detection of IgG, IgM, IgA in neonatal Guthrie card blood spots and prenatal IgG	1992–96	89,873	27	3.0 (1.5–5.0)

Key:

$One case mother treated, four cases mother untreated.

$$Observed for women seroconverting between 10 and 37 weeks of gestation (mean period of observation 213 days, SD 31); four spontaneous abortions with confirmed congenital toxoplasmosis.

£All women untreated.

Note: confidence intervals derived from Poisson distribution.

cord blood, which is reported to be present in about 80% of congenitally infected infants born to untreated women (E. Petersen, pers. commun.; Pinon et al. 1996). In the remaining 30% with undetectable IgM or IgA in early infancy, a diagnosis of congenital toxoplasmosis can only be made by persistence of IgG beyond the age of 12 months (Lebech et al. 1996). Conversely, congenital toxoplasmosis can only be excluded by the absence of *T. gondii* IgG, usually by 6 months of age, when maternal antibodies have declined (Alford et al. 1974).

Other limitations of the studies listed in Table 8.1 are that, with the exception of Switzerland, they relate to northern Europe or north America, and may not reflect the situation in other areas. In three studies (Conyn van Spaendonck 1991; Berger et al. 1995; Lappalainen et al. 1995*b*), some women were treated for toxoplasmosis during pregnancy. Nevertheless, these studies provide the best estimate available of the birth prevalence of congenital toxoplasmosis of 1–5/10,000 liveborns in northern European or USA populations. This compares with HIV infection in 7/10,000 liveborns in south east England (Holland et al. 1994) and herpes simplex virus infection in 1.65/100,000 liveborns in the UK (Forsgren 1990; Tookey & Peckham 1996).

Risk of symptoms due to congenital toxoplasmosis

Information on the risk of symptoms or disability is extremely limited. Most studies identify small numbers of congenitally infected children and, in general, report the presence of lesions attributable to toxoplasmosis which may not necessarily be manifest clinically rather than the presence of symptoms, such as visual impairment or neurodevelopmental delay. Most congenitally infected infants are asymptomatic at birth and some do not develop symptoms until adolescence (Koppe et al. 1986). Few long-term follow-up studies have been conducted.

Early symptoms

Foetal loss or perinatal death may be due to congenital toxoplasmosis, and clinical manifestations in surviving infants apparent at birth or in infancy are more likely to lead to impairment, disability or death. Most commonly reported are hydrocephalus, or generalized systemic symptoms associated with hepatosplenomegaly, jaundice and intrauterine growth retardation in the newborn. *Toxoplasma gondii* has a tropism for neural tissue and rarely gives rise to the classic triad of clinical signs considered to be pathognomic for congenital toxoplasmosis (Lebech et al. 1996): hydrocephalus, intracranial calcification and retinochoroiditis.

Desmonts and Courvreur (1984) reported that foetal loss or perinatal death occurred in up to 11/500 (2.2%) infected women and 7% (11/166) of congenital infections. This is an upper estimate because it is based on a referred population which is more likely to include severely affected foetuses and children. In addition, excess foetal loss attributable to congenital toxoplasmosis has never been assessed because few studies provide adequate confirmation of infection status in the foetus, and such losses may reflect spontaneous foetal loss rates unrelated to toxoplasma infection. For example, in unselected women with a viable pregnancy at 7–14 weeks gestation, approximately 2.5% would be expected to spontaneously abort (Heckerling & Verp 1991).

Estimates of the risk of early symptoms attributable to congenital toxoplasmosis derived from cohort studies are given in Table 8.2. To our knowledge, evidence derived from population-based, prospective cohort studies is limited to five studies (Koppe et al. 1986; Conyn van Spaendonck 1991; Guerina et al. 1994; Lappalainen et al. 1995*b*; Lebech et al. 1999) involving a total of 87 infected children of whom 38 had clinical signs. Hydrocephalus was reported in only 1 of the 38 children followed and none had generalized symptoms in the newborn period. These figures contrast with those of Desmonts who estimated that 10% of congenitally infected children had symptoms detectable at delivery or in infancy (Desmonts & Couvreur 1984).

Further sources of information about the size of the problem of symptomatic congenital toxoplasmosis are population-based, cross-sectional surveillance studies. In an attempt to estimate the birth prevalence of early symptoms attributable to congenital toxoplasmosis in infants in the UK, Hall reviewed all the laboratory reports of possible congenital toxoplasmosis to the Public Health Laboratory Service and cases of newly diagnosed congenital toxoplasmosis reported by paediatricians throughout the British Isles to The British Paediatric Surveillance Unit, an active monthly reporting scheme with 90% compliance (Hall 1992). There were 14 definite or probable cases detected in the 1989–1990 birth cohort of 680,000 in England and Wales, not all severely affected. These findings may be an underestimate but are nevertheless in marked contrast to previous projections of 50–70 severely affected cases in England and Wales, based on assumptions about the maternal infection rate, mother-to-child transmission rate, and a 10% rate of severe symptoms in congenitally infected babies.

Late symptoms

Information on late sequelae usually relates to eye lesions rather than visual impairment or other ocular symptoms. Eye lesions attributable to congenital toxoplasmosis are common and in the studies listed in Table 8.2, retinochoroidal lesions were detected in 25–80% of infected children, and intracranial calcifications in approximately one-sixth. New retinochoroidal lesions can occur as late as 18 years of age (Koppe et al. 1986) and detection is more likely with more sensitive examination and longer follow-up. However, the risk of retinochoroidal lesions appearing for

Table 8.2. Risk of signs and symptoms in live-born children with congenital toxoplasmosis

Study and country	Study design	Total number with congenital toxoplasmosis	Number with lesions (% of total)	H	ICC	RC	Symptoms and length of follow-up
				Number with specific lesions			
Koppe et al. (1986) The Netherlands	Prospective cohort of women seroconverting after 12 weeks of gestation. No postnatal treatment in 7 with no lesions initially, of whom 4 developed lesions by 18 years. Not treated prenatally. 1/12 lost to follow-up.	11	9 (82%)	0	0	9	3/9 children with lesions had severe unilateral visual impairment. Follow-up 20 years. Follow-up 20 years lesions detected at birth, 4/9 at 7 years and 9/9 at 20 years.
Conyn van Spaendonck (1991) The Netherlands	Prospective cohort of women seroconverting after first trimester. Of 44 infected women (1/44 lost to follow-up), 12 children were infected: 3 born to treated women, and 9 born to untreated women infected in the 3rd trimester. Infected children not treated.	12	3 (25%)	0	1	2	At follow-up beyond 1 year no neurological sequelae detected. Strabismus presents in 1 child.
Guerina et al. (1994) USA	Prospective cohort of congenitally infected neonates identified by detection of toxoplasma IgM on Guthrie card blood spots. Postnatal treatment only; 11/50 lost to follow-up after 1 year.	48	19 (38%)	1	9	12	8/12 retinochoroidal lesions involved the macula and were likely to be associated with visual impairment. Strabismus reported in 1 child. Hemiplegia in 1 child with calcified cystic intracranial lesion. Follow-up 1–6 years.
Lappalainen et al. (1995b) Finland	Prospective cohort study of women with seroconversion or low IgG avidity. Prenatal and postnatal treatment.	7	4 (58%)	0	1	4	Symptoms not described. Follow-up 4–5 years.
Lebech et al (1999) Denmark	Prospective cohort of congenitally infected infants identified by retrospective identification of women seroconverting between 12 and 38 weeks gestation. 1 lost to follow-up.	27	4 (15%)	0	2	3	Symptoms in 2 children: 1 with intracranial calcification and mental retardation; 1 with severe unilateral visual impairment. Follow-up 1–3 years.

Key:
H = hydrocephalus.   ICC = intracranial calcification.   RC = retinochoroiditis.

the first time in a congenitally infected child with normal ophthalmological examinations during infancy is uncertain. Guerina et al. (1994) reported that, of 12 children with retinochoroidal lesions, in three lesions appeared for the first time after one year, but early examinations had been unsatisfactory. In a study of 54 children with retinochoroidal lesions attributed to congenital toxoplasmosis, Mets et al. reported new lesions in two children with previously unaffected retinas after three to ten years of age (Mets et al. 1996). In contrast, Koppe et al. found new lesions in five children (four of seven definitely congenitally infected and one of ten dubiously infected) during later childhood and adolescence (Koppe et al. 1986; Koppe & Rothova 1989). More reliable information on the risk of new lesions in children with no detectable lesions in early childhood is important if we are to determine whether long-term ophthalmological follow-up is justifiable in congenitally infected children with no detectable lesions.

Symptoms of permanent visual impairment are rarely sufficiently severe to be noticed during infancy. Lesions involving the macula can cause unilateral or rarely bilateral, permanent visual impairment, but more commonly symptoms are due to the reactivation of retinochoroidal lesions manifest as episodes of transient visual impairment. Redness of the conjunctiva, and photophobia may also be present (Rothova 1993). These episodes resolve spontaneously within 6–8 weeks but the duration and severity of symptoms may be attenuated by treatment (Rothova 1993; Mets et al. 1996). In the study by Guerina et al. (1994) six of the 12 children with retinochoroidal lesions were reported to have minor, permanent, unilateral visual impairment after 1–5 years follow-up. The risk of acute episodes of visual symptoms attributed to the reactivation of latent toxoplasma cysts and a feature of *T. gondii* eye disease in adulthood was not reported in any of the cohort studies (see Table 8.2).

In an attempt to determine the incidence of eye symptoms in all age ranges presenting to ophthalmologists and attributable to toxoplasmosis – though not necessarily due to congenital infection – a surveillance study was conducted in South Greater London (Gilbert et al. 1995). Twenty-eight cases of symptomatic eye disease were detected, giving an estimated incidence of 0.4/100,000 person years for people born in Britain. However, over half the cases occurred in people born outside the UK. The incidence was approximately 100-fold higher for people born in West Africa than for people born in Britain. These findings have since been confirmed in a four-region study in the UK involving 87 cases (Gilbert et al. 1999). The authors calculate a cumulative incidence of symptomatic toxoplasmic retinochoroiditis of 18/100,000 up to 60 years of age. In other words, 75–178 individuals born each year in Britain will develop symptoms attributable to toxoplasmic retinochoroiditis, mostly associated with unilateral and transient visual impairment. In marked contrast to findings in the cohort studies of congenitally infected children, only two of the 87 patients reported having any signs or symptoms before ten years of age. This suggests that a substantial proportion of these individuals may have acquired the disease postnatally.

The long-term risk of neurodevelopmental impairment attributable to dilated ventricles or intracranial calcification is not known. Overall, impairment has rarely been reported in congenitally infected children and several studies have reported normal neurodevelopmental outcomes in young children with intracranial calcification (Berrebi et al. 1994; Guerina et al. 1994; Lappalainen et al. 1995b; Roizen et al. 1995; Lebech et al. 1999). Patel et al. (1996) reported that the majority of calcified intracranial lesions either diminish or resolve completely by one year of life, but whether this occurs spontaneously or as a result of treatment is not known.

In summary, estimates of the risk of congenital toxoplasmosis in northern Europe or north America are in the range of 1–5/10,000 births. Approximately 25–80% of congenitally infected children develop lesions attributable to congenital toxoplasmosis, most commonly retinochoroiditis, and roughly half of these have some degree of unilateral visual impairment during childhood. Reliable estimates of the risks of symptoms and impairment are not available, but neurodevelopmental impairment appears to be rare.

Potential benefits of prenatal screening

Prenatal screening aims to reduce the risk of symptomatic congenital toxoplasmosis through the identification of women who acquire a primary infection during pregnancy. Those infected can:

1 be offered treatment to reduce the risk of foetal infection or to reduce the risk of organ damage in infected foetuses and subsequent postnatal clinical manifestations;

2 avoid the birth of infants damaged by congenital toxoplasmosis by terminating the pregnancy;

3 undergo investigations to identify newborns at risk of infection who may benefit from clinical assessment and treatment during infancy.

Although all women should be offered information prior to or early in pregnancy about how to avoid infection, prenatal screening provides an opportunity to reinforce this message in susceptible women.

Identification and treatment of women who acquire primary infection during pregnancy

Foetal infection occurs in women who acquire a primary infection during pregnancy and has rarely been reported to occur following the reactivation of latent toxoplasma infection in immunocompetent women (Fortier et al. 1991; Holliman 1994; Hennequin et al. 1997). Primary toxoplasma infection is usually asymptomatic although a substantial minority of women (Babill Stray-Pedersen, personal communication) are reported to develop nonspecific symptoms of fever, malaise, myalgia or lymphadenopathy. The acquisition of toxoplasma infection in pregnancy can therefore only reliably be detected by serological testing. Two strategies are involved.

Serological tests

Detection of seroconversion

Toxoplasma gondii antibody-negative women are tested throughout pregnancy to identify those who seroconvert (become IgG and/or IgM positive). Retesting is carried out each month in France and Switzerland, and 3-monthly in Austria, Germany, Norway and Italy (Aspock & Pollak 1992; Hengst 1992; Thulliez 1992). Monthly testing has the advantage of earlier identification and in theory increases the opportunities for treatment before transmission of infection from mother to foetus. However, frequent testing has the disadvantage of lowering the detection rate with each additional test (as demonstrated below), increasing the number of women falsely identified as positive, increasing the number of prenatal visits and increasing costs.

In a recent national study of all women in France who were tested for toxoplasma infection during 1 week in 1995, 46% of 13,459 women were *T. gondii*-antibody-negative (assumed to be at their first visit) (Ancelle et al. 1996). The incidence of maternal infection during pregnancy, based on what the authors described as 'certain' diagnoses of seroconversion, was 32/6442 or approximately 5/1000 *T. gondii* antibody-negative pregnant women (assumed to have been tested over approximately 6 months of pregnancy; i.e. 0.83/1000 per month and 7.5/1000 per 9-month pregnancy). If these figures are extrapolated to 780,000 pregnant women (the number each year in France), 358,800 would be *T. gondii* antibody negative and 2,691 would acquire infection during pregnancy. Table 8.3 shows the estimated number of true positives and false positives (pregnant women with and without infection respectively) resulting from one, two or three serological tests for IgG or IgM carried out on a single serum sample from a *T. gondii* antibody-negative pregnant woman at monthly intervals. According to French law, a minimum of two tests is required on a single sample to confirm infection.

Table 8.3. Probability of toxoplasma infection in *T. gondii*-antibody-negative women found to seroconvert at each monthly test according to the number of tests performed on a single sample

Number of tests conducted on a single sample in 358,000 nonimmune French women/year	Number of truly infected women detected each month	Number of women falsely identified as infected	Risk of toxoplasma infection given 1, 2 or 3 positive test results on each monthly serum sample (%)
One test positive	299	17,885	1.6
Two tests positive	299	894	25
Three tests positive	299	45	87

Note:
If tested 3 monthly instead of monthly, 897 women would be truly positive, giving a risk of toxoplasma infection after 1 test of 5%. The high rate of false positives illustrates the importance of confirmation of infection by a reference laboratory where a range of tests are used.

We have assumed that each of the tests used is 100% sensitive (which is unlikely), and 95% specific (well within the range for IgG and IgM tests in routine practice) and that the performance of each test does not depend on that of the other.

Retest interval for screening for seroconversion

In the past, regional differences in *T. gondii* antibody prevalence and the incidence of maternal infection were used as a justification for monthly retesting in France compared with 3 monthly in Austria and elsewhere. Monthly retesting is costly, but when screening was first introduced in France, only 13% of pregnant women were *T. gondii*-antibody-negative and required monthly testing, compared with at least 60% elsewhere in Europe. In addition, the incidence of infection in *T. gondii*-antibody-negative women was high: 60/1000 nonimmune women according to studies reviewed by Remington et al. (1995, pp. 161–6). However, the risk of exposure to toxoplasma infection has decreased substantially throughout Europe over the last 20–30 years with the result that regional differences are now much less marked. Recent estimates from population-based studies suggest that 46% of French women are *T. gondii*-antibody-negative (Ancelle et al. 1996), compared with 90% in South Yorkshire in the UK (Walker et al. 1992) and Norway (Stray-Pedersen & Jenum 1992), 73% in Denmark (Lebech & Petersen 1992), 70% in Austria (Aspock & Pollak 1992) and 58% in southern Italy (Buffolano et al. 1994). Further evidence of a reduction in the prevalence and incidence of infection over the past two to three decades is provided by incidence estimations derived from age- and time-specific modelling of seroprevalence data (Bornand & Piguet 1991; Forsgren et al. 1991; Ades & Nokes 1993; Nokes et al. 1993).

Comparisons of incidence estimates of primary maternal *T. gondii* infection from different studies should be interpreted with caution (see Table 8.4). Unless based on a geographically defined population, incidence rates are easily exaggerated by the referral of infected women to specialist centres. In addition, few studies are explicit about the delay between negative and positive IgG tests or take account of these in the rates reported (Ades 1992). Thirdly, the tests and titres used to define maternal infection, high titre, rising titre or seroconversion, can substantially alter the chance of being classified as infected or not (Koppe et al. 1974; Sever et al. 1988). Given these concerns, recent estimates in Table 8.4 are restricted to those derived from population-based studies including only seroconverting women in the numerator. Despite the similarity of these figures (Table 8.4) screening is not recommended in the Netherlands and Finland (or in the UK), whereas neonatal screening occurs in Denmark and monthly prenatal screening is mandatory in France.

Identification of women with evidence of recent infection at the first prenatal test

All prenatal screening programmes involve tests designed to identify those women who acquired primary toxoplasmosis infection after conception but before the first pregnancy booking test. This is because the risk of foetal damage in infected foetuses is highest in early pregnancy (see 'Risk of symptomatic congenital toxoplasmosis'). *T. gondii* IgG-positive samples from the first prenatal test are subjected to additional tests for recent infection, such as specific IgM, high or rising IgG titre, IgG avidity, IgA or a combination of these. However, none of these tests can reliably distinguish between infection acquired before and after conception. Test combinations vary between centres. One of the most promising single-sample tests for recent infection is IgG avidity (Joynson et al. 1990; Lappalainen et al. 1993), which appears to have moderate specificity for infection within the past 3 months. In some centres, IgG- and IgM-positive women are retested 1 month later, and only those with a rising *T. gondii* IgG titre are considered to be at sufficient risk of post conception infection to justify treatment. In southern Italy, women may be treated or even offered termination on the basis of a positive IgM and IgG result (Buffolano et al. 1994).

One of the consequences of the low specificity of tests for infection acquired between conception and the first prenatal test is that a disproportionately high proportion of pregnant women identified in early pregnancy are offered antiparasitic treatment and amniocentesis. For example, in two French studies 55% or more pregnant women were infected during the first trimester (Hohlfeld et al. 1994; Pratlong et al. 1994;) (see Table 8.5).

Table 8.4. Incidence of maternal *T. gondii* infection during pregnancy derived from population-based studies of women with seroconversion, low IgG avidity or 'certain' primary infection during pregnancy

Study	Years	Number of nonimmune pregnant women (% of all pregnant women)	Number of *T. gondii* infected women	Observation period	Estimated incidence (/1000) *T.gondii* antibody-negative pregnant women (over 9 months)
Conyn van Spaendonck (1989, 1991) The Netherlands	1987	15,427 (55%)	55	Mean 5.9 months	5.4
Lappalainen et al. (1995b)[2] Finland	1988–89	13,336 (80%)	28	Approx. 25 weeks	3.4
Lebech et al. (1999) Denmark	1992–1994	29,585 (72%)	76	Mean 30 weeks	3.4
Ancelle et al. (1996)[1] France	1995	6442 (46%)	32	6 months assumed	7.5

[1] Only 'certain' diagnoses of primary infection included.
[2] Only women with seroconversion or low IgG avidity included.

Table 8.5. Risk of mother-to-foetus transmission of toxoplasma infection according to trimester at maternal infection

| Study | Years | Trimester at maternal infection Number infected/number exposed (%) | | |
		I	II	III
Desmonts & Couvreur (1984)[4,6] France	Before 1977	11/120 (9.1%)	68/241 (28%)	66/128 (52%)
Pratlong et al. (1994)[5] France	1985–1991	4/102 (4%)	12/70 (17%)	8/15 (53%)
Hohfeld et al. (1994)[5] France	1983–1992	52/1498 (3.4%)	123/745 (16%)	11/38 (29%)
Conyn van Spaendonck (1991)[6] South Netherlands	1987–1988	0	2/21 (9.5%)	10/23 (43%)
Koppe et al. (1974)[1,2,3,6] The Netherlands	1964–1966		12/38 (32%)	
Lebech et al. [1,2,6] (1999) Denmark	1992–1994		12/76 (14%)	

Key:
[1]Data combined for 2nd and 3rd trimester.
[2]No prenatal treatment.
[3]IgG titre of 1 in 256.
[4]Mix of treated and untreated women.
[5]Diagnosis of infection based on seroconversion or rising IgG.
[6]Diagnosis of infection based on seroconversion.

Early treatment to reduce the risk of foetal infection

The increase in mother-to-foetus transmission of infection with increasing gestation at maternal infection is a consistent finding (see Table 8.5). Estimates of the risk of mother-to-foetus transmission are much less consistent and appear to be lowest in those studies where women did not receive treatment (Koppe et al. 1974; Lebech et al. 1999). Such differences between studies are difficult to interpret as they may reflect differences in the tests and cut-offs used to define maternal infection and nonimmunity, differences in the methods used to estimate length of gestation at maternal infection, treatment differences, biases introduced during selection and follow-up and, possibly, regional differences in exposure to infection.

Mother-to-foetus transmission of toxoplasma infection is thought to occur during the parasitaemic phase following acquisition of primary infection. The delay between maternal and foetal infection creates a 'window of opportunity' when treatment with spiramycin may reduce transmission risk. However, it is not known how long this 'window of opportunity' lasts, nor how it varies with gestation (Remington et al. 1995). Retesting schedules, at regular monthly or 3-monthly intervals throughout pregnancy, are based on the assumption that transmission of *T. gondii* infection is delayed long enough in at least a proportion of women to allow treatment to be effective.

In most countries, treatment strategies to reduce the risk of foetal infection vary with gestation. Treatment is started immediately (or sometimes before) primary infection is confirmed and in most European referral centres consists of spiramycin, a macrolide antibiotic which concentrates in the placenta. An alternative but uncommon strategy is to use more potent antiparasitic agents during the early phase before encystment takes place in the foetus. For example, pyrimethamine and sulphadiazine (together with folinic acid) can be prescribed for 1 month after confirmation of primary maternal infection, at any point after 16 weeks of gestation (A. Pollak, personal communication). Pyrimethamine and sulphadiazine are not prescribed before 16 weeks because of a theoretical teratogenic risk (see 'Treatment to reduce the risk of foetal damage'). Much more common is routine treatment with pyrimethamine and sulphadiazine for maternal infection acquired in the third trimester, in view of the high risk of foetal infection (R. E. Gilbert, unpublished data from the European Multicentre Study on Congenital Toxoplasmosis).

The duration of therapy to prevent foetal infection also varies. In most centres, spiramycin is continued throughout pregnancy, even if infection occurred in the first trimester, due to a perceived risk of delayed transmission. Reports of delayed transmission come from studies in animals (Remington et al. 1995). In humans, direct evidence of delayed transmission would be provided by the absence of infection early in pregnancy (demonstrated by polymerase chain reaction, PCR, analysis of amniotic fluid) in foetuses who are found to be infected later in pregnancy or at birth, or by detection of *T. gondii* infection in the placenta of an uninfected baby. Such cases are rare (Couvreur et al. 1988; Hohlfeld et al. 1994) and may be due to delayed transmission of infection from the placenta to the foetus or to false-positive prenatal tests or false-negative postnatal tests. Given the low, or nonexistent risk of delayed transmission, continuation of treatment throughout pregnancy is controversial. However, few centres stop spiramycin after 1 month in the absence of foetal infection (personal communication, Babill Stray-Pedersen).

Reducing the risk of damage in infected foetuses

Identification of infected foetuses

Diagnosis of foetal infection is frequently based on PCR detection of toxoplasma DNA in amniotic fluid. The widespread availability and low cost of amniocentesis, which can be undertaken after 15 weeks gestation, has dramatically changed the management of toxoplasma infection during the second trimester. Previously, foetal infection could only be diagnosed by cordocentesis after 20–22 weeks gestation in a limited number of specialist centres and was associated with at least 1–2% risk of foetal loss due to the procedure, but this is now rarely offered. In contrast, the risk of foetal loss associated with amniocentesis is 0.9% (95% confidence interval: 0–1.9%) (Tabor et al. 1986).

When undertaken by specialist centres, PCR appears to be highly sensitive and specific (Hohlfeld et al. 1994). However, the performance of this technique under less rigorously controlled conditions is a cause for concern (Guy et al. 1996), because false-positive results are a recognized problem with PCR tests and could lead to unnecessary treatment or termination.

Identification of foetuses with lesions due to congenital toxoplasmosis

A variety of ultrasound findings have been reported in foetuses with congenital toxoplasmosis, the most commonly reported being intracranial calcification and hydrocephalus (Hohlfeld et al. 1991). These lesions are rarely detectable until after 22–24 weeks of gestation. The degree of calcification or hydrocephalus predictive of symptoms or disability is not known. Many children with these signs appear to be asymptomatic (Berrebi et al. 1994; Mets et al. 1996) and intracranial lesions appear to resolve or diminish in the majority of children treated postnatally (Patel et al. 1996). However, in many centres, infected women undergo regular foetal ultrasound, monthly or even 2 weekly, to detect abnormalities which might be attributable to congenital toxoplasmosis. There is general consensus about the offer of late termination if foetal infection and ultrasound abnormalities are confirmed.

Treatment to reduce the risk of foetal damage

Once foetal infection is diagnosed treatment is changed from spiramycin to pyrimethamine and sulphadiazine or pyrimethamine and sulphadoxine (Fansidar™) together with folinic acid. Both combinations of drugs cross the placenta into the foetal circulation and can lead to bone marrow suppression, liver damage as well as milder adverse effects such as rashes, nausea and vomiting in the mother. They also have a theoretical teratogenic effect because of their antifolate action. In view of these adverse effects, in most centres these regimens are usually limited to proven cases of foetal infection or to women infected in late pregnancy in the absence of foetal diagnosis (R. E. Gilbert, European Multicentre Study on Congenital Toxoplasmosis, unpublished data).

Evidence for treatment efficacy

To our knowledge, no controlled trials have been published comparing the effects of prenatal antiparasitic treatments with those of no treatment on the risks of foetal infection, or clinical signs or symptoms in congenitally infected children. In studies in which women were treated, the risks of congenital infection and clinical manifestations appeared to be similar or worse than those in studies in which women were not treated (see Tables 8.2 and 8.5). Such comparisons are essentially uninterpretable due to differences in definition of infection, lack of adjustment for gestation, and the selection and follow-up biases referred to earlier. The exception is the study by Desmonts and Couvreur (1984), who compared treated and untreated women and claimed that spiramycin reduced the risk of foetal infection by 50%. However, this finding may have been due to the way the study was carried out. The untreated women were ascertained retrospectively, increasing the risk of selection bias (Rothman & Greenland 1998). In other words, infected women with infected babies and particularly those with symptomatic babies would be more likely to be tested than infected women with healthy, uninfected babies. In addition, no account was taken of the fact that untreated women were infected later in pregnancy (Desmonts & Couvreur 1984). These problems are discussed by Couvreur et al. (1988) in a reanalysis of past case series, using isolation of *T. gondii* from the placenta as a proxy for congenital infection.

Termination of pregnancy

Pregnancy may be terminated for maternal infection alone or following the diagnosis of foetal infection or the detection of foetal abnormalities. Termination rates depend on gestation at diagnosis (early termination may be preferable to late termination), local regulations relating to abortion and cultural attitudes. The favourable clinical outcomes in congenitally infected children seen in recent studies have led to a shift away from therapeutic termination, even in proven foetal infection, except where intracranial abnormalities are demonstrable on foetal ultrasound. However, clinical policies in referral centres may not reflect local practice. According to anecdotal reports, the termination of pregnancy for maternal toxoplasma infection alone undoubtedly occurs in many European countries (Buffolano et al. 1994).

Identification of congenitally infected infants who may benefit from follow-up and treatment during infancy

A potentially important benefit of prenatal screening is to identify children at risk of congenital infection so that those children known to be infected may benefit from treatment and clinical follow-up during infancy. The vast majority of congenitally infected infants (at least 90%) are asymptomatic in early infancy and would be missed by routine paediatric examinations. Even where newborn screening operates, prenatal screening would identify a significant minority of infected infants missed by neonatal tests which appear to be only 80% sensitive (Pinon et al. 1996; Lebech et al. 1999). Based on a small number of infants missed by the Massachusetts newborn screening programme, it has been suggested that congenitally infected infants who have no detectable IgM antibodies are more likely to have acquired infection early in the pregnancy, and therefore to have lesions and symptoms, than IgM-positive infants (Guerina et al. 1994).

The benefits of prenatal compared with neonatal screening depend on: (1) the reduction in the risk of mother-to-child transmission of *T. gondii* infection achieved by prenatal treatment; (2) the reduction in the risk of symptoms in congenitally infected children achieved by prenatal and postnatal treatment compared with postnatal treatment alone in children detected by both screening strategies; and (3) the reduction in the risk of symptoms achieved by prenatal and postnatal treatment in the 30% missed by neonatal screening compared with postnatal treatment given after clinical manifestations become apparent. None of these effects have been assessed in studies with comparable treated and untreated patients.

Risk of symptomatic congenital toxoplasmosis

Women who acquire infection during pregnancy must decide whether to undergo further investigations, treatment, termination or to take no action. In order to make this decision, they need to know the risk of giving birth to a child who will develop clinical symptoms due to congenital toxoplasmosis, the nature of these symptoms and how much this risk can be reduced by treatment. These risks are not known with any certainty. The risk of symptoms due to congenital toxoplasmosis is a function of the risk of mother-to-child transmission, which increases with gestation at maternal acquisition of infection, and the risk of symptoms in infected children, which decreases with gestation (Dunn et al. 1999).

Table 8.6 represents these risks based on upper estimates derived from studies by Desmonts and Couvreur (1984). These data include a mix of retrospectively and prospectively ascertained women, are based on a referral centre caseload and have limited information about methods of selection, loss to follow-up and clinical symptoms. Such biases are likely to overestimate the risk of significant signs and symptoms. A recent study in Lyon, France showed that the risk of clinical signs in congenitally infected infants was highest if infection occurred at 24–30 weeks of gestation, falling to 5% in women infected in the first trimester or just before delivery (Dunn et al. 1999).

The figures in Table 8.6 provide an upper estimate of the risk of significant clinical manifestations in infected women. Between 2.5% and 6% of women (or 1 in

Table 8.6. Estimated risks of congenital toxoplasmosis and significant signs and symptoms of congenital toxoplasmosis according to gestation at acquisition of maternal infection (upper estimates derived from Desmonts & Couvreur 1984)

Risk in infected women	Trimester I	Trimester II	Trimester III
Liveborn with congenital toxoplasmosis	9% (11/120)	28% (68/241)	52% (66/128)
Liveborn with significant signs and symptoms[*]	6% (7/120)	2.5% (6/241)	0% (0/128)[**]

Key:
[*]Excludes mild signs such as peripheral retinochoroidal lesions.
[**]95% confidence interval = 0–3%.

40 to 1 in 17) who undergo diagnostic amniocentesis and treatment or termination are predicted to have a child who develops significant symptoms or signs due to congenital toxoplasmosis. These estimates are based on studies in which most women were treated. The lack of information about treatment efficacy means that we cannot assess the risk associated with not giving antiparasitic treatment.

Identification of susceptible women who may benefit from information about how to avoid infection

There is general consensus that, in addition to providing information about how to avoid toxoplasma infection before or early in pregnancy, prenatal testing provides the opportunity to reinforce this advice to nonimmune pregnant women (Ho-Yen et al. 1995). However, the quality of information given is variable and it is not known whether giving health information to pregnant women has any effect on the risk of toxoplasma infection (Newton & Hall 1995). Typically women are advised to cook meat thoroughly, avoid contact with cat faeces, wash their hands after handling soil, wash vegetables thoroughly and avoid cured meat products (Ho-Yen et al. 1995; Buffolano et al. 1996). One study showed a small change in the incidence of infection over time when health information was given, but this effect cannot be separated from random chance or secular trends (Foulon et al. 1988). No studies have been undertaken to determine whether women who know that they are susceptible to infection, and have this reinforced by repeated serological tests during pregnancy, are more likely to avoid sources of toxoplasma infection than pregnant women given information without testing. In a French study, only 17% of women who knew they were susceptible and had received health information reported taking any action to avoid infection (Wallon et al. 1994).

Potential harms of prenatal screening

Virtually all health-care interventions involve a trade-off between potential harms and benefits. Decisions will vary depending on individual's values about possible outcomes and how likely these are to occur. Before deciding whether to undergo screening tests for toxoplasma infection, women need to be informed about the chances of harm as well as benefit. Moreover, judging by women's responses when asked about other screening tests, they want to be more informed (Oliver et al. 1996; Dodds 1997).

Psychological effects

The potential psychological harmful effects of prenatal screening programmes in general have been reviewed by Green and Statham (1996). Harmful effects relating specifically to prenatal screening for toxoplasmosis include: anxiety generated by delays between screening and diagnostic tests, anxiety associated with false-positive tests and anxiety generated by the anticipation of late onset of symptoms in congenitally infected children.

Evidence from studies on screening for Down syndrome suggests that the high levels of anxiety generated by false-positive results do not resolve immediately when subsequent testing shows no signs of diseases (Marteau et al. 1992), and may leave the parents asking, 'If the baby doesn't have Down's, what does it have?'. Similar concerns are likely to affect the large number of women falsely identified as infected with *T. gondii*. For women with confirmed *T. gondii* infection, anxiety is likely to be even more prolonged, because of the poor sensitivity of tests for foetal infection: a negative PCR test of amniotic fluid still leaves the theoretical possibility of transplacental transmission of infection later in pregnancy – and many centres continue treatment throughout pregnancy for this reason. Each test is associated with delays and difficult choices between treatment, termination or no intervention.

Similar anxieties affect the parents and child after birth. Negative tests cannot rule out congenital infection until late infancy, and infected but asymptomatic children are labelled as at risk of eye disease, or even mental impairment, reinforced by yearly examinations throughout childhood.

Clinical effects in mothers, foetuses and children
Mother and foetus

One of the principle harmful effects of toxoplasma screening is the risk of termination of uninfected or unaffected foetuses and the risk of foetal loss as a result of amniocentesis undertaken for foetal diagnosis. Women with confirmed infection during pregnancy usually undergo amniocentesis to detect foetal infection. The procedure related foetal loss rate is 0.9%. Consequently, for every 100 women infected during the second trimester and undergoing amniocentesis one foetus will be lost as a result of the procedure and 28 infected foetuses would be identified, of whom two to three would develop significant signs or symptoms (based on upper estimates in Table 8.5), and an unknown proportion, if any, would benefit from treatment. The risk of foetal loss is at least two times higher following cordocentesis, leading to an approximately equal risk of losing a foetus due to cordocentesis.

Termination of pregnancy carries a considerable risk of clinical and psychological harms which are likely to vary with the length of gestation. The chance of terminating a normal foetus is high at all gestations, and particularly in the absence of confirmed foetal infection. When foetal infection is confirmed, false-positive PCR detection of toxoplasma DNA in amniotic fluid is a concern in some centres. However, even where tests have been shown to be highly specific, it is not possible to determine which babies are destined to develop symptoms. In the example above, 28 infected foetuses would be terminated for every two to three symptomatic babies prevented. In view of these figures, termination is usually recommended only in the presence of confirmed foetal infection and intracranial abnormalities which cannot be detected by foetal ultrasound until 22–24 weeks gestation. Although the presence of such abnormalities reduces the risk of terminating an asymptomatic foetus, the psychological effects of late termination may be greater than for early termination.

Other adverse clinical effects for the mother include repeated blood tests, the discomfort of amniocentesis and adverse effects of drug therapy. Adverse effects include bone marrow suppression, which is common but rarely sufficient to discontinue therapy, and gastrointestinal disturbance.

Children

Investigations All children exposed to maternal infection experience the distress and discomfort of repeated examinations and investigations. They are subjected to approximately six blood tests during the first year of life, repeated clinical examinations, at least one ophthalmological examination, and skull radiograph or cranial ultrasound scan on at least one occasion. For children with confirmed congenital toxoplasmosis, even in the absence of symptoms, investigations are repeated at least annually for years, possibly until adolescence.

Drug effects Some children born to infected women are given antiparasitic treatment with spiramycin for at least the first 2–3 months or until there is evidence of a decline in maternal IgG antibody titre. Adverse effects of spiramycin are minimal apart from the distress of administration of the drug itself. Young infants with confirmed or suspected congenital toxoplasmosis are treated with pyrimethamine and sulphadiazine (or sulphadoxine) for 12 months in most centres and up to 24 months in some. The principle adverse effects of such treatment include bone marrow suppression, rashes and gastrointestinal disturbance. The risk of bone marrow suppression generates the need for blood tests to monitor leucocyte counts every 3–6 weeks. Anecdotal reports suggest that clinicians frequently have to lower drug dosages because of falling leucocyte counts. Permanent or temporary discontinuation of therapy due to adverse side-effects has been reported in 10–35% of children (Guerina et al. 1994; Mombro et al. 1995).

There is a theoretical but yet unknown possibility of rare or long-term adverse effects of treatment *in utero* or early childhood, given the small number of children followed-up long term. Pyrimethamine and sulphadiazine, or sulphadoxine (Fansidar™) have a profound depressive effect on IgG production and it is not clear whether this has any effect on childhood response to infective agents. Toxic shock syndrome (Lyells disease) is a rare, potential adverse effect of Fansidar™.

Legal considerations

Fears about legal action in the event of a symptomatic child whose mother was not detected and treated in pregnancy appears to be a major incentive for aggressive testing and treatment by clinicians. Such fears, and the legal cases themselves, reinforce the perception that treatment can reduce or even prevent symptoms in infected children, despite the lack of empirical evidence of the benefits of treatment. Complaints about the harmful effects of screening and subsequent interventions rarely result in litigation or even publicity (Anonymous 1991). However, both these bases for complaint and legal action, namely the failure to detect and treat and unnecessary investigation and treatment, could be avoided if women were fully informed about the potential harms and benefits before they decided whether or not to undergo screening and subsequent interventions.

Costs

Given the universal pressures to contain health-care costs, the incremental cost effectiveness – the extra cost of one programme compared with that of preventing another symptomatic child– is likely to be the principle determinant of policy. However, such information is not yet available and, in particular, there are no clear answers to two key questions: what is the risk of symptoms due to congenital toxoplasmosis and how much is this risk reduced by treatment? Sensitivity analyses can be used to test the effect of a range of risk estimates and treatment effects but, to date, the scope of economic analyses of preventive strategies for congenital toxoplasmosis is too limited to be useful for policy decisions. Many studies have failed to adequately explore the combined effect of different absolute risks of symptoms and treatment efficacy on the outcomes of prenatal screening, and the costs of the large number of women falsely identified as positive (Henderson et al. 1984; Thorp et al. 1988; Roberts & Frenkel 1990; Lappalainen et al. 1995a). In view of the considerable costs and uncertain benefits, several reports have called for further research, including randomized controlled trials of prenatal treatment, before prenatal screening is implemented further (Jeannel et al. 1990; Multidisciplinary Working Group 1992; Eskild et al. 1996).

In view of the lack of evidence about the relative effectiveness of treatment during pregnancy or infancy, no economic analyses have yet been carried out to determine the incremental cost-effectiveness (how much additional cost per symptomatic case prevented) of prenatal compared with newborn screening and/or primary prevention. However, the comparatively low cost of newborn screening has generated pressure for demonstrable benefits of prenatal over newborn screening. Crude estimates of the cost of serological testing alone for 780,000 pregnant women (the approximate number per year in France and UK) are approximately £32 million in France (Petithory et al. 1993) for prenatal screening with monthly retesting and £3 million for the same number based on Danish costs for neonatal blood spot screening (to detect neonatal toxoplasma IgM) (E. Petersen, personal communication).

Decisions about prenatal screening for toxoplasmosis

The existence of tests to detect foetal problems creates pressures to use technology. Studies show that obstetricians routinely use tests that they consider to be inaccurate (Green & Statham 1996) and, although women can in theory decide to accept or decline an offer of a screening test, in France this would disqualify them from state maternity benefit. Tymstra (1989) suggests that women are driven by 'anticipated decision regret', 'I would never forgive myself if . . .', and this motivation, together with the expectation that the very existence of a test makes an implicit statement that the test is of proven benefit (Green & Statham 1996), may make it difficult to weigh uncertain harms and benefits of screening even if the information were available. The extent of shock and surprise expressed at the extremely low risk of one normal foetus terminated for every 200 abnormal foetal ultrasounds resulting in termination reinforces the view that women do not expect harmful outcomes when offered screening (Oliver et al. 1996).

Given the lack of evidence about the effect of antiparasitic treatment on the risk of foetal infection or damage, the offer of prenatal screening implies benefits which are unknown, and is unethical unless undertaken in the context of controlled studies. Where women request testing, the uncertain benefits make it imperative that women are fully informed about the potential benefits and harms in order to decide whether to opt for screening and subsequent interventions or not. However, women's decisions are not solely determined by the risk of harms of benefits. Their trade-off of a potential reduction in the risk of a symptomatic child afforded by treatment versus the risk of adverse drug effects, or of terminating a normal foetus compared with a damaged one, are also affected by their values of these different outcomes. For example, some women may be willing to forego a small risk of mild visual impairment in return for avoiding treatment associated with a low and unquantified risk of foetal damage and unknown long-term risks. Exceptionally, women may be willing to undergo termination for a one in ten risk (odds of symptoms in infected children born to women infected during the second trimester – see Table 8.5) that the baby will develop significant symptoms such as unilateral visual impairment in later life.

Because of such extreme cases, it is difficult to refuse prenatal testing on request, although compulsory testing is not justifiable. The provision of services to support on-request testing needs to balance the benefits of choice with the harms and costs of testing, diagnosis and treatment. Where testing is requested, it is the role of the clinician to inform the woman about the risks of harms and benefits and to find out what outcomes she values most in order to help her decide. However, anecdotally it appears that clinicians advising women are often not well informed, and, based on their beliefs that the law penalizes only missed cases (and not unnecessary intervention), feel obliged to encourage the woman to agree to testing and treatment. In such circumstances, informed decision-making by women is likely to be the exception rather than the rule.

REFERENCES

Ades, A. E. (1992). Methods for estimating the incidence of primary infection in pregnancy, a reappraisal of toxoplasmosis and cytomegalovirus data. *Epidemiology and Infection*, **108**, 367–75.

Ades, A. E. & Nokes, D. J. (1993). Modeling age- and time-specific incidence from seroprevalence, toxoplasmosis. *American Journal of Epidemiology*, **137**, 1022–34.

Alford, C. Jr., Stagno, S. & Reynolds, D. W. (1974). Congenital toxoplasmosis, clinical, laboratory, and therapeutic considerations, with special reference to subclinical disease. *Bulletin of the New York Academy of Medicine*, **50**, 160–81.

Ancelle, T., Goulet, V., Tirard-Fleury, V. et al. (1996). La Toxoplasmose chez la femme enceinte en France en 1995. Resultats d'une enquete nationale perinatale. *Bulletin Epidemiologique Hebdomadiare*, **51**, 227–9.

Anonymous (1991). Controversy breeds ignorance. *British Medical Journal*, **302**, 973–4.

Aspock, H. & Pollak, A. (1992). Prevention of prenatal toxoplasmosis by serological screening of pregnant women in Austria. *Scandinavian Journal of Infectious Diseases Supplement*, 84, 32–7.

Berger, R., Merkel, S. & Rudin, C. (1995). Toxoplasmose und Schwangerschaft-Erkenntnisse aus einem Nabelschnurblut-Screening von 30 000 Neugeborenen. *Schweizerische Medizinische Wochenschrift*, 125, 1168–73.

Berrebi, A., Kobuch, W. E., Bessieres, M. H. et al. (1994). Termination of pregnancy for maternal toxoplasmosis. *Lancet*, 344, 36–9.

Bornand, J. E. & Piguet, J. D. (1991). Toxoplasma infestation, prevalence, risk of congenital infection and development in Geneva from 1973 to 1987. *Schweizerische Medizinische Wochenschrift*, 121, 21–9.

Buffolano, W., Sagliocca, L., Fratta, D., Tozzi, A., Cardone, A. & Binkin, N. (1994). Prenatal Toxoplasmosis screening in Campania region, Italy. *Italian Journal of Gynaecology and Obstetrics*, 3, 70–4.

Buffolano, W., Gilbert, R. E., Holland, F. J., Fratta, D., Palumbo, F. & Ades, A. E. (1996). Risk factors for recent toxoplasma infection in pregnant women in Naples. *Epidemiology and Infection*, 116, 347–51.

Conyn van Spaendonck, M. A. E. (1989). Prevention of congenital toxoplasmosis, experience in The Netherlands. *International Ophthalmology*, 13, 403–6.

Conyn van Spaedonck, M. A. E. (1991). Prevention of congenital toxoplasmosis in the Netherlands [Thesis]. *National Institute of Public Health and Environmental Protection*.

Couvreur, J., Desmonts, G. & Thulliez, P. (1988). Prophylaxis of congenital toxoplasmosis. Effects of spiramycin on placental infection. *Journal of Antimicrobial Chemotherapy*, 22 [Suppl. B], 193–200.

Desmonts, G. & Couvreur, J. (1984). Toxoplasmose congenitale. Etude prospective de l'issue de la grossesse chez 542 femmes atteintes de toxoplasmose acquise en cours de gestation. *Annales de Pediatrie*, 31, 806–9.

Dodds, R. (1997). *The Stress of Tests in Pregnancy*. Summary of a National Childbirth Trust antenatal screening survey. Oxford: National Childbirth Trust.

Dunn, D., Wallon, M., Peyron, F. et al. (1999). Mother to child transmission of toxoplasmosis: risk estimates for clinical counselling. *Lancet*, 353, 1824–33.

Eskild, A., Oxman, A., Magnus, P. et al. (1996). Screening for toxoplasmosis in pregnancy, what is the evidence of reducing a health problem? *Journal of Medical Screening*, 3, 188–94.

Forsgren, M. (1990). Genital herpes simplex virus infection and incidence of neonatal disease in Sweden. *Scandinavian Journal of Infectious Diseases Supplement*, 69, 37–41.

Forsgren, M., Gille, E., Ljungstrom, I. & Nokes, D. J. (1991). *Toxoplasma gondii* antibodies in pregnant women in Stockholm in 1969, 1979, and 1987 [letter]. *Lancet*, 337, 1413–14.

Fortier, B., Aissi, E., Ajana, F. et al. (1991). Spontaneous abortion and reinfection by *Toxoplasma gondii* [letter]. *Lancet*, 338, 444.

Foulon, W., Naessens, A., Lauwers, S. et al. (1988). Impact of primary prevention on the incidence of toxoplasmosis during pregnancy. *Obstetrics and Gynecology*, 72, 363–6.

Gilbert, R. E., Stanford, M. R., Jackson, H., Holliman, R. E. & Sanders, M. D. (1995). Incidence of acute symptomatic toxoplasma retinochoroiditis in south London according to country of birth. *British Medical Journal*, 310, 1037–40.

Gilbert, R. E., Dunn, D., Lightman, S. et al. (1999). Incidence of symptomatic toxoplasma eye disease: aetiology and public health implications. *Epidemiology and Infection*, 123, 283–9.

Green, J. & Statham, H. (1996). Psychological aspects of prenatal screening and diagnosis. In *The Troubled Helix. Social and Psychological Implications of the New Human Genetics*, 1st edn, ed. T. Marteau, M. Richards. Cambridge: Cambridge University Press, pp. 140–63.

Guerina, N. G., Hsu, H. W., Meissner, H. C. et al. (1994). Neonatal serologic screening and early treatment for congenital *Toxoplasma gondii* infection. *New England Journal of Medicine*, 330, 1858–63.

Guy, E. C., Pelloux, H., Lappalainen, M. et al. (1996). Interlaboratory comparison of polymerase chain reaction for the detection of *Toxoplasma gondii* DNA added to samples of amniotic fluid. *European Journal of Clinical Microbiology and Infectious Diseases*, 15, 836–9.

Hall, S. M. (1992). Congenital toxoplasmosis. *British Medical Journal*, 305, 291–7.

Heckerling, P. S. & Verp, M. S. (1991). Amniocentesis or chorionic villus sampling for prenatal genetic testing, a decision analysis. *Journal of Clinical Epidemiology*, 44, 657–70.

Henderson, J. B., Beattie, C. P., Hale, E. G. & Wright, T. (1984). The evaluation of new services, possibilities for preventing congenital toxoplasmosis. *International Journal of Epidemiology*, 13, 65–72.

Hengst, P. (1992). Screening for toxoplasmosis in pregnant women, presentation of a screening programme in the former "East" Germany, and the present status in Germany. *Scandinavian Journal of Infectious Diseases Supplement*, 84, 38–42.

Hennequin, C., Dureau, P., N'Guyen, L. et al. (1997). Congenital toxoplasmosis acquired from an immune woman. *Pediatric Infectious Disease Journal*, 16, 75–7.

Ho-Yen, D. O., Dargie, L., Chatterton, J. M. W. & Petersen, E. (1995). Toxoplasma health education in Europe. *Health Education Journal*, 54, 415–20.

Hohlfeld, P., MacAleese, J., Capella-Pavlovsky, M. et al. (1991). Fetal toxoplasmosis, ultrasonographic signs. *Ultrasound in Obstetrics and Gynecology*, 1, 241–4.

Hohlfeld, P., Daffos, F., Costa, J.-M., Thulliez, P., Forestier, F. & Vidaud, M. (1994). Prenatal diagnosis of congenital toxoplasmosis with a polymerase-chain reaction test on amniotic fluid. *New England Journal of Medicine*, 331, 695–9.

Holland, F. J., Ades, A. E., Davison, C. F. et al. (1994). Use of anonymous newborn serosurveys to evaluate antenatal HIV screening programmes. *Journal of Medical Screening*, 1, 176–9.

Holliman, R. E. (1994). Clinical sequelae of chronic maternal toxoplasmosis. *Reviews in Medical Microbiology*, 5, 47–55.

Jeannel, D., Costagliola, D., Niel, G., Hubert, B. & Danis, M. (1990). What is known about the prevention of congenital toxoplasmosis?. *Lancet*, 336, 359–61.

Joynson, D. H., Payne, R. A. & Rawal, B. K. (1990). Potential role of IgG avidity for diagnosing toxoplasmosis. *Journal of Clinical Pathology*, 43, 1032–3.

Kimball, A. C., Kean, B. H. & Fuchs, F. (1971). Congenital toxoplasmosis, a prospective study of 4,048 obstetric patients. *American Journal of Obstetrics and Gynecology*, 111, 211–18.

Koppe, J. G. & Rothova, A. (1989). Congenital toxoplasmosis. A long-term follow-up of 20 years. *International Ophthalmology*, 13, 387–390.

Koppe, J. G., Kloosterman, G. H., de Roever-Bonnet, H., et al. (1974). Toxoplasmosis and pregnancy, with a long-term follow-up of the children. *European Journal of Obstetrics, Gynaecology and Reproductive Biology*, 4/3, 101–10.

Koppe, J. G., Loewer-Sieger, D. H. & Roever-Bonnet, H. D. (1986). Results of 20-year follow-up of congenital toxoplasmosis. *Lancet*, 1, 254–6.

Lappalainen, M., Koskela, P., Hedman, K. et al. (1992). Incidence of primary toxoplasma infections during pregnancy in southern Finland, a prospective cohort study. *Scandinavian Journal of Infectious Diseases*, 24, 97–104.

Lappalainen, M., Koskela, P., Koskiniemi, M. et al. (1993). Toxoplasmosis acquired during pregnancy: improved serodiagnosis based on avidity of IgG. *Journal of Infectious Diseases*, 167, 691–7.

Lappalainen, M., Sintonen, H., Koskiniemi, M. et al. (1995a). Cost-benefit analysis of screening for toxoplasmosis during pregnancy. *Scandinavian Journal of Infectious Diseases*, 27, 265–72.

Lappalainen, M., Koskiniemi, M., Hiilesmaa, V. et al. (1995b). Outcome of children after maternal primary Toxoplasma infection during pregnancy with emphasis on avidity of specific IgG. *Pediatric Infectious Diseases Journal*, 14, 354–61.

Lebech, M. & Petersen, E. (1992). Neonatal screening for congenital toxoplasmosis in Denmark; presentation of the design of a prospective study. *Scandinavian Journal of Infectious Diseases*, 84 [Suppl.], 75–9.

Lebech, M., Joynson, D. H. M., Seitz, H. M. et al. (1996). Classification system and case definitions of *Toxoplasma gondii* infection in immunocompetent pregnant women and their congenitally infected offspring. *European Journal of Clinical Microbiology and Infectious Diseases*, 15, 799–805.

Lebech, M., Andersen, O., Christensen, N. C. et al. (1999). Feasibility of neonatal screening for toxoplasma infection in the absence of prenatal treatment. Danish Congenital Toxoplasmosis Study Group. *Lancet*, 353, 1834–7.

Marteau, T. M., Cook, R., Kidd, J. et al. (1992). The psychological effects of false positive results in prenatal screening for fetal abnormality, a prospective study. *Prenatal Diagnosis*, 12, 205–14.

Mets, M. B., Holfels, E., Boyer, K. M. et al. (1996). Eye manifestations of congenital toxoplasmosis. *American Journal of Ophthalmology*, 122, 309–24.

Mombro, M., Perathoner, C., Leone, A. et al. (1995). Congenital toxoplasmosis, 10-year follow-up. *European Journal of Pediatrics*, 154, 635–9.

Multidisciplinary Working Group (1992). Prenatal screening for toxoplasmosis in the UK. London: Royal College of Obstetricians and Gynaecologists.

Newton, L. H. & Hall, S. M. (1995). A survey of health education material for the primary prevention of congenital toxoplasmosis. *Communicable Disease Reports*, 5, R21–R27.

Nokes, D. J., Forsgren, M., Gille, E. & Ljungstrom, I. (1993). Modelling toxoplasma incidence from longitudinal seroprevalence in Stockholm, Sweden. *Parasitology*, 107, 33–40.

Oliver, S., Rajan, L., Turner, H. et al. (1996). Informed choice for users of health services, views on ultrasonographers. *British Medical Journal*, 313, 1251–5.

Patel, D. V., Holfels, E., Vogel, N. et al. (1996). Resolution of intracranial calcifications in infants with treated congenital toxoplasmosis. *Radiology*, 199, 433–40.

Petithory, J. C., Garin, J. P. & Milgram, M. (1993). Serologie de la toxoplasmose. Aspect actuels a travers le controle de qualite nationel en parasitologie en France. In *Formation Continue Conventionelle des Directeurs de Laboratoires Prives d'Analyses de Biologie Medicale 1992*. Paris: Bioforma, pp. 25–51.

Pinon, J. M., Chemla, C., Villena, I. et al. (1996). Early neonatal diagnosis of congenital toxoplasmosis, Value of comparative enzyme-linked immunofiltration assay immunological profiles and anti-*Toxoplasma gondii* immunoglobulin M (IgM) or IgA immunocapture and implications for postnatal therapeutic strategies. *Journal of Clinical Microbiology*, **34**, 579–83.

Pratlong, F., Boulot, P., Issert, E. et al. (1994). Fetal diagnosis of toxoplasmosis in 190 women infected during pregnancy. *Prenatal Diagnosis*, **14**, 191–8.

Remington, J. S., McLeod, R. & Desmonts, G. (1995). In *Infectious Diseases of the Foetus and Newborn*, 4th edn., ed. J. S. Remington, J. Klein. Philadelphia: WB Saunders, pp. 140–267.

Roberts, T. & Frenkel, J. K. (1990). Estimating income losses and other preventable costs caused by congenital toxoplasmosis in people in the United States. *Journal of the American Veterinary Medical Association*, **196**, 249–56.

Roizen, N., Swisher, C. N., Stein, M. A. et al. (1995). Neurologic and developmental outcome in treated congenital toxoplasmosis. *Pediatrics*, **95**, 11–20.

Rothman, K. J. & Greenland, S. (1998). *Modern Epidemiology*, 2nd edn. Philadelphia: Lippincott-Raven Publishers.

Rothova, A. (1993). Ocular involvement in toxoplasmosis. *British Journal of Ophthalmology*, **77**, 371–7.

Sever, J. L., Ellenberg, J. H., Ley, A. C. et al. (1988). Toxoplasmosis, maternal and pediatric findings in 23,000 pregnancies. *Pediatrics*, **82**, 181–92.

Stray-Pedersen, B. & Jenum, P. (1992). Economic evaluation of preventive programmes against congenital toxoplasmosis. *Scandinavian Journal of Infectious Diseases Supplement*, **84**, 86–96.

Tabor, A., Madsen, M., Obel, E. B. et al. (1986). Randomised controlled trial of genetic amniocentesis in 4606 low-risk women. *Lancet*, i, 1287–93.

Thorp, J. M., Seeds, J. W., Herbert, W. N. P. et al. (1988). Prenatal management and congenital toxoplasmosis. *New England Journal of Medicine*, **319**, 372–3.

Thulliez, P. (1992). Screening programme for congenital toxoplasmosis in France. *Scandinavian Journal of Infectious Diseases Supplement*, **84**, 43–5.

Tookey, P. A. & Peckham, C. (1996). Neonatal herpes simplex virus infections in the British Isles. *Paediatric and Perinatal Epidemiology*, **10**, 432–42.

Tymstra, T. (1989). The imperative character of medical technology and the meaning of anticipated decision regret. *International Journal of Technology Assessment in Health Care*, **5**, 207–13.

Walker, J., Nokes, D. J. & Jennings, R. (1992). Longitudinal study of Toxoplasma seroprevalence in South Yorkshire. *Epidemiology and Infection*, **108**, 99–106.

Wallon, M., Mallaret, M. R., Mojon, M. & Peyron, F. (1994). Congenital toxoplasmosis, assessment of prevention policy. *Presse Medicale*, **23**, 1467–70.

9

Newborn screening for congenital toxoplasma infection

R. B. Eaton, R. Lynfield, H.-W. Hsu and G. F. Grady

Newborn Toxoplasmosis Screening Program, State Laboratory Institute, Jamaica Plain, USA

Introduction

Congenital transmission of *Toxoplasma gondii*, accompanied by severe pathology, was recognized over a half century ago (Wolf et al. 1939). Medical communities around the world have struggled with how best to respond to this threat. Even though an impressive amount of knowledge of *T. gondii* has been accumulated, some of the most basic questions required to set public health policies regarding congenital toxoplasmosis have yet to be answered.

In the midst of such uncertainty, and under influences unique to each region of the globe, three philosophical approaches to the detection of congenitally infected babies have evolved:

1 universal prenatal screening of mothers to identify those who seroconvert to produce *T. gondii* antibody during pregnancy;
2 universal newborn screening to identify infants with *T. gondii* specific IgM; and
3 no universal programme.

It is doubtful that any one of these may presently be unequivocally deemed the approach of choice for all communities.

In 1986, The New England Newborn Screening Programme, currently operating under the University of Massachusetts Medical School, was the first centre to choose the second option, newborn screening, on a universal scale. In January 1999, countrywide newborn screening was implemented in Denmark. Newborn screening for congenital toxoplasmosis is also being performed in parts of Brazil and France (Marseilles region), and pilot programmes have been initiated in other countries.

This chapter describes the experiences of the New England programme. We hope that the information will be particularly useful to those centres in the process of re-evaluating ongoing programmes or considering implementation of a screening programme for congenital *T. gondii* infection, and will be of general interest to readers of this volume.

The philosophy

Appropriateness of newborn screening

Before newborn screening may be considered a viable option for detecting congenital *T. gondii* infection in a particular community, one needs to ask whether newborn screening is ever appropriate for this medical situation. Newborn screening was first implemented in 1961 to detect an inborn error of phenylalanine metabolism. Endocrine disorders were added to many programmes in the 1970s, and haemoglobinopathies were added more recently. However, infectious diseases have generally not been included in the list of conditions tested for by newborn screening programmes.

CORN (the USA Council of Regional Networks for Genetic Services) provided guidelines regarding the issues that should be considered before adding a new test to a newborn screening programme. Briefly, 'incidence data and population statistics must indicate that screening for the disorder will result in detection of a reasonable number of cases. Additionally, the laboratory protocol proposed must be sufficiently sensitive to serve as a viable method for use with the specimens of interest. These specimens must be economically and technically feasible to collect, transport, and analyse. Screening should be initiated only if intervention is accessible to all affected individuals.' (Therrell et al. 1992). Each of these issues deserves our attention.

Sufficient incidence

The incidence of *T. gondii* infection for a given community is generally not known because the majority of affected infants are not identified at birth (Desmonts & Couvreur 1974). Estimates may be derived by conducting a pilot study of the age-specific seroprevalence of *T. gondii* antibodies in childbearing women, calculating the expected frequency of primary infections during pregnancy, and estimating the expected maternal–foetal transmission rate. In 1986 a pilot study conducted on specimens from 100,000 Massachusetts newborns suggested a 0.1–0.2% annual rate of new infections among pregnant women in Massachusetts (Hsu et al. 1992). Unfortunately, published estimates of maternal–foetal transmission rate vary widely even when allowance is made for gestational times (Desmonts & Couvreur 1974; Jeannel et al. 1988; Henri et al. 1992) and estimates of congenital infection rates vary accordingly. Even assuming an average transmission rate of only 10% (the low end of estimates), the expected rate of *T. gondii* infection in our population is about ten per 100,000. This incidence is clearly sufficient to warrant a newborn screening test when compared to the more standard newborn screening test for phenylketonuria (PKU). In this same population, the rate of detection of PKU in 1992 was about eight per 100,000.

Sufficiently sensitive protocol

The New England Newborn Screening Programme began universal newborn screening of the approximately 92,000 annual Massachusetts births in the January of 1986, and added the approximately 15,000 annual New Hampshire births in the July of 1988. As of January 1 2000, we are aware of 118 cases of congenital toxoplasma infection among the 1.6 million babies screened; 115 of these 118 babies were positive by screening for IgM. Only six of the 118 were identified clinically by routine examination at birth (although several others had been identified from mother's prenatal history).

The screening protocol is, therefore, sufficiently sensitive to detect 112 congenitally infected babies who would not have been identified from clinical signs at birth; the superior sensitivity of detections compared with 'no screening' is clear.

The absolute sensitivity of IgM newborn screening cannot be determined from the New England experience alone, because infected babies with normal screens and who do not come to clinical attention may remain uncounted. Informal speculations of very low sensitivities (for detectable IgM in the newborn period) are voiced frequently enough at various scientific meetings to warrant a few notes of caution to such speculations. First, the rate of specific IgM antibody in infected newborns cannot be determined in a population where most infections are treated prenatally, since the treatment itself lowers the presence of IgM antibody. Second, the sensitivity of the IgM antibody assay is of course very crucial to the data. A newborn screening programme must set its detection limit to be highly sensitive, even at some expense to specificity; diagnostic testing interpretations are not appropriate for application to newborn screening, yet they have been used to estimate rates of IgM antibody positivity in the newborn period. Third, predictions of IgM antibody positivity rates in infected newborns have usually been calculated from serum antibody, even though over 10% of the congenitally infected newborns detected in New England had no detectable *T. gondii*-specific IgM in the serum when first follow-up serum was obtained (usually within 2 weeks of birth). Rates of *T. gondii*-specific IgM in the mothers of babies with elevated screening results suggest that the newborn screening specimen (usually drawn within 3 days of birth), analysed by an assay with cut-offs set with appropriately high sensitivity (for the screening function for which the test is designed), may detect traces of maternal *T. gondii*-specific IgM in some babies who have not formed detectable IgM antibody themselves. Nonetheless, the babies are detected by newborn screening through the serum follow-up of mothers (who do have detectable levels of IgM) and careful follow-up of all babies born to mothers known to be IgM positive at childbirth. Fourth, predictions of how many congenitally infected infants 'should' be detected in a population rely heavily on poorly defined factors used in the calculation. Thus, calculations based upon age-specific seroconversion rates in

Massachusetts, and a transmission rate of 30%, predict that in New England we should see three times the cases that we actually detect. By simply changing the estimated vertical transmission rate from 30% to the 10% actually reported among untreated seroconverting pregnant women in an extensive Belgian study (Henri et al. 1992), the predicted incidence of congenital infection in Massachusetts becomes one per 10,000, a number very close to our observed rate. Finally, studies by Dr. Petersen in Denmark produced the firmest data to date on the subject, and indicated that, in their laboratory, newborn screening identified 75–80% of infected newborns (Lebech et al. 1999).

Economic and technical feasibility of specimen collection and analysis

Our Toxoplasma Screening Division tests the same newborn filter paper specimen used to screen for 30 other conditions (see 'The technical operation', below). This linkage allows specimen collection to be economically and technically feasible. The microtitre enzyme-linked immunosorbent assay format allows for feasible analysis, and is discussed further below.

Availability of effective intervention

Newborn screening offers little opportunity to affect the pathology already present at birth. However, significant new pathology may develop after birth, including chorioretinitis, cerebral calcifications (Desmonts & Couvreur 1974), and hydrocephalus (Wilson et al. 1980). Studies concerning the efficacy of the treatment of mild or subclinical congenital toxoplasma infection are compromised by difficulties in case identification, ethical restrictions regarding untreated (or placebo) control groups, the scarcity of data regarding the natural history of untreated congenital infection [and the differences among results from the studies that have been reported (Wilson et al. 1980; Koppe et al. 1986)], and a variable natural history, with a latency period frequently extending for years before the development of sequelae. The studies that are available suggest that treated babies do better than untreated babies (Wilson et al. 1980; Couvreur et al. 1984; Hohlfeld et al. 1989; Remington & Desmonts 1990; Guerina et al. 1994). Although the data are incomplete, the unanimous recommendation arising from these studies is to treat infants with proven *T. gondii* infection regardless of clinical presentation. Antitoxoplasma therapies are discussed further in Chapters 10 and 13.

Is newborn screening appropriate for congenital toxoplasmosis? Questions remain concerning protocol sensitivity; however, even the *detected* incidence of congenital toxoplasma infection meets conventional incidence criteria, and long-term studies teach us that nearly all of these children will eventually develop adverse sequelae if left untreated (Wilson et al. 1980; Koppe et al. 1986). The technical issues of specimen collection and analysis are feasible. The appropriateness of newborn screening for congenital toxoplasma infection remains viable according to standard criteria.

Biological considerations

If one accepts that newborn screening for congenital *T. gondii* infection may be appropriate under the right circumstances, one may return to the question of whether newborn screening should be favoured over other options in a given community. Biologically, it would seem that newborn screening has an advantage over no screening since the latter would largely depend upon the detection of the small minority who are discovered by clinical presentation alone.

A comprehensive system of prenatal screening, as was initiated in France (Jeannel et al. 1988; Thulliez 1992) and adopted in some other European countries (Aspöck & Pollak 1992; Hengst 1992), coupled with an aggressive system for diagnosing foetal infection (Desmonts et al. 1985; Daffos et al. 1988), has biological advantages over newborn screening (see also Chapter 8). It should be noted, however, that even with good prenatal screening, the date of maternal exposure (the best indicator of foetal risk) cannot always be established with certainty.

Early detection of maternal infection allows for spiramycin treatment, which may reduce the rate of transmission of infection to the foetus (Desmonts & Couvreur 1974; Desmonts et al. 1985; Aspöck & Pollak 1992; Stray-Pedersen 1992). Prenatal foetal diagnosis, including protozoan isolation, allows for informed decisions regarding the initiation of additional antiparasitic drugs (Daffos et al. 1988; Hohlfeld et al. 1989). Recent advances in utilizing polymerase chain reaction (PCR) technology promise to significantly shorten the delay in obtaining proof of infection (Cazenave et al. 1992a, 1992b), although the sensitivity and specificity of *T. gondii* PCR varies considerably among laboratories (Guy et al. 1996).

Earlier intervention is not the only biological advantage of prenatal screening. Some congenital infections detectable by prenatal screening might be missed by newborn screening alone, for example when an infection occurs so early in gestation that the IgM is not present at birth. To date we have seen three cases of clinically detected congenital toxoplasmosis with negative newborn IgM filter paper screens. A second possible situation when prenatal screening may detect congenital infection missed by newborn screening is when transmission of an infection to the foetus occurs too late for IgM to be produced by the newborn. A third (theoretical) possibility is an undetectable IgM response due to the suppressive effect of passively transmitted maternal IgG antibody. Note that in all three of these situations whereby the baby may fail to produce detectable IgM, the baby's infection may still be detected by newborn screening if trace levels of maternal IgM leak into the baby perinatally, and appropriate follow-up measures are in place.

There are several reports of congenitally infected babies that are negative for

T. gondii-specific IgM; this is of concern even if one allows for the possible insensitivity of some assays (Foulon et al. 1984; Daffos et al. 1988; Hohlfeld et al. 1989; Berger et al. 1992). We suspect that in our population, more than the three cases noted above may have occurred during the first 12 years of our screening programme.

Realization of the full benefits of prenatal screening assumes a comprehensive system involving early IgG and IgM antibody testing of all pregnant women, and monthly follow-up testing of antibody-negative women until delivery. In addition, prenatal diagnostics are performed on foetuses of women who were positive for *T. gondii*-specific IgM at the initial screen, as well as on foetuses of all seroconverting women. Some centres begin antiparasitic treatment without foetal diagnosis when maternal seroconversion occurs late in pregnancy.

'Cutting corners' in a prenatal serology system transfers some biological advantages to a newborn IgM screen approach. Thus, if prenatal IgG screening is not accompanied by IgM screening, detectable IgG at the first prenatal visit would be interpreted as evidence of exposure before pregnancy, and follow-up may not be pursued. Another possibility, particularly if the first prenatal visit is late, is that the IgG represents production due to a recent exposure during pregnancy. Similarly, if repeat screens are not continued until delivery, a woman infected late in her pregnancy may be negative for *T. gondii*-specific IgG antibody at her last screen. We have seen seven newborns (6% of our series of cases) who may fit this category of very recent congenital toxoplasma infection. All seven newborn samples were negative for *T. gondii*-specific IgG antibody, despite being positive for *T. gondii*-specific IgM. The follow-up serum samples of five of these seven babies were IgG negative, and indeed three of the mothers' sera were still negative for *T. gondii*-specific IgG at this time. All seven babies later developed IgG antibodies.

In theory, newborn screening would also have a biological advantage in the case of a baby born to a mother with an immunodeficiency that prevents her from mounting an IgG antibody response (see Chapters 5 and 6 for discussions on toxoplasma infection in HIV-positive and transplant patients, respectively). A final biological advantage of newborn screening is that it directly detects infected infants, not infected women who have a statistical chance of transmitting the infection to the foetus.

Sociological considerations

The philosophy chosen for screening for congenital toxoplasma infection must take into consideration the various sociological factors prevailing in that particular community. In the United States, there is currently no universal social or private health-care system. In 1990 it was estimated that 8% of Massachusetts residents carried no health insurance of any kind, and the figure for the United States at large was 13% (Blendon et al. 1990). In such a situation, there is no mechanism to ensure equal access to or entry into any prenatal screening programme. By contrast, our state-mandated newborn screening programme already succeeds in collecting blood specimens from virtually 100% of babies at birth.

Another sociological factor that may be relevant to the acceptability of a government-sponsored programme is the political environment surrounding abortion as a consideration when acute prenatal infection is detected.

Newborn screening programmes incur sociological costs in terms of increased anxiety to families who receive false-positive screening results. In Massachusetts, carefully designed reporting and follow-up procedures seem to limit, but certainly do not eliminate, such anxiety.

Economic considerations

When coupled with other ongoing newborn screening programmes, the laboratory costs of newborn screening for congenital *T. gondii* infection would compare favourably with those of prenatal screening programmes requiring multiple testing of *T. gondii*-antibody-seronegative mothers. The costs of prenatal screening programmes are highest in communities with low *T. gondii* antibody prevalence. In Massachusetts, *T. gondii* prevalence among women giving birth is so low (less than 15%) that over 85% of pregnant women would require serological follow-up. It may also be noted that if the cost of a prenatal programme is kept to a minimum by increasing the interval between serological follow-ups, the advantage of increased therapeutic options decreases proportionately. Prenatal programmes become much more expensive when linked with the prenatal diagnosis of foetuses of seroconverting women. These procedures (serology on foetal blood samples, protozoan isolation and PCR) are all sophisticated, invasive and costly. In addition, prenatal diagnostics carry significant risks to the foetus.

Conclusions

In Massachusetts, prenatal screening carries significant economic and sociological disadvantages relative to newborn screening. In such an environment, which may be shared by many communities or countries, the only philosophical alternative to doing nothing may be newborn screening.

The technical operation

In our newborn screening programme, a blood sample obtained from a heel prick of every baby born in participating New England states is collected onto a filter paper card, dried and sent to the central laboratory operated by The New England Newborn Screening Programme, University of Massachusetts Medical School. Although the particular tests performed for each of the participating states vary somewhat, each sample from babies born in Massachusetts (currently 84,000 births per year) is tested for the following analytes (for the indicated diseases): phenylalanine (PKU), galactose (galactosemia), leucine (maple syrup urine disease), methionine (homocystinuria), biotinidase (biotinidase deficiency), thyroxine and, if warranted, thyroid stimulating hormone (for congenital hypothyroidism), irregular electrophoretic mobility of haemoglobin (for sickle cell disease and other haemoglobinopathies), 17-hydroxyprogesterone (for congenital adrenal hyperplasia), acylcarnitine profile (for medium chain acyl CoA dehydrogenase deficiency, MCAD), and *T. gondii*-specific IgM antibody. Screening is also offered (but parents may opt out) as part of two pilot studies for:

1 immunoreactive trysinogen/PCR (for cystic fibrosis); and
2 a panel of analytes designed to detect an additional 19 rare metabolic disorders by tandem mass spectrometry. The *T. gondii*-specific IgM test is also performed on samples from babies born in New Hampshire (about 15,000 births per year).

The assay

The IgM capture enzyme immunoassay is an in-house modification of an IgM assay developed for serum specimens (Naot et al. 1981). The single 6-mm filter paper disk from the newborn filter paper sample is eluted overnight with 0.2 ml of a PBS-TWEEN-milk buffer; 0.1 ml of eluate is then removed and added to wells precoated with goat antihuman IgM. A source of toxoplasma antigen is added (soluble saline extract from sonicated parasites grown in mouse cell cultures), followed by alkaline-phosphatase-conjugated rabbit antitoxoplasma antibodies and substrate. Each microtitre plate contains standards and controls to allow the identification of newborn samples with elevated reactions. The sensitivity is purposefully set high at some expense to specificity, so that elevated results may be examined carefully with appropriate follow-up testing on the original sample.

Strategy for requesting a follow-up serum sample

Our programme's strategy for requesting follow-up serum samples is summarized in Table 9.1. Newborn filter paper samples which result in an optical density (OD) ≥0.080 are retested in duplicate for specificity, once in a well that includes the toxoplasma antigen at the appropriate step, and once in a well into which buffer alone is added in place of the toxoplasma antigen. In addition, the sample is tested for IgG antibody concurrently with the IgM specificity retest. If the difference between the two IgM assay wells (well with toxoplasma antigen minus well without toxoplasma antigen) is ≥0.100, the IgM screen is considered positive and a follow-up serum specimen is requested from the baby and its mother.

Occasionally (with a good-quality conjugate, in less then 0.01% of the samples), the reactivity in the well without antigen is ≥ 0.100. We are uncomfortable to con-

Table 9.1. Strategy for requesting serum follow-up samples, based upon filter paper screening result

Filter paper result for toxoplasma IgM			Filter paper result for toxoplasma IgG	Follow-up sample requested
Positive[a]	Nonspecific negative[b]	Negative		
√			(+)	Serum
√			(−)	Filter paper
	√		(+)	Serum
	√		(−)	None
		√	ND[c]	None

Key:
[a]Includes all filter papers for which the difference between the wells 'with antigen' minus 'without antigen' is ≥0.100, regardless of the optical density (OD) of the 'without antigen' sample.
[b]Filter papers for which the OD in the well 'without antigen' ≥0.100, and the difference between the wells 'with antigen' minus that 'without antigen' is <0.100. Very rare (<0.01%) when good-quality conjugate is used.
[c]Not done: toxoplasma IgG antibody is not routinely tested when the IgM screen is negative.

sider those screens with OD differences <0.100 as normal if the well without antigen is ≥ 0.100 ('nonspecific negative'). Such nonspecific activity may often be inhibited by adding excess heat-aggregated human gamma globulin (this removes interference by rheumatoid factor, but does not affect the reactivity of specific antibodies).

A second troublesome serological profile is one in which the IgM filter paper screen is positive, but the IgG test is negative. Even if the baby has not produced its own IgG antibody, in a true congenital infection one would expect to find passively transferred IgG antibody elicited by the mother's ongoing infection. Usually (but not always), a positive *T. gondii*-specific IgM in the absence of *T. gondii*-specific IgG is due to a borderline false-positive IgM antibody screen. Follow-up samples are required to identify the occasional IgG-negative baby who is truly infected (6% of cases).

After many years' experience, we have never found a congenitally infected baby whose *T. gondii*-specific IgM became negative before the *T. gondii*-specific IgG became positive. Recently we have requested only a follow-up filter paper specimen in such cases (rather than a liquid blood sample from baby and mother) because this generally elicits less anxiety in the family and is simpler for the paediatrician. Filter papers are monitored until the sample becomes negative for both *T. gondii*-specific IgM and IgG antibodies. Of course, the development of toxoplasma-specific IgG would be diagnostic of infection.

Table 9.2. Strategy for recommendations concerning clinical follow-up, based upon results obtained on sera requested because filter paper IgM screen is positive

Toxoplasma antibody results in serum				
Baby		Mother		
IgM	IgG	IgM	IgG	Recommendations
(+)	(+)	(+)	(+)	Evaluate clinically; treat all
(+)	(−)	(+)	(−)	Verify serology; evaluate clinically, treat
(−)	(+)	(+)	(+)	Evaluate[a], follow serology
(−)	(+)	(−)	(+)	Follow serology
(−)	(−)	(−)	(−)	False (+) screen; no action

Key:

[a]Treat if the clinical evaluation (physical, neurological and ophthalmological examinations; cranial CT scan, lumbar puncture) leads to a diagnosis of congenital toxoplasma infection, or if toxoplasma IgG antibody in baby persists.

Follow-up

The role of a newborn screening programme does not end with the notification of the primary physician of a positive toxoplasma antibody result. Our programme also provides the primary care physician with medical consultation, educational materials, recommended treatment protocols and referral to a network of paediatric infectious disease specialists to assist the doctor with the care of babies we identify. Finally, a follow-up programme is in place to monitor the progress of identified infants.

Typically, in cases of congenital toxoplasma infection the baby's and mother's sera are both positive for both IgM and IgG antitoxoplasma antibodies. Occasionally other serological profiles present themselves and carry varying degrees of suspicion. Table 9.2 summarizes clinical recommendations based upon the final results of the follow-up serum tests.

If a diagnosis of congenital *T. gondii* infection is made, we recommend that the baby should receive a full blood analysis, and physical, neurological and ophthalmological examinations, a cranial CT scan and a lumbar puncture (for cells, protein and glucose) (Guerina et al. 1994). Treatment is initiated regardless of the results of these examinations, and consists of a 1-year course of pyrimethamine with folinic acid, and sulphadiazine. In addition, the baby's serology is followed through the year of treatment, and a final specimen is obtained after treatment has been stopped for at least 1 month.

Occasionally, the baby's serum follow-up is negative but we discover that the mother has a positive IgM. This situation is particularly suspicious because IgM antibody had been detected on the infant's filter paper screened at birth. We recommend that such babies be evaluated clinically, and that the serology be followed through the first year to verify whether the IgG disappears. A baby with clinical findings of toxoplasmosis or a rising IgG antibody is treated.

If the mother and baby both have negative IgM antibody levels in the serum follow-up, the baby is considered to be uninfected. Toxoplasma-specific IgG antibody may be monitored until it becomes undetectable.

Clinical impact of the programme

The ultimate goal of a toxoplasma newborn screening programme is to decrease morbidity due to congenital toxoplasmosis in the programme's population. Summaries of the clinical assessments are reported elsewhere (Guerina et al. 1994). Only 10% of congenitally infected babies were clinically apparent. However, more detailed examination revealed abnormalities in either the retina or the central nervous system (including elevated CNS protein) in 40% of the remaining infected babies. Up to 10% of infected babies may have developed new retinal lesions postnatally. Only 1 of 46 infected children had a lasting neurological deficit, which was a mild hemiparesis attributable to a large cerebral lesion present at birth. Not surprisingly, this cohort of babies identified through newborn screening appeared to have a better clinical outcome (5 year) than cohorts identified clinically. Evaluation of a 10-year follow-up of the New England cohort is in preparation. Reports from other centres (Wilson et al. 1980; Koppe et al. 1986) make it clear that clinical follow-up studies of congenital toxoplasmosis must continue until the children are over 10 years of age.

Summary

The implementation of the Massachusett's Newborn Screening programme is described and the scientific, technical and economic requirements delineated. The appropriateness and feasibility of newborn screening *vis à vis* prenatal screening is discussed. It is stressed that newborn screening does not end with the notification of a positive result but is structured to include treatment protocols, educational materials, paediatric support and a follow-up programme to monitor the progress of infected infants.

REFERENCES

Aspöck, H. & Pollak, A. (1992). Prevention of prenatal toxoplasmosis by serological screening of pregnant women in Austria. *Scandinavian Journal of Infectious Diseases, Supplementum,* **84,** 32–8.

Berger, R., Sturchler, D. & Rudin, C. (1992). Cord blood screening for congenital toxoplasmosis: detection and treatment of asymptomatic newborns in Basel, Switzerland. *Scandinavian Journal of Infectious Diseases, Supplementum,* **84,** 46–50.

Blendon, R. J., Donelan, K., Thorpe, K. E., Dailey, T. E., Taylor, H., Bass, R., Frankel, M., Belodoff, J. D. & Lucas, C. V. (1990). *Final Report: A Household Survey of the Health Insurance Status of Massachusetts Residents.* A comprehensive survey conducted for the Commonwealth of Massachusetts Department of Medical Security by the Harvard School of Public Health Boston.

Cazenave, J., Broussin, B., Cambeilh, C. & Discamps, G. (1992a). Détection rapide de toxoplasmes par la "polymerase chain reaction": un apport au diagnostic antenatal. *La Presse Medicale,* **21,** 221.

Cazenave, J., Forestier, F., Bessieres, M. H., Broussin, B. & Begueret, J. (1992b). Contribution of a new PCR assay to the prenatal diagnosis of congenital toxoplasmosis. *Prenatal Diagnosis,* **12,** 119–27.

Couvreur, J., Desmonts, G. & Aron-Rosa, D. (1984). Le pronostic oculaire de la toxoplasmose congenitale: rôle du traitment. *Annales de Pédiatrie,* **31,** 855–8.

Daffos, F., Forestier, F., Capella-Pavlovosky, M., Thulliez, P., Aufrant, C., Valenti, D. & Cox, W. L. (1988). Prenatal management of 746 pregnancies at risk for congenital toxoplasmosis. *New England Journal of Medicine,* **318,** 271–5.

Desmonts, G. & Couvreur, J. (1974). Congenital toxoplasmosis: a prospective study of 378 pregnancies. *The New England Journal of Medicine,* **290,** 1110–16.

Desmonts, G., Daffos, F., Forestier, F., Capella-Pavlovsky, M., Thulliez, P. & Chartier, M. (1985). Prenatal diagnosis of congenital toxoplasmosis. *The Lancet,* **i,** 500–4.

Foulon, W., Naessens, A., Volckaert, M., Lauwers, S. & Amy, J. J. (1984). Congenital toxoplasmosis: a prospective survey in Brussels. *British Journal of Obstetrics and Gynaecology,* **91,** 419–23.

Guerina, N. G., Hsu, H. W., Meissner, H. C., Maguire, J. H., Lynfield, R., Stechenberg, B., Abroms, I., Pasternack, M. S., Hoff, R., Eaton, R. B., Grady, G. F., Cheeseman, S. H., Mcintosh, K., Medearis, D. N., Robb, R. & Weiblen, B. J. (1994). Neonatal serologic screening and early treatment for congenital *Toxoplasma gondii* infection. *New England Journal of Medicine,* **330,** 1858–63.

Guy, E. C., Pelloux, H., Lappalainen, M. (1996). Interlaboratory comparison of polymerase chain reaction for the detection of *Toxoplasma gondii* DNA added to samples of amniotic fluid. *European Journal of Clinical Microbiology and Infectious Disease,* **15,** 836–9.

Hengst, P. (1992). Screening for toxoplasmosis in pregnant women: presentation of a screening programme in the former "East"-Germany, and the present status in Germany. *Scandinavian Journal of Infectious Diseases, Supplementum,* **84,** 38–42.

Henri, T., Jacques, S. & Rene, L. (1992). Twenty-two years screening for toxoplasmosis in pregnancy: Liege – Belgium. *Scandinavian Journal of Infectious Diseases, Supplementum,* **84,** 84–85.

Hohlfeld, P., Daffos, F., Thulliez, P., Aufrant, C., Couvreur, J., MacAleese, J., Descombey, D. & Forestier, F. (1989). Foetal toxoplasmosis: outcome of pregnancy and infant follow-up after *in utero* treatment. *The Journal of Pediatrics*, 115, 765–9.

Hsu, H.-W., Grady, G. F., Maguire, J. H., Weiblen, B. J. & Hoff, R. (1992). Newborn screening for congenital toxoplasma infection: five years experience in Massachusetts, USA. *Scandinavian Journal of Infectious Diseases, Supplementum*, 84, 59–64.

Jeannel, D., Niel, G., Costagliota, D., Danis, M., Travore, B. M. & Gentilini, M. (1988). Epidemiology of Toxoplasmosis among pregnant women in the Paris Area. *International Journal of Epidemiology*, 17, 595–602.

Koppe, J. G., Loewer-Sieger, D. H. & de Roever-Bonnet, H. (1986). Results of 20-year follow-up of congenital toxoplasmosis. *The Lancet*, 1, 254–6.

Lebech, M., Andersen, O., Christensen, N. C., Hertel, J., Nielsen, H. E., Peitersen, B., Rechnitzer, C., Larsen, S. O., Norgaard-Pedersen, B. & Petersen, E. (1999). Feasibility of neonatal screening for toxoplasma infection in the absence of prenatal treatment. Danish Congenital Toxoplasmosis Study Group. *The Lancet*, 353, 1834–7.

Naot, Y. N., Desmonts, G. & Remington, J. S. (1981). IgM enzyme-linked immunosorbent assay test for the diagnosis of congenital Toxoplasma infection. *The Journal of Pediatrics*, 98, 32–6.

Remington, J. S. & Desmonts, G. (1990). Toxoplasmosis. In *Infectious Diseases of the Fetus and Newborn Infant*, 3rd edn., ed. J. S. Remington & J. O. Klein, pp. 89–195. Philadelphia: W. B. Saunders Company.

Stray-Pedersen, B. (1992). Treatment of toxoplasmosis in the pregnant mother and newborn child. *Scandinavian Journal of Infectious Diseases, Supplementum*, 84, 23–31.

Therrell, B. L., Panny, S. R., Davidson, A., Eckman, J., Hannon, W. H., Henson, M. A., Hillard, M., Kling, S., Levy, H. L., Meaney, F. J., McCabe, E. R. B., Mordaunt, V., Pass, K., Shapira, E. & Tuerck, J. (1992). U.S. newborn screening system guidelines: statement of the Council of Regional Networks for Genetic Services. *Screening*, 1, 135–47.

Thulliez, P. (1992). Screening programme for congenital toxoplasmosis in France. *Scandinavian Journal of Infectious Diseases, Supplementum*, 84, 43–5.

Wilson, C. B., Remington, J. S., Stagno, S. & Reynolds, D. W. (1980). Development of adverse sequelae in children born with subclinical congenital toxoplasmosis infection. *Pediatrics*, 66, 767–74.

Wolf, A., Cowen D. & Paige, B. H. (1939). Human toxoplasmosis: occurrence in infants as an encephalomyelitis. Verification by transmission to animals. *Science*, 89, 226–7.

10

Infections in neonates and infants

J. Couvreur

Institute de Puériculture de Paris, ADHMI, Laboratoire de Serologie et de Recherche sur la Toxoplasmose, Paris, France

History

The important milestones that led to the full knowledge of congenital toxoplasmosis were the discovery of 'parasitic cysts' in the retina of a child who died with coloboma and hydrocephaly by Janku in Czechoslovakia (1923), the identification of this organism as toxoplasma by Levaditi in Paris (1928), the discovery of an encephalitozoic infantile granulomatosis associated with toxoplasma and evidence of its prenatal transmission by Wolf et al. (1939). The clinical pattern was delineated first in studies of a large series of patients investigated retrospectively (Feldman 1953; Couvreur & Desmonts 1962) and later in prospective studies (Desmonts & Couvreur 1974a).

Epidemiology

The prevalence of congenital toxoplasma infection in a given community is directly related to the rate of acquired infection in pregnant women adjusted by the 40% rate of materno–foetal transmission. Any evaluation of the prevalence of infection in newborns requires routine screening for seroconversion in the pregnant population and thorough study of their newborn infants. This prevalence can vary over years and it is influenced by preventive measures. This explains why it decreased in Paris from 3 to less than 1 per 1000 live births within 20 years (Remington & Desmonts 1990). The prevalence of neonatal infection has been reported as 0.6 to 2 per 1000 in Alabama, 2 per 1000 in Brussels, 0.25 to 0.7 per 1000 in London and 2 per 1000 in Melbourne. Frenkel (1974b) has proposed a mathematical epidemiological model for such evaluations.

Clinical manifestations

Following the recognition of toxoplasma foetal infection, the symptoms and signs of congenital toxoplasmosis were first documented in series of patients identified

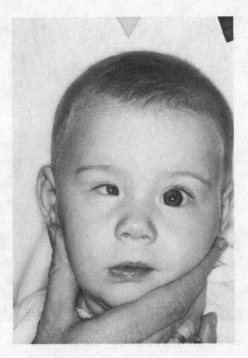

Figure 10.1 Microphthalmy

retrospectively (Feldman 1953; Couvreur & Desmonts 1962; Remington et al. 2001). Four clinical signs were thus considered as representative of the disease: hydrocephaly or microcephaly, retinochoroiditis, cerebral calcifications and neuro-logical injury. This clinical spectrum, which represents some of the late sequelae of infection, was later enlarged with a variety of acute signs: hydrops foetalis, eryth-roblastosis and jaundice with hepatosplenomegaly. A child with congenital toxo-plasmosis and eyeball atrophy is shown in Figure 10.1. It was not until the prospective follow-up of infants born to mothers infected during pregnancy was done that the full range of clinical presentation of the disease was elicited. Thus, three points will be considered – an analytical inventory of the presenting signs, the clinical syndromes observed and their relative frequency.

Clinical signs

Ocular disease

Focal retinochoroiditis is the most frequent sign of congenital toxoplasmosis found in 76% of cases (Couvreur & Desmonts 1962). It has been estimated to be respon-sible for up to 4% of blindness in children. Presenting features can be strabismus or nystagmus. On ophthalmic examination, the characteristic lesion is a focal

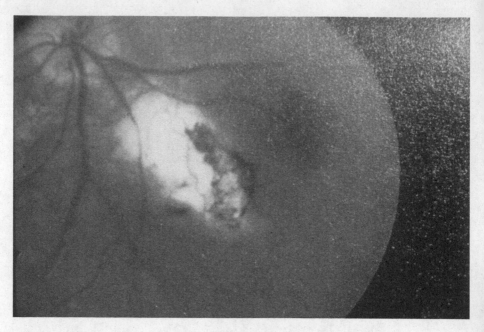

Figure 10.2 Macular retinochoroiditis in a 7-year-old girl with congenital toxoplasmosis

necrotizing retinitis (Figure 10.2). Recent lesions appear as a white yellowish focus with oedema of the retina. Vitreous inflammatory exudate can impede fundoscopic examination. Within several weeks these lesions appear as glial scars with a punched-out pattern, a depigmented central area and peripheral pigment deposits. The lesion is one or two times the papillar diameter; it can be solitary or associated with other smaller lesions of various ages. It can mimic a coloboma. The distinguishing features of retinochoroiditis in congenital toxoplasmosis include the affinity for the macular area, the frequency of bilateral involvement, the normal pattern of retina and vasculature surrounding the lesion and the tendency for relapses. The retinochoroiditis can be seen at birth or can occur much later in a previously normal retina.

Inflammatory involvement of the anterior uvea, iris and ciliary bodies with subsequent synechiae (namely fibrous retractions following an inflammatory process) and possibly cataract, microphthalmy, small cornea and optic atrophy may be observed.

Neurological signs

The clinical spectrum of neurological involvement has no specific features and ranges from important signs of localization to subtle signs and symptoms related to anatomical lesions of the brain which can be at best delineated by computed tomography.

Hydrocephalus

As a rule hydrocephalus is related to obstruction of the aqueduct of Sylvius. It can be the sole clinical manifestation or be associated with other signs. A personal experience of 21 cases with a follow-up of 6 months to 15 years has revealed three types of presentation: detection *in utero* by sonography in foetuses at risk (probably the most common presentation nowadays), primary hydrocephalus in infancy and recognition in patients with known congenital toxoplasmosis. Hydrocephalus developed within 4 months in 71% of patients. In two cases it occurred as late as 14 and 17 years of age. A shunting procedure was necessary in 90.5%. Spontaneous stabilization occurred in 9.5%. Hydrocephalus was associated with retinochoroiditis in 78%, neurological signs in 43% and an intelligence quotient (IQ) below 100 in 57% of the patients.

Transfontanellar sonography is mandatory for detecting hydrocephalus in any infant at risk of congenital toxoplasmosis and computed tomography is of prognostic value in investigating brain injury. A wide pattern of lesions from discrete granulomatosis to multicystic aspect or almost total cerebral atrophy are detected by these techniques.

Microcephaly

Microcephaly reflects severe brain damage but it is not specific for the disease.

Intracerebral calcifications

Two types are observed. Small nodular deposits 1–3 mm or more in diameter may be found scattered in the white matter and most frequently seen in the periventricular areas and curvilinear streaks lining the ventricles or located in the basal ganglia (Figure 10.3). Calcifications may also be found in the caudate nucleus, choroid plexus and meninges and these are associated with a poor prognosis. Disseminated calcifications can be observed in patients without any neurological or intellectual impairment.

Convulsions

These occur in about 50% of patients with clinically apparent disease. When isolated and of late occurrence, without any sign of cerebral injury either clinically or on radiological imaging, they present a diagnostic challenge. They can be associated with a subtle brain injury or be a sign of encephalomyelitis relapse or be purely coincidental. The discovery of local synthesis of antitoxoplasma antibodies in the cerebrospinal fluid is diagnostic of their relationship with toxoplasma infection.

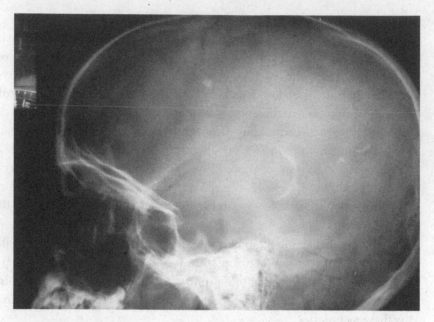

Figure 10.3 Cerebral calcifications. Nodular deposits. Curvilinear periventricular streaks

Mental retardation

Congenital toxoplasmosis with neurological injury is often associated with mental retardation. However, this can also be observed in children with subclinical toxoplasmosis. It is difficult to determine to what extent congenital toxoplasmosis is responsible for mental retardation in children. Retrospective studies have provided contradictory results, ranging from those which show no significant association to those which found that toxoplasma was implicated in 4–20% of cases. Prospective controlled studies will be required to make an accurate evaluation of a causative relationship, particularly in the field of minimal cerebral dysfunction.

Cerebrospinal fluid abnormalities

Cerebrospinal fluid (CSF) examination must be one of the investigations performed on babies with suspected congenital toxoplasmosis. A high protein content is the most frequent abnormality encountered in infected infants, found in 34% of cases; indeed, it may be the only finding (8% in otherwise subclinical patients) (Couvreur et al. 1984a). A raised CSF protein content as high as 800 mg/ml may be found. White blood cells in the CSF are rare, and when present are a nonspecific finding. Toxoplasma can be isolated from CSF in the first weeks of life (Desmonts & Couvreur 1974b), and the presence of toxoplasma nucleic acid can be demonstrated by polymerase chain reaction (PCR).

Other organ manifestations

These are less frequent and are generally part of a severe postnatally progressing disease. Jaundice is related to liver damage associated with haemolysis. Toxoplasmosis was present in 2.2% of a personal series of 225 patients with neonatal jaundice (Couvreur et al. 1984*b*). It was associated with hepatosplenomegaly. Liver calcifications were found rarely, but when present they frequently progressed into cirrhosis. Purpuric petechiae and echymosis were related to severe thrombocytopaenia. Erythroblastosis and hydrops foetalis were observed. A nephrotic syndrome was associated with histologically apparent lesions and the presence of toxoplasma in glomeruli (Couvreur et al. 1984*b*). Subclinical interstitial pneumonia has been documented histopathologically. Toxoplasma has a great affinity for the myocardium, where it is found regularly in fatal cases with interstitial lesions. Myocardial involvement is always subclinical.

Prematurity – intrauterine growth retardation

Premature birth has been reported in 17.7% of a series of patients with congenital toxoplasmosis studied prospectively, which is much higher than the rate in the general community (Couvreur et al. 1984*a*).

Toxoplasmosis in twins

A personal experience of 14 pairs of twins (Couvreur et al. 1976) and a review of the published reports revealed that there is a distinct difference between dizygotic and monozygotic twins. Monozygotic twins always have a similar clinical pattern. Conversely, in dizygotic twins, discrepancies in clinical patterns are usual (Figure 10.4). For instance, subclinical infection can occur in one twin and a severe involvement in the other. In three sets, two bichorial and biamniotic and one monochorial and biamniotic, only one infant of each set was infected (Couvreur et al. 1976). These discrepancies between monozygotic and heterozygotic twins illustrate the importance of the placenta in the pathophysiology of materno–foetal transmission of toxoplasma.

Syndromes

Almost all cases of congenital toxoplasmosis observed in clinical practice present as one of the following patterns.

Severe neonatal disease

This form is severe with several of the following features reflecting a multivisceral progressive disease: prematurity, jaundice, purpura with thrombocytopaenia,

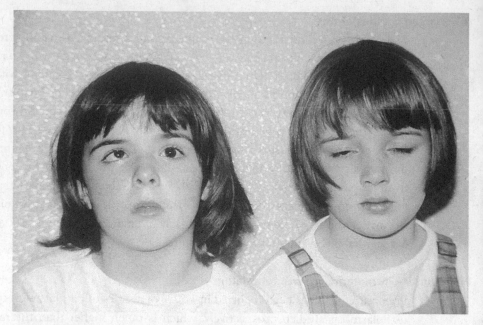

Figure 10.4   Five-year-old dizygotic twins. Left: Congenital toxoplasmosis: strabismus and macular retinochoroiditis in the right eye. Right: uninfected girl

anaemia, signs of hydrops foetalis, neurological signs, bulging of the fontanelle, high CSF protein content and ventricular dilation (Figure 10.5). Prognosis is poor when there are signs of brain injury on clinical and/or imaging grounds or a very high CSF protein content. Conversely, prognosis can be good when there is no neurological involvement. However, it must be emphasized that in such cases severe central nervous system involvement (hydrocephalus, encephalitis, progressing eye lesions) can occur after several weeks or months, a fact which warrants protracted treatment.

Symptomatic infection with signs of brain injury

Hydrocephalus, neurological signs, developmental retardation and convulsions are the presenting signs. They are usually associated with other signs such as retinochoroidal scars and cerebral calcifications.

Mild infection

There are isolated signs, mainly mild retinochoroiditis or a few cerebral calcifications without any clinical evidence of cerebral damage and a normal intellectual and neurological development.

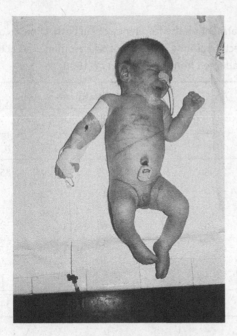

Figure 10.5 Systemic neonatal disease: jaundice,
hepatosplenomegaly purpura, thrombocytopenia,
bilateral evolutive retinochoroiditis and severe
neurological injury

Subclinical infection

Prospective studies of mothers infected during pregnancy have revealed that this
pattern is the most common form of congenital toxoplasmosis. Accurate diagnosis
requires that two conditions are fulfilled. Congenital infection should be well documented on laboratory data (toxoplasma identification in placental tissue, specific
IgM and/or the persistence of IgG, i.e. antibody synthesis in the neonate).
Thorough physical examination and appropriate ancillary investigations (fundoscopic examination, radiography of the skull, transfontanellar sonography, CSF
examination) should be performed in order to exclude signs of disease.

Delayed signs of congenital infection

This important feature of congenital toxoplasmosis is characterized by the development of ophthalmological and/or neurological symptoms at several months or
years of age.

Secondary retinochoroiditis is recognized as a complication of pre-existing congenital ocular injury as well as in patients with previously normal retina. One prospective study has suggested that 66% of patients followed from birth to 15 years of

Table 10.1. Effect of spiramycin treatment on the frequency of stillbirth, clinical congenital toxoplasmosis, and subclinical infection among offspring of 542 women who acquired toxoplasmosis during pregnancy (adapted from Couvreur *et al.* 1988).

| | Treatment | | | | | |
| | No | | Yes | | Total | |
Outcome in offspring	*n*	(%)	*n*	(%)	*n*	(%)
No. with congenital toxoplasmosis	60	39	297	77	357	66
Congenital toxoplasmosis:						
subclinical	64	41	65	17	129	24
mild	14	9	13	3	27	5
severe	7	5	10	2	17	3
Stillbirth or perinatal death	9	6	3	1	12	2
Total	154	100	388	100	542	100

age develop late-onset retinochoroiditis (Koppe et al. 1986). In a series of 13 USA children with subclinical infection at birth who developed primary lesions between 1 month and 9.3 years of age, 85% developed late-onset retinochoroiditis (Wilson et al. 1980). Twenty-seven percent of 48 infants, followed from 10 months to 4 years of age (Ladadie & Hazeman 1984) and 8% in a personal series of 172 patients who were initially treated (119 with subclinical infection) had late-onset retinochoroiditis at between 2 and 11 years of age (Couvreur et al. 1984*c*) (Table 10.1).

Late-onset neurological involvement has been noted, but is often subtle since the lesions are probably self-limiting and it is not easy to demonstrate mild damage when a brain biopsy sample has not been obtained. It has been documented in some selective cases, for instance by the late occurrence of hydrocephalus. In a personal series of 21 cases of hydrocephaly with a mean follow-up of 6.1 years, two patients developed impaired neurological function and required surgery at 13 and 17 years of age respectively.

The late development of humoral antibodies (*T. gondii* IgG titre rise) as well as the local synthesis of antibodies in the aqueous humour or CSF provide further evidence of late-onset disease. During the first year of life, the humoral IgG antibody titre decreases in most congenitally infected infants particularly in those treated with active antiparasitic drugs. In our personal experience, a significant rise in *T. gondii* IgG was observed in 70% of the patients followed from 2 to 19 years of age. There is a maximum frequency during the second year of life (52%) and this decreases to 5–9% between 3 and 10 years of age but rises again to 15% during the

12th year. It is exceptional for this to occur after this age (J. Couvreur, unpublished data). There is no significant correlation between these rebound phenomena and an increased risk of secondary ocular flare-ups, although this does occur in some cases.

Local synthesis of IgG antibodies in the aqueous humour of the eye was demonstrated by Desmonts (1973) when he studied 2000 patients aged 5 to 60 years of age with retinochoroiditis, most of whom were congenitally infected. He pointed out that the aqueous humour/serum antibody titre ratio was greater than 2 in 34% of the patients with a peak in frequency between 15 and 20 years of age. Similarly, local synthesis of antibodies in CSF (serum/CSF ratio ≥4) was observed in 19 out of 46 (41%) patients 2–27 years old (Couvreur et al. 1984*d*) This percentage rose to 61.5% in patients with recent clinical activity, mostly ocular flare-ups. Also, sequential determinations in 13 patients with hydrocephalus 1–14 years following a shunting procedure revealed a significant ratio (4/37) in 11 patients. In five patients it correlated well with progress of the disease (unpublished data).

Diagnosis

Laboratory diagnosis is mandatory, particularly in subclinical infection. It is based on the demonstration of a specific humoral response in the infant and detection of the parasite in the placenta or the newborn infant. Inoculation of placental tissue into mice is the most rewarding method of isolating the parasite. Correlation between positive culture in mice and foetal disease is excellent. The organism was isolated from the placentas of infected babies in 90% of cases in untreated women, in 73% in mothers treated with spiramycin (Couvreur et al. 1988) and in 50% in mothers treated with pyrimethamine-sulphonamide drugs (Couvreur et al. 1991).

Toxoplasma gondii can be isolated from the blood of infected newborn babies. Parasitaemia is not observed after 4 weeks of age. Specific IgM antibodies in the serum of a newborn is diagnostic of congenital infection. The detection of *T. gondii*-specific IgM in cord blood should be confirmed a few days later by testing a sample from the infant to rule out maternal contamination of cord blood produced by birth trauma. The result is positive in 25% of infected babies when the IgM indirect fluorescent antibody test (IFA) is used and in 70% with the immunosorbent agglutination assay (ISAGA) method. Positive or negative results are not related to the clinical condition. IgM antibodies may disappear within a few weeks or persist for months.

Whenever parasitological investigations are negative and specific IgM antibodies are lacking, the only way to confirm congenital infection is to test the baby's blood monthly for *T. gondii*-specific IgG antibodies. Passively transmitted maternal *T. gondii* IgG usually disappears by 10–12 months of age or earlier depending on the initial titre. Congenital *T. gondii* infection is confirmed when *T. gondii* IgG persists for more than 10–12 months or earlier if an initial decrease in *T. gondii* antibody titre is followed by a significant rise in titre. Antibody synthesis can be inhibited by early treatment.

In summary, when a clinician deals with a newborn thought to be at risk (i.e. when the mother was definitely infected during pregnancy) there are three diagnostic possibilities:

1 The diagnosis is definite when one or several of the following criteria apply: *in utero* diagnosis positive during pregnancy, infection confirmed postnatally by laboratory tests and the presence of specific signs (retinochoroiditis, cerebral calcifications).

2 The diagnosis, although probable, is not definite when signs of congenital infection are not specific, e.g. prematurity, jaundice, hepatosplenomegaly, haematological signs, high CSF protein content and late maternal infection (up to 90% risk of transmission after 36 weeks).

3 No conclusion can be drawn when there are no clinical signs of foetal disease, the baby has not produced any specific antibodies and maternal infection occurred early in pregnancy.

In these two last situations a careful follow-up of the baby for *T. gondii* antibody is mandatory up to 12 months of age to confirm or rule out the diagnosis.

Pathology of congenitally infected foetuses

Placenta

Chronic inflammatory reactions in the decidua capsularis are most commonly found along with focal reactions in the villi, intravillous and perivillous infiltrates with lymphocytes and other mononuclear cells. Histopathological identification of parasites is time-consuming and the best way to achieve a parasitological diagnosis is by inoculation into mice.

Central nervous system

Extensive vasculitis with glial nodules and necrotic areas are usually found. These can progress to form cystic cavities containing homogenous eosinophilic material or calcifications. Areas of calcification are found either as broad bands or as diffusely scattered foci. Both tachyzoites and cysts are found in and adjacent to necrotic foci or glial nodules, in perivascular regions and in noninflammatory areas of cerebral tissue. Periventricular and periacqueductal vasculitis with necrosis may be extensive. Ependymitis can result in obstruction of the aqueduct of Sylvius and hydrocephaly. There is often cellular infiltration of the leptomeninges.

Heart

Toxoplasma gondii has a great affinity for heart muscle and appears as cysts in the myocardial fibres with or without an inflammatory reaction, or as focal areas of infiltration sometimes with necrosis.

Lung

An interstitial lymphocytic and mononuclear inflammatory infiltrate which affects the walls of small vessels as well is usually found. Parasites are rarely identified within the endothelial cells of the alveolar septa.

Liver

Inflammatory reactions and parasites are seldom found. Clusters of erythroblasts mimicking foetal erythroblastosis can be observed, in some cases mimicking true erythroblastosis. Hepatic cirrhosis and calcifications are infrequent.

Kidney

Focal glomerulitis with areas of necrosis can extend into adjacent tubules and in severe cases to collecting tubules in the medulla: tachyzoites can be found. Nephrotic syndrome is rarely observed, but, when present, lesions of immune complex nephritis or alterations of the basement membrane and glomerular deposits of IgM may be found (Couvreur et al. 1984*b*).

Eye

The lesions mainly involve the retina and choroid. According to the stage of the lesion, one can see inflammation of the retina with vitreous exudate, inflammation of the choroid, or a healing process with proliferation of the pigment surrounding the inflammatory area. Retina and choroid can be bound together by connective tissue.

Prognosis

Once the diagnosis of maternal infection is made, it is important not only to treat the mother, and later the baby, but also to determine the frequency of follow-up considering the considerable risk of late sequelae such as retinochoroiditis. It would be useful to identify patients who are at an increased risk of late sequelae in order to follow them more closely. In an attempt to identify babies with a higher risk of developing late sequelae, 85 congenitally infected babies were studied prospectively. There were two groups: 30 children who subsequently developed retinochoroiditis and 55 who did not develop ocular lesion after birth, after a mean follow-up of

52 months (range 2–27 years). Comparison between these two groups revealed that there was an increased risk of late-onset retinochoroiditis in babies whose mothers were infected before 26 weeks of pregnancy, and in those babies born with cerebral calcifications, neurological injury, bilateral ocular lesions and *T. gondii* antibody synthesis in the CSF. In addition, the mean serum *T. gondii*-specific IgG titre on birth was twofold higher in patients who developed secondary retinochoroiditis than in those who did not (unpublished data).

Pathogenesis

The sequence of events leading to foetal damage are maternal infection during pregnancy resulting in parasitaemia, which leads to infection of the placenta with local multiplication of the parasite and spread of the organism in the foetal circulation. However, several questions must be answered. Why is congenital toxoplasmosis clinically so protean, with infection producing a range of outcomes between death *in utero* and subclinical infection? Why is the humoral antibody response so variable from one child to another? Why is there a lack of correlation between the foetal or postnatal immunological response and the extent of congenital damage? Lastly, what is the significance of the secondary progress of the disease? The following data are of importance in attempting to answer these questions.

The timing of maternal infection

This is an important determinant both for the rate of materno–foetal transmission and for the congenital damage produced in the baby. Materno–foetal transmission is rare, about 1% when maternal infection occurs during the first 4 weeks. It increases then progressively to reach 90% for infection in the last few weeks of pregnancy. This risk is 14%, 29% and 59% when maternal infection occurs at the end of the first trimester, during the second and during the third trimester, respectively (Desmonts & Couvreur 1974*a*).

Four clinical patterns are found in the foetuses and babies:

1 fatal disease (foetal wastage or neonatal death);
2 severe multisystems disease with neurological signs;
3 mild disease without evidence of neurological involvement; and
4 subclinical infection.

Foetal damage is more often very severe in early pregnancy and almost always absent when maternal infection occurs in late pregnancy (see Chapter 7). It seems that the 26th week of pregnancy marks a turning-point in foetal risk. Infants born to mothers infected before this date are at risk of a severe disease while infants whose mothers are infected later have a much lower risk of developing symptomatic infection. However, this is not always the case. On the whole, the risk of materno–foetal transmission increases steadily throughout the pregnancy, while conversely the risk of severe foetal damage is greatest in early infection and is markedly decreased after the 26th week of pregnancy.

Placental infection

Whenever parasitological investigation of the placenta is positive, the infant is also almost invariably infected. However, *T. gondii* may not always be found in the placenta of infected infants, particularly when the mother has been treated.

Spiramycin treatment given to infected mothers significantly reduces infection of the placenta (Couvreur et al. 1988) (Table 10.2). If given orally for 1 month or more as a daily dose of 2–3 g there is a 50% reduction in the number of congenitally infected babies. However, spiramycin does not affect the clinical pattern in infected foetuses (Desmonts & Couvreur 1975). The pyrimethamine–sulphadiazine combination given to mothers with seroconversion has been said to reduce by 70% the risk of materno–foetal transmission (Kraübig 1963).

Delay between placental and foetal infection

Transmission of infection from the placenta to the foetus can be delayed for weeks or even months. Evidence for this is gleaned from the similarity of the clinical pattern in monozygotic twins and the discrepancies observed in dizygotic twins, a fact which suggests that the transmission does not occur at the same time when there are two placentas (Couvreur et al. 1976). Also, parasitological investigation of the foetus and placenta after the termination of at-risk pregnancies has revealed that the placenta can be infected while the foetus is not (Remington & Desmonts 1990).

Latent infection and clinical relapses

Clinical, ophthalmological and biological data show that congenital toxoplasma infection can progress for a lengthy period after birth extending to childhood, adolescence and even adulthood. The mechanism of these long-term relapses has been a matter of debate, particularly as far as ocular relapses are concerned. Several theories have been proposed:

1 Cyst rupture has been observed histologically. In animal experiments, the coexistence of large and small cysts has been thought to be the consequence of cyst rupture generating satellite cysts. The possibility of a leak of antigen material from the cyst has also been evoked. This leakage might provide an inflammatory process involving previously committed lymphocytes able to release lymphokines and catabolic enzymes that can disrupt the cyst wall.

2 Long-term intracellular persistence of the parasite as a pseudocyst is thought probable (Frenkel 1974a). It might produce recurrent or persistent parasitaemia.

Table 10.2. Incidence of secondary retinochoroiditis in four series of patients with congenital toxoplasmosis

Author	Patients (n)	Follow-up	Treated	Untreated	Patients with new ocular lesions n (%)
Wilson et al. 1980	13*	2.5–17.2 years	7***	6	11 (85)
Koppe et al. 1986	12*	15 years	5***	7	7 (58)
Ladadie et al. 1984	60**	0.10–4 years	0	60	17 (28)
Couvreur et al. 1984c	172*	2–11 years	172****	0	14 (8)

*Diagnosis on birth following prospective study of maternal infection.

**Retrospective diagnosis through routine dye test at 10 months of age.

***One or two short courses of pyrimethamine–sulpha drug treatment before 12 months of age.

****Two to four 3-week courses of pyrimethamine–sulpha drug treatment before 12 months of age.

3 Recurrent retinochoroiditis has been ascribed to cyst rupture with ensuing multiplication of tachyzoites. A hypersensitivity phenomenon has also been hypothesized.

4 According to the theory of immunological tolerance, maternal IgG antibodies may inhibit antibody formation in the foetus in response to *T. gondii*. They may impede extracellular dissemination but favour intracellular multiplication and cyst formation. The protective effect of humoral maternal antibodies is however limited and transitory. It is limited because immunity against toxoplasma is mainly cell-mediated, and transitory because it ceases with the disappearance of passively transmitted IgG. Recognition of toxoplasma antigen by foetal cells is impaired and consequently the development of humoral and cellular immunity in the foetus is postponed. A specific tolerance state is induced. This tolerance depends on an equilibrium between the titre of specific IgG and the degree of antigenic stimulation. Active antibody synthesis indicates the end of this tolerance (Desmonts & Couvreur 1975).

In summary the interval between placental infection and transmission of the parasite to the foetus probably plays a key role in the pattern of foetal disease. It is severe if this delay is short. Conversely, if the interval is long the foetus is protected by maternal IgG antibodies and an immunological tolerance is established with minimal signs or subclinical infection after birth. Any intermediary pattern can be observed between these two extremes. However, once the protective effect of maternal antibodies has waned, the patient will remain under a life-long antigenic stimulus as witnessed by marked antibody titre fluctuations and possibly clinical relapses.

Treatment

Drugs

Pyrimethamine

This folic acid antagonist has a parasitostatic cytopathogenic effect on *T. gondii*. Its half-life is 64 ± 12 hours. In infants the mean serum level 4 hours after a daily dose of 1 mg/kg is 1.3 µg/ml and 0.7 µg/ml when the same dose is given every other day. In infants less than 1 month old, serum concentrations do not differ from values obtained in older children on the same dosage. Concentrations in the CSF are 10–25% of concomitant serum values, but they proved effective *in vitro* against *Toxoplasma gondii* (McLeod et al. 1992). The current dosage is 1 mg/kg in a once-daily dose by the oral route. Haematological tolerance must be checked every week while treatment is being given.

Sulphonamides

The most widely used is sulphadiazine in a dosage of 50–80 mg/kg per day in two or three divided doses.

Pyrimethamine–sulphonamide combination

Pyrimethamine activity is increased six- to eightfold by combination with sulpha drugs. However, experience with AIDS patients suggests that pyrimethamine has some activity when given alone on a higher dosage whenever sulphonamide treatment had to be discontinued because of its side-effects.

Pyrimethamine–sulphadoxine combination

It seems to have effects similar to the pyrimethamine–sulphadiazine combination. It is available as tablets (pyrimethamine 25 mg, sulphadoxine 500 mg, Fansidar™) and is given at a dosage of half a tablet per 10 kg body mass every 7 to 10 days. Administration before 12 months of age is not recommended because of the risk of potential side-effects (Lyell syndrome). It must be permanently discarded if a rash occurs.

Spiramycin

Given to infected mothers on a daily dose of 3 g in two or three divided doses, spiramycin treatment is associated with a significant reduction of foetal infection (23% versus 61% in untreated women) (Desmonts & Couvreur 1974a). In maternal treatment, the foetal serum concentration is 47% of the maternal serum values between 20 and 24 weeks. At birth, the placental concentration is four times the average blood concentration in the mother and 6.5 times that in cord blood (Forestier et al. 1987). Positive parasitological investigation of the placenta in infected newborns is also reduced from 90% to 75% (Couvreur et al. 1988). However, despite its preventive effects on materno–foetal transmission of the parasite, spiramycin does not alter the clinical pattern in infected foetuses and its clinical efficacy in the postnatal treatment of infected infants has not been demonstrated.

Other drugs

The risk of toxoplasma infection in AIDS and the frequent occurrence of side-effects with pyrimethamine or sulpha drugs in involved patients has fostered research for new drugs, particularly for those which might have activity against cysts. When reviewing progress in this matter (Couvreur & Leport 1998), it appears that some of them that reached clinical trials gave interesting results, mostly when given in combination with pyrimethamine, and that some might be used in congenital toxoplasmosis. The most interesting are macrolides (clindamycin, clarithromycin, azithromycin, a hydroxynaphthoquinone derivative, atovaquone, folate inhibitors, piritrexim, trimetrexate) but other drugs such as arprinocid, dapsone, pentamidine and, lastly, gamma interferon and interleukin 12 also have some effect (see Chapter 13).

Adjuvant therapy

Folinic acid (5–10 mg by oral or intramuscular route every 2–4 days) can prevent the side-effects of pyrimethamine (granulocytopaenia, thrombocytopaenia and megaloblastic anaemia), a risk that warrants weekly blood tests at the beginning of treatment.

Steroid therapy can be used whenever there is an inflammatory process such as progressive retinochoroiditis or high CSF protein level. Prednisone or methylprednisone must be continued on full dosage until the process has subsided. The dosage is then progressively reduced until it is discontinued.

Indications

The pyrimethamine–sulphadiazine combination remains the mainstay of all the regimens proposed. It has been widely used by the author as three to four courses of 21 days during the first year of life. The efficacy of this regimen was proved by a significant lowering of *T. gondii* antibodies titres at 1 year of age in treated patients (Couvreur et al. 1984*a*) and a trend to limit the frequency of ocular secondary recurrences (Couvreur et al. 1984*c*). These results were significantly improved using a more aggressive treatment. The Chicago Collaborative Treatment Trial (McAuley et al. 1994) recommends continuous treatment during the first 12 months after birth. Pyrimethamine is given at a loading dose of 2 mg/kg per day for 2 days, then 1 mg/kg per day for 6 months and later at 1 mg/kg three times a week for the next 6 months together with sulphadiazine (100 mg/kg per day) in two divided doses. Calcium leukovorin (folinic acid) is given at an initial dosage of 5 mg three times a week, increasing to 10 mg at 1 month of age when the weight reaches 4.5 kg. It is increased to 5–20 mg/day in cases of neutropaenia. An alternative to this regimen of leukovorin is daily treatment for 2 months and then three times a week for 10 months. This treatment, which was used mainly in patients with overt disease, gave good results; for example, acute signs of active retinochoroidal disease became quiescent within 2 weeks, or visual loss did not occur or worsen in most of the patients. Almost all infants with hydrocephalus developed IQs of 85 to 140. Half of the patients who underwent a shunting procedure developed normally (McAuley et al. 1994; Swischer et al. 1994; Roizen et al. 1995). The frequency of ocular relapses was reduced (Mets et al. 1996) and intracranial calcifications had diminished or resolved in 75% of the patients by 1 year of age (Patel et al. 1996).

The commonest side-effect of pyrimethamine is neutropaenia. Blood counts with platelet and haematocrit values must checked twice a week during the first month of treatment. Later, neutrophil counts can be made once a week and haematocrit and platelet values every 2–4 weeks. A neutrophil count below 1000/mm^3 warrants an increased dosage of calcium leukovorin to 10–20 mg three times a week. A count below 500/mm^3 implies a temporary discontinuation of pyrimethamine. A rash or pancytopaenia may be ascribed to sulphonamides and can result in their permanent withdrawal. After interruption of the treatment because of haematological side-effects, recommencing first with pyrimethamine alone and then adding sulphadiazine may help to identify which of the two drugs is responsible for the side-effects. If sulphadiazine cannot be tolerated, pyrimethamine should be used alone or possibly with one of the new drugs mentioned above. Spiramycin is no longer used for the curative treatment of congenital toxoplasmosis after birth.

Treatment of congenitally infected infants

Every case of congenital toxoplasmosis, even subclinical infection, must be treated. The pattern of the disease or difficulties in the initial diagnosis can, however, alter the suggested course of treatment (Figure 10.6):

1 Overt congenital toxoplasmosis. Continuous treatment for 1 year according to the Chicago protocol is mandatory.
2 Overt congenital toxoplasmosis with evidence of inflammatory processes (progressing retinochoroiditis, high CSF protein content, systemic infection and jaundice). Treatment should be the same as for overt toxoplasmosis but initially corticosteroids should be added until the inflammatory process has subsided.
3 Subclinical infection. The pyrimethamine–sulphadiazine combination for 2 months followed by a dose three times a week for 10 months seems the best regimen.
4 Apparently healthy babies whose laboratory data are not diagnostic (i.e. parasitological investigation negative and no antibody synthesis although maternal infection was definitely acquired during pregnancy). A course of pyrimethamine and sulphadiazine should be given for 1 month. Thereafter the regimen depends upon the findings of clinical and serological follow-up. It is mandatory to study repeatedly the antibody titre until 10 months of age (the utmost limit of persistency of passively transmitted maternal antibodies) even if parasitological investigation proved negative, if there is no specific IgM and if there was an initial decrease of specific IgG titre.
5 Healthy babies born to mothers whose date of acquired infection was undetermined. No treatment but very careful follow-up or as in number 4 if maternal infection seems to have occurred rather late in pregnancy (increased risk of materno–foetal transmission).

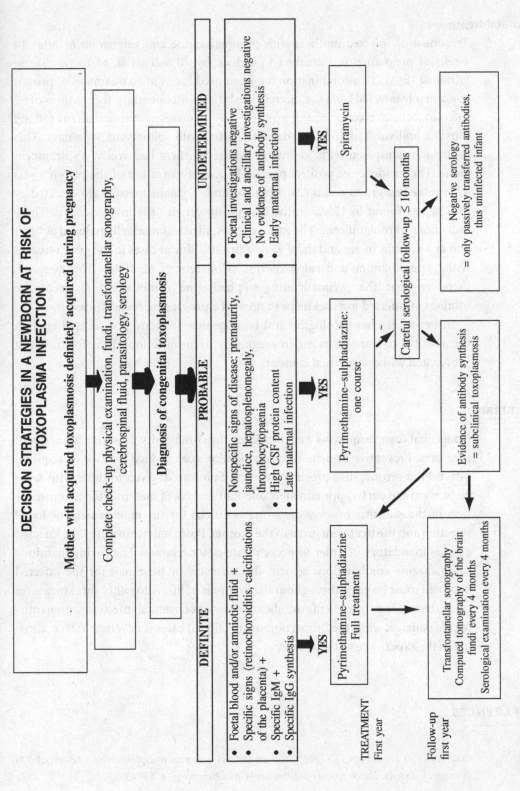

DECISION STRATEGIES IN A NEWBORN AT RISK OF TOXOPLASMA INFECTION

Mother with acquired toxoplasmosis definitely acquired during pregnancy

Complete check-up physical examination, fundi, transfontanellar sonography, cerebrospinal fluid, parasitology, serology

Diagnosis of congenital toxoplasmosis

DEFINITE	PROBABLE	UNDETERMINED
• Foetal blood and/or amniotic fluid + • Specific signs (retinochoroiditis, calcifications of the placenta) + • Specific IgM + • Specific IgG synthesis	• Nonspecific signs of disease: prematurity, jaundice, hepatosplenomegaly, thrombocytopaenia • High CSF protein content • Late maternal infection	• Foetal investigations negative • Clinical and ancillary investigations negative • No evidence of antibody synthesis • Early maternal infection
YES	YES	YES
Pyrimethamine–sulphadiazine: Full treatment	Pyrimethamine–sulphadiazine: one course	Spiramycin

Careful serological follow-up ≤ 10 months

Evidence of antibody synthesis = subclinical toxoplasmosis

Negative serology = only passively transferred antibodies, thus uninfected infant

TREATMENT
First year

Follow-up
first year

Transfontanellar sonography
Computed tomography of the brain
fundi every 4 months
Serological examination every 4 months

Figure 10.6 Decision strategies in the newborn at risk from toxoplasma infection

Prenatal treatment

Treatment of infected mothers with pyrimethamine and sulphadiazine after 14 weeks of pregnancy was claimed to reduce by 70% the risk of foetal disease (Kraübig 1963). This combination has been used for *in utero* treatment of proven congenitally infected babies (Couvreur et al. 1991). In one study, the mothers of 52 infected foetuses received one or several 3-week courses of pyrimethamine (50 mg plus 3 g oral sulphadiazine per day alternating with spiramycin 3 g a day). This group was compared with 51 infants whose mothers had received spiramcyin alone. The incidence of positive parasitological investigation of the placenta was 42% in the first group versus 83% in the second. *T. gondii*-specific IgM detected by ISAGA was found in 17.4% in the first group versus 68% in the second. These reductions were significant. The mean dye test titre was markedly reduced at birth and at 4 months of age and there were more subclinical cases in the group treated with pyrimethamine and sulphadiazine (Couvreur et al. 1991). This suggests, therefore, that the pyrimethamine–sulphadiazine combination given to the mothers of infected foetuses helps to prevent a progressive foetal disease.

However, its pharmacological and teratogenic effects are not yet well enough documented to warrant its use in pregnancy when infection of the foetus is not proven and without parental consent.

Summary

Congenital toxoplasmosis is a challenge for the community. It warrants a series of measures. Preventive hygiene recommendations can reduce the risk of acquired infection in seronegative pregnant women. Spiramycin given to those with seroconversion can cut by approximately one-half the risk of materno–foetal transmission of the parasite. *In utero* diagnosis is crucial for the management of foetal infection and the treatment given to the mother. Postnatal treatment of the infected child is mandatory in order to prevent late-onset relapses. The pyrimethamine–sulphadiazine combinations remain the mainstay of treatment for the infected baby and must be given throughout the first year of life. Altogether these measures can reduce to less than 2% the number of cases of congenital infection with neurological damage, while the proportion of subclinical cases is now over 70% according to the experience of the author.

REFERENCES

Couvreur, J. & Desmonts, G. (1962). Congenital and maternal toxoplasmosis. A review of 300 congenital cases. *Development Medicine and Child Neurology*, 4, 519–30.

Couvreur, J. & Leport, C. (1998). Toxoplasmosis. In *Antimicrobial Chemotherapy*, ed. V. L. Yu, T. Merigan & S. Barriere. Baltimore, MD: Williams and Wilkins.

Couvreur, J., Desmonts, G. & Girre, J. Y. (1976). Congenital toxoplasmosis in twins. A series of fourteen pairs of twins; absence of infection in one twin in two pairs. *Journal of Pediatrics*, **89**, 235–40.

Couvreur, J., Desmonts, G., Tournier, G. & Szusterkac, M. (1984*a*). Etude d'une série homogène de 210 cas de toxoplasmose congénitale chez des nourrissons de 0 à II mois et dépistés de façon prospective. *Annales de Pediatrie* (Paris), **31**, 815–19.

Couvreur, J., Alison, F. & Boccon-Gibod, L. (1984*b*). Rein et toxoplasmose. *Annales de Pediatrie (Paris)*, **31**, 847–52.

Couvreur, J., Desmonts, G. & Aron-Rosa, D. (1984*c*). Le pronostic oculaire de la toxoplasmose congénitale. Role du traitement. *Annales de Pédiatrie (Paris)*, **31**, 855–8.

Couvreur, J., Desmonts, G., Tournier, G. & Collin, J. (1984*d*). La production locale accrue d'immunoglobulines spécifiques G dans le liquide céphalorachidien au cours de la toxoplasmose congénitale. *Annales de Pédiatrie (Paris)*, **31**, 829–35.

Couvreur, J., Desmonts, G. & Thulliez, P. H. (1988). Prophylaxis of congenital toxoplasmosis. Effects of spiramycin on placental infection. *Journal of Antimicrobial Chemotherapy*, **22b**, 193–200.

Couvreur, J., Thulliez, P. H., Daffos, F., Gesquiere, A. & Desmonts, G. (1991). Foetopathie toxoplasmique: traitement "*in utero*" per association pyrimethamine-sulfamides. *Archives Françaises de Pédiatrie*, **48**, 397–403.

Desmonts, G. (1973). Toxoplasmose oculaire. Etude épidémiologique. (Bilan de 2000 examens d'humeur aqueuse). *Archives d'Ophtalmologie (Paris)*, **33**, 87–102.

Desmonts, G. & Couvreur, J. (1974*a*). Congenital toxoplasmosis: a prospective study of 378 pregnancies. *The New England Journal of Medicine*, **290**, 1010–16.

Desmonts, G. & Couvreur, J. (1974*b*). L'isolement du parasite dans la toxoplasmose congénitale. Intérêt pratique et théorique. *Archives Françaises de Pédiatrie*, **31**, 157–66.

Desmonts, G. & Couvreur, J. (1975). Toxoplasmosis: epidemiologic and serologic aspects of perinatal infection. In *Infections of the fetus and the newborn infant*, ed. S. Krugman & A. A. Gershon, Vol. 3. *Progress in Clinical and Biological Research*. New York: Alan Liss, pp. 115–132.

Feldman, H. A. (1953). Congenital toxoplasmosis. A study of one hundred and three cases. *American Journal of Diseases of Children*, **86**, 487–9.

Forestier, F., Daffos, F., Rainaut, M., Desnotte, J. F., Gaschard, J. C. (1987). Suivi thérapeutique foeto–maternel de la spiramycine au cours de la grossesse. *Archives Françaises de Pédiatrie*, **44**, 539–44.

Frenkel, J. K. (1974*a*). Pathology and pathogenesis of congenital toxoplasmosis. *Bulletin of the New York Academy of Medicine*, **50**, 182–91.

Frenkel, J. K. (1974*b*). Breaking the transmission chain of toxoplasma: a programme for the prevention of human toxoplasmosis. *Bulletin of the New York Academy of Medicine*, **50**, 228–35.

Janku, J. (1923). Die Pathogenese und pathologische Anatomie des sogenannten angeborenen Koloboms des gelben Fleckes im normal grossen sowie im mikrophthalmischen Auge mit Parasitenbefund in der Netzhaut [German translation]. *Ceska Parasitologie*, **6**, 9–56.

Koppe, J. G., Loewer-Siegler, D. H. & De Roever-Bonnet, D. H. (1986). Results of 20 years follow-up congenital toxoplasmosis. *The Lancet*, **1**, 254–6.

Kraübig, H. (1963). Erste praktische Erfahurungen mit des Prophylaxe der Konnatalen Toxoplasmose. *Medicine Klinische*, 58, 1361–1364.

Ladadie, M. D. & Hazeman, J. J. (1984). Apport des bilans de santé dans l'étude epidémiologique de la toxoplasmose congénitale. *Annales de Pédiatrie (Paris)*, 31, 823–8.

Levaditi, C. (1928). Au sujet de certaines protzooses héréditaires humaines a localisation oculaire et nerveuse. *Comptes Rendus de la Societe de Biologie*, 98, 297–9.

McAuley, J., Boyer, K., Patel, D., Mets, M., Swischer, C., Roizen, N., Wolters, W., Stein, L., Schey, W., Remington, J., Meir, P., Johnson, D., Heydeman, P., Holfels, E., Withers, S., Mack, D., Brown, C., Patton, D. & McLeod, R. (1994). Early and longitudinal evaluations of treated infants and children and untreated historical patients with congenital toxoplasmosis: The Chicago Collaborative Treatment Trial. *Clinical Infectious Diseases*, 18, 38–72.

McLeod, R., Mack, D., Foss, R., Boyer, K., Withers, S., Levin, S. & Hubbel, J. (1992). Levels of pyrimethamine in sera and cerebrospinal and ventricular fluids from infants treated for congenital toxoplasmosis. *Antimicrobial Agents and Chemotherapy*, 36, 1040–8.

Mets, M. B., Holfels, E., Boyer, K. M., Swisher, C. M., Roizen, N., Stein, L., Stein, M., Hopkins, J., Withers, S., Mack, D., Luciano, R., Patel, D., Remington, J. S., Meier, P. & McLeod, R. (1996). Eye manifestations of congenital toxoplasmosis. *American Journal of Ophthalmology*, 122, 309–24.

Patel, P. V., Holfels, E. M., Vogel, N. P., Boyer, K. M., Mets, M. B., Swisher, C. N., Roizen, N. J., Stein, L. K., Stein, M. A., Hopkins, J., Witters, S. E., Mack, D. G., Luciano, R. A., Meier, P., Remington, J. S. & McLeod, R. (1996). Resolution of intracranial calcifications in infants with treated congenital toxoplasmosis. *Radiology*, 199, 433–40.

Remington, J. S. & Desmonts, G. (1990). Toxoplasmosis. In *Infectious Diseases of The Foetus and Newborn Infant*, 3rd edn. ed. J. S. Remington & J. O. Klein, pp. 143–263. Philadelphia: WB Saunders.

Remington, J. S., McLeod, R., Thulliez, P & Desmonts, G. (2001). Toxoplasmosis. In *Infectious Diseases of the Fetus and Newborn Infant*, 5th edn. ed. J. S. Remington & J. O. Klein. Philadelphia: WB Saunders.

Roizen, N., Swisher, C. N., Stein, M. A., Hopkins, J., Boyer, K. M., Holfels, E., Mets, M. B., Stein, L., Pattet, D., Meir, P., Whitters, S., Remington, J. S., Mack, D., Heydemann, P., Patton, D. & McLeod, R. (1995). Neurologic and developmental outcome in treated congenital toxoplasmosis. *Pediatrics*, 95, 11–20.

Swischer, C. N., Boyer, K. M. & McLeod, R. (1994). The Toxoplasmosis Study Group. Congenital toxoplasmosis. *Seminars in Pediatric Neurology*, 1, 4–25.

Wilson, C. B., Remington, J. S., Stagno, S. & Reynolds, D. W. (1980). Development of adverse sequelae in children born with subclinical toxoplasma infection. *Pediatrics*, 66, 767–74.

Wolf, A., Cowen, D. & Paige, B. H. (1939). Human toxoplasmosis. Occurrence in infants as an encephalomyelitis. Verification by transmission to animals. *Science*, 89, 226–7.

11

Ocular infection

G. N. Dutton

Tennet Institute of Ophthalmology, Gart Naval General Hospital, Glasgow, Scotland

Introduction

Focal retinochoroiditis is the most frequent outcome of infection of the eye by *Toxoplasma gondii* (Figure 11.1). The natural history of the disease is for an acute inflammatory lesion of the retina to slowly resolve, leaving a focus of retinochoroidal scarring.

The normal retina is transparent. Beneath this, the choroid is filled with blood, which is responsible for the red appearance. (As seen in the pupils when using flash photography.) Initially, the inflammatory cell infiltrate whitens the retina and may involve the overlying vitreous gel. As the inflammation regresses, focal destruction of the choroid reveals the underlying white sclera. The surrounding brown pigmentation of a healed lesion is due to replication of melanin-containing cells, which contribute to the healing process.

History

The first reported case in which the parasitic cysts of *T. gondii* were found within the retina was that of a child who died with hydrocephalus. Histology of the eyes revealed parasitic cysts in the retina adjacent to a 'congenital coloboma' of the macula (Janku 1923). However, the original basis for the statement that focal retinochoroidal scarring is due to *T. gondii* was the work of Koch et al. (1943), who reported the condition in six infected children and the pathology of three infected eyes. Vail et al. (1943) also described the condition in association with positive serological tests for *T. gondii* in older children and adults.

In 1952 organisms indistinguishable from *T. gondii* were discerned by Wilder in the retina in the eyes of 53 adults. Apart from three exceptions, in which a diagnosis of syphilis had originally been made by the pathologists, the majority of these eyes had been ascribed a clinical and pathological diagnosis of tuberculous choroiditis. Twenty-one of these patients were all subsequently found to have *T. gondii* antibody in their sera (Jacobs et al. 1954). Not surprisingly few such eyes have been

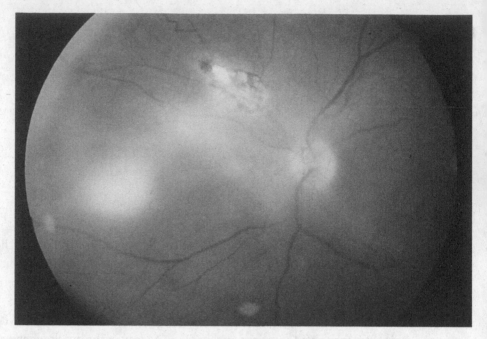

Figure 11.1   Retinal photograph showing the typical focal retinochoroidal scarring pattern of toxoplasmic retinochoroiditis, with an adjacent focus of inflammatory activity

removed since the publication of these seminal papers. It is, therefore, these historical data which allow the ophthalmologist to diagnose toxoplasmic retinochoroiditis in most cases, primarily on the basis of the clinical picture.

Epidemiology

The presence of *T. gondii* antibody in serum indicates previous systemic infection. Worldwide, the prevalence of Toxoplasma infection varies from 97%, in those over 50 years old in El Salvador (Remington et al. 1970), to 0% amongst Icelanders and Eskimos, where the low temperature presumably destroys the organisms (Frenkel 1971), and amongst those living on Pacific atolls where there are no cats (Wallace 1969). In general, however, *T. gondii* antibody prevalence in humans in the Western World approximates to the age of the population studied (Schlaegel 1978). In countries such as France, the penchant for eating undercooked meat has been ascribed as the cause of earlier acquisition of the disease and its greater prevalence.

As toxoplasmic retinochoroiditis may be asymptomatic, there are few data available concerning its incidence and prevalence. In one survey of a community in the

United States, five (0.6%) out of 852 people were found to have asymptomatic retinal lesions typical of the disorder (Smith & Ganley 1972).

Toxoplasmic retinochoroiditis is considered, in most cases, to be the result of recrudescence of retinal parasitization, originally acquired *in utero*. The rationale for this statement has been succinctly summarized by Perkins (1981):

1 Most cases show evidence of old scars indicating previous activity.
2 There is rarely any history of recent systemic disease compatible with systemic infection.
3 *Toxoplasma gondii* antibody titres do not suggest recent infection.
4 The incidence of ocular lesions does not rise with age as would be expected from the known increase in *T. gondii* antibody prevalence with age.
5 Retinochoroiditis is a rare complication of known acquired systemic disease (2–3%).

These statements are based primarily upon his earlier work (Perkins 1961, 1973). An observation that is in accordance with these statements is that a woman suffering from recurrent ocular toxoplasmosis during pregnancy will not transmit the infection to her foetus (O'Connor 1983).

Epidemiological studies in southern Brazil suggest that the remarkably high incidence of toxoplasmic retinochoroiditis in that country is related to acquired, rather than congenital disease (Glasner et al. 1992). In Brazil a number of sibships have been reported with recurrent necrotizing retinochoroiditis, which has been said to lend weight to this observation (Silveira et al. 1988). A single infection by *T. gondii* confers immunity upon the host to subsequent exposure; therefore, a mother would not be expected to have more than one child with toxoplasmic retinochoroiditis. However, other such sibships have been reported (Lou et al. 1978; Stern & Romano 1978; Asbell et al. 1982), and have been attributed by these authors to persistent *T. gondii* cysts within the uterine muscle, which release their contents into the foetal circulation during pregnancy or labour.

There is no apparent congenital predisposition to developing ocular toxoplasmosis, and males and females are affected equally. No relationship has been found between this type of uveitis and HLA antigens (Ohno et al. 1977; Bloch-Michel et al. 1979).

An apparently higher incidence of the disease in white people as compared with blacks in the United States has been attributed to the protective effect of the high prevalence of *T. gondii* antibody amongst immigrants from West Africa (Schlaegel 1978).

Henderson et al. (1982) reviewed the epidemiological data for the UK concerning congenital toxoplasmosis. From this information, they estimated that the annual incidence of visual handicap caused by *T. gondii* in the UK ranged from 40 to 400 with a central estimate of 120 (six being blind, and 114 with moderate visual handicap). More recent studies have shown that toxoplasmic retinochoroiditis is fortunately an unusual cause of blindness in children (Grey et al. 1989; Thompson et al. 1989; Goggin & O'Keefe 1991).

Overall in the UK congenital toxoplasmosis is the cause of blind registration in 0.1–0.2% of patients (Sorsby 1972; Ghafour 1983).

Pathogenesis

The risk to the foetus of developing toxoplasma infection appears to be related to the time when maternal infection occurs. If the disease is acquired during the last month of pregnancy, the protozoon is most likely to be transmitted to the foetus, but the infection will initially be subclinical in infancy. However, if the mother is infected earlier, the transmission to the foetus will occur less often but more severe disease may result.

Parasitization of the retina

Parasitization of a cell is followed by intracellular replication of the organism with resultant cyst formation. Ultrastructural studies in a murine model of congenital toxoplasmic retinochoroiditis have shown that each mature cyst is surrounded by what appears to be viable host cell tissue (McMenamin et al. 1986) (Figure 11.2).

In the majority of cases, intraretinal cyst formation probably occurs as a sequel to perinatal parasitaemia. These cysts may then remain dormant within the retina. It has also been proposed that organisms may gain access to the eye by passage along the optic nerve (Levaditi et al. 1928; Berengo & Frezzotti 1962). Remington and Desmonts (1976) have postulated that the release of organisms elsewhere in the body later in life could also result in retinal parasitization. This hypothesis is based on the observation that parasitaemia may occur during chronic infection in Man (Siegel et al. 1971). It has been argued that the barrier to passive diffusion of antibodies presented by the cerebral and retinal vasculature results in persistent cysts in the brain and retina (Frenkel 1961), but tissues such as cardiac and skeletal muscle may also contain parasitic cysts. A feature common to all the tissues in which cysts are found is the absent or low cell turnover rate.

Retinal parasitization as a result of acquired disease is thought to be an unusual but recognized event (Perkins 1973; Montoya & Remington 1996). However, it has been suggested that retinochoroiditis associated with acquired toxoplasma infection may be more common than previously supposed (Holland 1999).

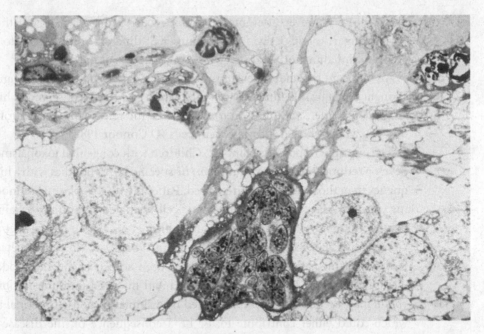

Figure 11.2 Electron micrograph of a *T. gondii* cyst within the ganglion cell layer of mouse retina. The disposition of the cyst suggests that it is incorporated within a Müller cell, which is one of the glial supporting cells of the retina (×3000)

The acute inflammatory episode

The most commonly advanced hypothesis is that cyst rupture is the precipitating event for an acute inflammatory episode (Frenkel 1958). This may be precipitated by the demise of a host cell, resulting in the release of free parasites seeking to penetrate adjacent cells, with a view to reestablishing their encysted state. The release of free parasites probably results in a number of damaging effects.

Toxic damage has been proposed. The intravitreal inoculation of a soluble non-viscous dialysable toxin derived from a murine peritoneal exudate containing virulent *T. gondii* causes severe retinal disruption (Hogan et al. 1971). (The inoculum could, however, have contained host cell tissue components which could have contributed to the pathological process.) Necrotizing retinitis due to *T. gondii* has been reported in an immunosuppressed patient with a negative dye test titre and it was argued that the retinal damage resulted from a cytolytic and necrotizing action of the parasite (Yeo et al. 1983). Thus, in the absence of a normal host immune response, the parasites may give rise directly to retinal damage.

Hypersensitivity to *T. gondii* antigen has been ascribed as the cause of the characteristic granulomatous inflammatory response which may be observed (Frenkel

1958, 1961). However, attempts to induce recurrent inflammatory pathology by inoculating *T. gondii* antigens by a number of different routes failed to produce recurrent inflammatory pathology in animal models of the disease.

An innocent bystander mechanism, in which damage to the normal anatomy is brought about by inflammatory cell infiltration and lysis, is observed in histopathological specimens, and has been ascribed to the release of acid hydrolases and other enzymes which destroy adjacent cells (O'Connor 1982).

The immune response is complex. Children with congenital toxoplasmosis who develop retinochoroiditis exhibit *T. gondii*-specific IgE antibodies with a higher frequency than those whose eyes are spared. Patients with toxoplasmic retinochoroiditis may display both humoral and cell-mediated immunity against both toxoplasmal and retinal antigens (Nussenblatt et al. 1980*a*, *b*; Wyler et al. 1980; Gregerson et al. 1981; Abrahams & Gregerson 1982, 1983; Nussenblatt et al. 1989). Similar cell-mediated responses have also been seen in a murine model of the disease (Hay et al. 1985). A cell-mediated and humoral immune response to *T. gondii* may, therefore, be complemented by a similar response to retinal antigens, which could either contribute to, or be a consequence of, the disease process. However, Kijistra et al. (1990) were unable to identify any differences in the humoral and cellular responses to retinal antigens between patients with active toxoplasmic retinochoroiditis and patients with uveitis of other causes.

The effects of persistent parasitization

In animal models of congenital toxoplasmic retinochoroiditis and in naturally occurring disease in animals, two prominent features are commonly observed. *Toxoplasma gondii* cysts are found in the apparently normal retina, with little if any surrounding inflammatory response (Figure 11.2). However, retinal vasculitis and photoreceptor destruction is commonly observed, remote from the organism (Figure 11.3).

Frenkel (1955) documented photoreceptor cell loss in a golden hamster chronically infected with *T. gondii* and Piper et al. (1970) described the same phenomenon occurring in a wide range of infected animals. Kramar and Vrabec (1960), Vainisi and Campbell (1969), Yoshizumi (1976), Ashton (1979), and Dutton et al. (1986*a*, *b*) have all reported such features in the eyes of *T. gondii*-infected rats, cats, rabbits, wallabies and mice respectively. In each of these reports, the photoreceptor damage, which was either described or illustrated, resembles closely the condition of experimental allergic uveo-retinitis. In this condition, destruction of the photoreceptors takes place as a sequel to the inoculation elsewhere in the body of retinal antigens, derived from photoreceptors.

In Man, focal retinochoroiditis, in association with unilateral extensive retinal destruction accompanied by a pattern of pigmentary retinopathy resembling retin-

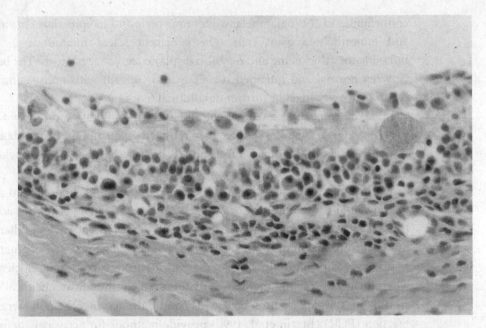

Figure 11.3   Light micrograph showing perivascular and subretinal inflammatory cell infiltration with marked depletion and damage of the photoreceptors (rods and cones). The *T. gondii* cyst is present within relatively undisturbed retina (×300) (Paraffin, Haematoxylin and Eosin)

itis pigmentosa, has been described in a small number of patients. The histopathology of this condition characteristically shows the absence of photoreceptors and it has been suggested that an analogous secondary autoimmune response directed against retinal antigens may be responsible for this process (Silveira et al. 1989). Patients with chronic *T. gondii*-induced scarring have never, to the author's knowledge, been assessed prospectively for the possible development of progressive visual dysfunction in the peripheral visual field, which would be the natural sequel to less severe, perhaps asymptomatic, variants of the same condition.

Pathology

The histopathological features of the disease, seen in enucleated adult eyes, have a characteristic pattern. The acute lesion produces a zonal granuloma with central coagulative necrosis and karolytic retinal cells. Lymphocytes, plasma cells, epithelioid cells and occasionally giant cells surround this region. *Toxoplasma gondii* organisms may be seen in the central and surrounding areas. Rarely, if ever, are organisms found in ocular tissues other than the retina (in the immunocompetent host). The underlying choroid is usually involved in the disease process and is either necrotic or replaced by epithelioid cells. Melanin from the necrotic pigment epithelium and choroidal melanocytes may be found in epithelioid macrophages and multinucleate giant cells. The subjacent sclera may undergo nodular inflammatory thickening and may also display coagulative necrosis. The boundary between normal and inflamed tissues is fairly abrupt with nonspecific chronic inflammatory changes in surrounding retinal tissues.

In the immunosuppressed patient, unchecked proliferation of *T. gondii* within the retina appears to give rise directly to retinal damage and the host inflammatory response is less in evidence (Toussaint & Wanderhaeghen 1975; Nicholson & Wolchok 1976; Yeo et al. 1983).

The histopathological features of the eyes of infants and children who succumb to congenital toxoplasmosis are similar to those described above, but additional features include microphthalmia, cataract and the persistence of a pupillary membrane. Intraretinal dystrophic calcification has occasionally been documented.

It may be difficult to distinguish the parasite from surrounding nuclear debris when tinctorial staining methods only are used. Immunohistochemical demonstration of *T. gondii* (Dutton et al. 1984) and more recently the polymerase chain reaction (PCR) (Brezin et al. 1990) provide methods for accurately defining the presence of *T. gondii* in ocular and other tissues.

Clinical features and diagnosis

Focal retinochoroidal scarring is commonly attributed to *T. gondii* as the causative agent. The original basis for this statement is the work of Koch et al. (1943), in which they demonstrated the parasites in three infected eyes which exhibited this feature.

Patients suffering from active toxoplasmic retinochoroiditis characteristically present with symptoms of blurred vision and floaters, which may be associated with pain and discomfort. On examination of the eye, these symptoms are found to be attributable to one or more foci of active retinal inflammation. Such foci may occur *de novo*, or may be adjacent to an area of retinochoroidal scarring.

Within the anterior chamber, signs of iritis may be seen. These include the presence of cells, a flare and keratic precipitates. In the posterior segment, precipitates may be deposited upon the posterior face of a vitreous detachment, and cells can be observed within the vitreous itself. Inflammatory foci may occur anywhere on the retina. Involvement of the retina adjacent to the optic disc causes juxtapapillary choroiditis and involvement of the optic nerve gives rise to papillitis (Folk & Lobes 1984).

When the macula is affected by the disease process, there is loss of central vision. Such inflammatory lesions may be discrete and short-lived, or they may extend and become chronic. In most cases the disease gradually resolves to leave a quiescent scar, whether or not the patient has received treatment. However, it has been shown that the greater the size of the focus of toxoplasmic retinochoroiditis, the longer the duration of the disease process (Rothova et al. 1989).

Further clinical signs which may develop include segmental periarteritis (O'Connor 1970), retinal and vitreous haemorrhage (Rieger 1952), choroidal or retinal neovascularization (Fine et al. 1981; Malbrel 1981; Gaynon et al. 1984), branch artery occlusion (Willerson et al. 1977; Braunstein & Gass 1980) and retinochoroidal anastomoses (Kennedy & Wise 1971; Owens et al. 1979) Persistent inflammation may give rise to intravitreal fibrosis with retinal tears and detachment, to secondary cataract and to glaucoma. Another morphological variant which was initially described by Friedman and Knox (1969), but which has subsequently been reported by Doft and Gass (1985), and Matthews and Weiter (1988) is that of deep punctate retinitis occurring in association with a clear vitreous. Such lesions may be multifocal and have a grey-white pattern with little or no associated overlying vitreous reaction. They tend to resolve to form fine granular white dots and presumably represent discrete inflammatory foci, due to the release of free parasites in the outer retina.

Patients who are immunosuppressed on account of infection, neoplasia or drug treatment may manifest more extensive inflammation, particularly in the posterior segment of the eye which may be associated with exudative retinal detachment. The differential diagnosis in such cases is difficult as the clinical picture is not specific and recourse is made to sampling intraocular fluids for serological and PCR analysis for cytomegalovirus, herpes simplex virus, varicella zoster virus and toxoplasma (de Boer et al. 1996).

When congenital ocular toxoplasmosis presents in childhood, the infection may have interfered with the development of the eye. A different spectrum of clinical signs may, therefore, be seen. Franceschetti and Bamatter (1953) reviewed the clinical signs in 243 cases of congenital ocular toxoplasmosis and found the following percentages: bilateral involvement, 66%; strabismus, 28%; optic atrophy, 27%; nystagmus (resulting either from impaired fixation or from involvement of the central nervous system) 23%; microphthalmia, 23%; cataract, 8%; iritis and posterior synaechiae, 8%; persistence of pupillary membrane, 4%; and vitreous changes, 11%.

The differential diagnosis of toxoplasmic retinochoroiditis includes such infectious diseases as tuberculous or syphilitic choroiditis, candidiasis, cytomegalic inclusion disease, neonatal herpes simplex, nocardiosis, cryptocaccosis, toxocariasis and presumed ocular histoplasmosis syndrome. Noninfectious diseases which may give rise to a similar clinical picture include Coats' disease, pigment epithelial hypertrophy, retinoblastoma, traumatic chorioretinal scarring and vitelliruptive macular dystrophy (Schlaegel 1978). Familial macular colobomata (Miller & Bresnick 1978) and Aicardi's syndrome (Hoyt et al. 1978) should also be considered.

Investigation

Apart from rare cases in which it is possible to isolate *T. gondii* from the eye, the diagnosis of toxoplasmic retinochoroiditis is presumptive and necessitates exclusion of the aforementioned diseases, usually on clinical grounds alone. Reliance is then placed upon the clinical characteristics, the presence of *T. gondii* antibody and, in certain cases, the response to treatment.

Unlike acute infections in which a rising serum *T. gondii* antibody titre is diagnostic, in patients with toxoplasmic retinochoroiditis, there is no relationship between the titre and disease severity, and a single positive serum antibody titre at any level is likely to be significant. Depending upon the investigation performed, negative or borderline antibody titres have also been documented in patients with proven disease (Zscheile 1964; Rothova et al. 1986).

Some immunocompromised patients (i.e. those with acquired immunodeficiency syndrome, AIDS) can present more of a diagnostic problem when retinal necrosis caused by *T. gondii* occurs in the absence of *T. gondii*-positive serology (Yeo et al. 1983). In this situation, any structure of the eye may be invaded by the parasite (Holland 1989). Fortunately however, toxoplasmic retinochoroiditis is an unusual complication of AIDS (Jabs et al. 1989; Sidikaro et al. 1991). Optic neuritis due to *T. gondii* has also been described in these patients (Grossniklaus et al. 1990). Under such circumstances, *T. gondii* antibodies should be sought in samples of aqueous humour. The *T. gondii* antibody titres obtained can be compared with those in the serum of the same patient, and the result expressed as a coefficient; a value of above 3.0 is considered significant (Kijlstra et al. 1989). *Toxoplasma gondii* DNA has also been detected by PCR in the aqueous humour of affected patients (Manners et al. 1994; de Boer et al. 1996). Details of the diagnostic methods used are described in Chapter 12.

Treatment

A number of chemotherapeutic agents have been used in the treatment of toxoplasmic retinochoroiditis.

Pyrimethamine and sulphonamides (the most commonly used sulphonamide being sulphadiazine) have been used since the early 1950s in the treatment of toxoplasmic retinochoroiditis. Pyrimethamine inhibits replication of *T. gondii* by interfering with folic acid metabolism. It, therefore, has toxic side-effects which mirror those of folate depletion. These effects may be overcome by the administration of folinic acid, which does not interfere with the therapeutic efficacy of pyrimethamine (Giles 1971).

Clindamycin has also been found to be an effective antitoxoplasma agent which reaches high intraocular concentrations (Tabbara & O'Connor 1975) and which is effective in treating rabbit eyes previously infected with *T. gondii* (Tabbara et al. 1979). Other reports at that time suggested that this drug is effective in the treatment of toxoplasmic retinochoroiditis (Chandra & Donaldson 1978; Tabbara & O'Connor 1980; Lakhanpal et al. 1983). Clindamycin must be used with caution, however, in view of the uncommon but serious side-effect of pseudomembraneous colitis (Swartzberg et al. 1977). The incidence of such complications necessitating the withdrawal of treatment is about 10% (Mittelviefhaus 1992). In addition, it is probably unwise to use this drug via a periocular route, as this may give rise to optic nerve damage (Tate & Martin 1977).

Uncontrolled trials document that a combination of trimethoprim and sulphamethoxazole is an effective treatment (Oprerneak et al. 1992). Minocycline has also been found to be effective in the treatment of experimental ocular toxoplasmosis in the rabbit (Rollins et al. 1982).

Spiramycin was initially described in an encouraging report to be 'the therapy of choice in ocular toxoplasmosis' (Chodos & Habegger-Chodos 1961), but three subsequent studies failed to confirm their findings (Fajardo et al. 1962; Leopold 1963; Heaton 1963).

A number of new agents for the treatment of toxoplasmosis are currently being developed and may well prove effective in the management of toxoplasmic retinochoroiditis in the future (Dutton 1989). Colin and Harie (1989) published a prospective randomized trial in which they compared the outcome of the treatment between clindamycin and pyrimethamine with sulphadiazine. No significant difference was found in the outcome between these treatment modalities with a mean healing time of 1.8 months. However, the incidence of side-effects with clindamycin was lower.

Rothova et al. (1989) were the first to carry out a prospective trial in which various combinations of chemotherapeutic agents (pyrimethamine/sulphadiazine/folinic acid/steroids, clindamycin/sulphadiazine/steroids and trimethoprim/sulphamethoxazole) were compared with the effects of no treatment. Central lesions threatening visual function were treated, while peripheral lesions were not. It was concluded that no significant therapeutic benefit accrued from any of these drug combinations. The pyrimethamine drug combination was accompanied by a smaller final lesion size, but this was a trend only. Whether any regime decreases the rate of recurrence, the size or depth of an inflammatory focus or decreases the incidence of oedema of the macula remains to be determined.

Few data are available concerning recurrence. The reported recurrence rate in patients treated with sulphadiazine and pyrimethamine varies between 13% and 17% (Ghosh et al. 1965; Canamucio et al. 1963), whilst that for clindamycin is reported as being just under 8% over an 8-year period (Lakanpal et al. 1983).

However, as the criteria for patient selection and assessment of the disease differ in many respects, such comparisons are solely empirical.

The macrolide antibiotic azithromycin has specific activity against toxoplasma. In one observational study in which 11 immunocompetent patients were treated with the drug for 5 weeks, the inflammation resolved within 4 weeks in seven cases (Rothova et al. 1998).

A phase-1 trial of atovaquone for the treatment of toxoplasmic retinochoroiditis in 17 immunocompetent patients has shown encouraging results with a favourable response being observed between 1 and 3 weeks of starting treatment in all patients and no adverse effects (Pearson et al. 1999).

The use of steroids in the treatment of toxoplasmic retinochoroiditis is controversial. In one controlled trial involving 20 patients, no difference could be found when the results of using pyrimethamine and steroids were compared with those of placebo and steroids (Acers 1964). Immunosuppression potentiates replication of *T. gondii*. On this basis a number of authors warn against the use of steroids as the sole therapeutic agent (Nicholson & Wolchok 1976; O'Connor & Frenkel 1976; Sabates et al. 1981; Bosch-Driessen & Rothova 1998). Most clinicians supplement specific antimicrobial treatment with steroids with the intention of diminishing the risk of inflammatory cell damage to the macula and optic nerve, but there is no published evidence that these objectives are realized. It is not known whether the use of steroids influences the recurrence rate of the disease in any way.

Both photocoagulation and cryotherapy have also been used in the treatment of toxoplasmic retinochoroiditis. Spalter et al. (1966) reported successful results following the application of photocoagulation around active foci of toxoplasmic retinochoroiditis in 24 patients. In a controlled trial Saari et al. (1984) found that such treatment significantly reduced the recurrence rate. Ghartey and Brockhurst (1980) obtained satisfactory resolution in four out of five patients following direct photocoagulation of the retinochoroidal lesion. Cryotherapy has also been claimed to give rise to a more rapid resolution than when medical treatment alone is used (Dobbie 1968).

The rationale for using either of these techniques is that both encysted and free parasites are susceptible to extremes of temperature (Jacobs et al. 1960).

Inflammatory debris in the vitreous humour causes shadow formation on the retina, which is seen as a floater across central vision. This is commonly the first sign of recurrent disease. Usually, gradual spontaneous clearance of vitreous inflammation takes place, but in cases in which inflammatory debris persists and gives rise to significant impairment of vision, surgical removal of the vitreous humour (vitrectomy) is occasionally performed (Werry & Honegger 1987).

There is no wholly satisfactory means of treating ocular toxoplasmosis and it is evident that further research is required to establish optimum modalities and regimens of treatment.

Summary

Toxoplasmic retinochoroiditis is the commonest form of posterior uveitis. The majority of infants infected *in utero* will eventually go on to develop the disorder but this may be many years later. Acquired infection by the parasite can also rarely cause an acute episode of the disease. The organism resides in the retina and acute inflammation is thought to result from the release of free parasites. Treatment with antitoxoplasma agents with additional steroid medication when central retinal function is threatened is indicated in symptomatic cases. The dynamics of the host–parasite interaction in the eye and the development of optimal treatment strategies require further investigation.

REFERENCES

Abrahams, W. I. & Gregerson, D. S. (1982). Longitudinal study of serum antibody responses to retinal antigens in acute ocular toxoplasmosis. *American Journal of Ophthalmology*, 93, 224–31.

Abrahams, W. I. & Gregerson, D. S. (1983). Longitudinal study of serum antibody responses to bovine retinal S-antigen in endogenous granulomatous uveitis. *British Journal of Ophthalmology*, 67, 681–84.

Acers, T. E. (1964). Toxoplasmic retinochoroiditis: a double blind therapeutic study. *Archives of Ophthalmology*, 71, 58–62.

Asbell, P. A., Vermund, S. H. & Hofeldt, A. J. (1982). Presumed toxoplasmic retinochoroiditis in four siblings. *American Journal of Ophthalmology*, 94, 656–63.

Ashton, N. (1979). Ocular toxoplasmosis in wallabies (*Macropus rufogriseus*). *American Journal of Ophthalmology*, 88, 322–32.

Berengo, A. & Frezzotti, R. (1962). Active neuro-ophthalmic toxoplasmosis: a clinical study on nineteen patients. *Advances in Ophthalmology*, 12, 265–343.

Bloch-Michel, E., Campinchi, R., Muller, J. Y., Binaghi, M. & Sales, J. (1979). HLA antigens and uveitis with special reference to Behcet's disease chronic herpes simplex, toxoplasmosis, and recurrent acute anterior uveitis. In *Immunology and Immunopathology of the Eye*, ed. M. A. Silverstein & G. R. O'Connor. New York: Masson.

Bosch-Driessen, E. H. & Rothova, A. (1998). Sense and nonsense of corticosteroid in the treatment of ocular toxoplasmosis. *British Journal of Ophthalmology*, 82, 858–60.

Braunstein, R. A. & Gass, J. D. M. (1980). Branch artery occlusion caused by acute toxoplasmosis. *Archives of Ophthalmology*, 98, 512–13.

Brezin, A. P., Edwuagu, C. E., Burnier, M., Silveira, C., Mahdi, R. M., Gazzinelli, R. T., Belfort, R.

& Nusenblatt, R. B. (1990). Identification *of Toxoplasma gondii* in paraffin-embedded sections by the polymerase chain reaction. *American Journal of Ophthalmology*, 110, 599–604.

Canamucio, C. J., Hallet, J. W. & Leopold, I. H. (1963). Recurrence of treated toxoplasmic uveitis. *American Journal of Ophthalmology*, 55, 1035–43.

Chandra, J. & Donaldson, E. J. (1978). Clindamycin in human ocular toxoplasmosis: a preliminary report. *Australian Journal of Ophthalmology*, 6, 135–42.

Chodos, J. E. & Habegger-Chodos, H. E. (1961). The treatment of ocular toxoplasmosis with spiramycin. *AMA Archives of Ophthalmology*, 65, 401–9.

Colin, J. & Harie, J. C. (1989). Chorioretinites presumees toxoplasmiques. Etude comparative des traitements par pyrimethamine et sulfadiazine ou clindamycine. *Journal Francais d'Ophtalmologie*, 12, 161–5.

de Boer, J. H., Verhagen, C., Bruinenberg, M., Rothova, A., deJong, P. T., Baarsma, G. S., Vander Leiij, A., Ooyman, F. M., Bollameijar, J. G., Derhaag, P. J. & Kijlstra, A. (1996). Serologic and polymerase chain reaction analysis of intracocular fluids in the diagnosis of infectious uveitis. *American Journal of Ophthalmology*, 121, 650–8.

Dobbie, J. G. (1968). Cryotherapy in the management of Toxoplasma retinochoroiditis. *Transactions of the American Academy of Ophthalmology and Otolaryngology*, 72, 364–73.

Doft, B. H. & Gass, J. D. M. (1985). Punctate outer retinal toxoplasmosis. *Archives of Ophthalmology*, 103, 1332–6.

Dutton, G. N. (1989). Recent developments in the prevention and treatment of congenital toxoplasmosis. *International Ophthalmology*, 13, 407–13.

Dutton, G. N., Hay, J. & Ralston, J. (1984). The immunocytochemical demonstration of Toxoplasma within the retina of congenitally infected mice. *Annales of Tropical Medicine and Parasitology*, 78, 431–3.

Dutton, G. N., Hay, J., Hair, D. M. & Ralston, J. (1986a). Clinico-pathological features of a congenital murine model of ocular toxoplasmosis. *Von Graefe's Archive for Clinical and Experimental Ophthalmology*, 224, 256–64.

Dutton, G. N., McMenamin, P. G., Hay, J. & Cameron, S. (1986b). The ultrastructural pathology of congenital murine toxoplasmic retinochoroiditis. II. The morphology of the inflammatory changes. *Experimental Eye Research*, 43, 545–60.

Fajardo, R. A., Furgiuele, F. P. & Leopold, I. H. (1962). Treatment of toxoplasmosis uveitis. *AMA Archives of Ophthalmology*, 67, 712–20.

Fine, S. L., Owens, S. L., Haller, J. A., Knox, D. L. & Patz, A. (1981). Choroidal neovascularization as a late complication of ocular toxoplasmosis. *American Journal of Ophthalmology*, 91, 318–22.

Folk, J. C. & Lobes, L. A. (1984). Presumed toxoplasmic papillitis. *Archives of Ophthalmology*, 91, 64–7.

Franceschetti, A. & Bamatter, F. (1953). Diagnostic clinique, anatomique et histoparasitologique des affections toxoplasmiques. Primus Latinus Congressus Ophthalmologiae, June 1953, Rome, pp. 315–437. Societas Ophthalmologica Latina, Rome.

Frenkel, J. K. (1955). Ocular lesions in hamsters with chronic Toxoplasma and Besnoita infection. *American Journal of Ophthalmology*, 39, 203–25.

Frenkel, J. K. (1958). Ocular toxoplasmosis. Pathogenesis, diagnosis and treatment. *AMA Archives of Ophthalmology*, 59, 260–79.

Frenkel, J. K. (1961). Pathogenesis of toxoplasmosis with a consideration of cyst rupture in Besnoita infection. *Survey of Ophthalmology*, **6**, 799–825.

Frenkel, J. K. (1971). Toxoplasmosis. Mechanism of infection. Laboratory diagnosis and management. *Current Topics in Pathology*, **54**, 28–75.

Friedman, C. T. & Knox, D. L. (1969). Variations in recurrent active toxoplasmic retinochoroiditis. *Archives of Ophthalmology*, **81**, 481–93.

Gaynon, M. W., Boldrey, E. E., Strahlman, E. R. & Fine, S. L. (1984). Retinal neovascularization and ocular toxoplasmosis. *American Journal of Ophthalmology*, **98**, 585–9.

Ghafour, I. M. A. (1983). *Diabetic Eye Disease in the West of Scotland*. PhD Thesis. Glasgow University, pp. 1–234.

Ghartey, K. N. & Brockhurst, R. J. (1980). Photocoagulation of active toxoplasmic retinochoroiditis. *American Journal of Ophthalmology*, **89**, 858–64.

Ghosh, M., Levy, P. M. & Leopold, I. M. (1965). Therapy of toxoplasmosis uveitis. *American Journal of Ophthalmology*, **59**, 55–61.

Giles, C. L. (1971). Pyrimethamine (Daraprim) and the treatment of toxoplasmic uveitis. *Survey of Ophthalmology*, **16**, 88–91.

Glasner, P. D., Silveira, C., Kruszon-Moran, D., Martins, M. C., Burnier, M., Silveira, S., Camargo, M. E., Nussenblatt, R. B., Kaslow, R. A. & Belford, R. (1992). An unusually high prevalence of ocular toxoplasmosis in Southern Brazil. *American Journal of Ophthalmology*, **114**, 136–44.

Gregerson, D. S., Abrahams, W. I. & Thirkill, C. E. (1981). Serum antibody levels of uveitis patients to bovine retinal antigens. *Investigative Ophthalmology and Visual Science*, **21**, 669–80.

Grey, R. H. B., Burns-Cox, C. J. & Hughes, A. (1989). Blind and partial sight registration in Avon. *British Journal of Ophthalmology*, **73**, 88–94.

Goggin, M. & O'Keefe, M. (1991). Childhood blindness in the Republic of Ireland, a national survey. *British Journal of Ophthalmology*, **75**, 425–9.

Grossniklaus, H. E., Specht, C. S., Allaire, G. & Leavitt, J. A. (1990). *Toxoplasma gondii* retinochoroiditis and optic neuritis in acquired immune deficiency syndrome. *Ophthalmology*, **97**, 1342–6.

Hay, J., Dutton, G. N. & Hair, D. M. (1985). Blastogenic responses to splenic lymphocytes and to toxoplasmal and retinal antigens and T- and B-cell mitogens in mice with congenital ocular toxoplasmosis. *Annals of Tropical Medicine and Parasitology*, **79**, 113–15.

Heaton, J. M. (1963). Spiramycin in treatment of posterior uveitis. *British Journal of Ophthalmology*, **47**, 677–81.

Henderson, J. B., Beattie, C. P., Hale, E. G. & Wright, T. (1982). *The Evaluation of New Services: Possibilities for Preventing Congenital Toxoplasmosis*. Health Economics Research Unit Discussion Paper No. 02/82. Aberdeen.

Hogan, M. J., Moschini, G. B. & Zardi, O. (1971). Effects of *Toxoplasma gondii* toxin on the rabbit eye. *American Journal of Ophthalmology*, **72**, 733–42.

Holland, G. N. (1989). Ocular toxoplasmosis in the immunocompromised host. *International Ophthalmology*, **13**, 399–402.

Holland, G. N. (1999). Reconsidering the pathogenesis of ocular toxoplasmosis. *American Journal of Ophthalmology*, **128**, 502–5.

Hoyt, C. S., Billson, F., Ouvrier, R. & Wise, G. (1978). Ocular features of Aicardi's syndrome. *Archives of Ophthalmology*, **96**, 291–5.

Jabs, D. A., Green, R., Fox, R., Polk, B. F. & Bartlett, J. G. (1989). Ocular manifestations of acquired immune deficiency syndrome. *Ophthalmology*, **96**, 1092–9.

Jacobs, L., Cook, M. K. & Wilder, H. C. (1954). Serologic data on adults with histologically diagnosed toxoplasmic chorioretinitis. *Transactions of The American Academy of Ophthalmology*, **58**, 193–200.

Jacobs, L., Remington, J. S. & Melton, M. L. (1960). The resistance of the encysted form of *Toxoplasma gondii*. *Journal of Parasitology*, **46**, 11–21.

Janku, J. (1923). Pathogenes a pathologicka anatomie tak nazvaneho kolobomu zlute skvyrny v oku nomalne velikem a mikrophthalmickem s nalexem parazitu v sitnici. *Casopis Lekaruceskych*, **62**, 1021–27, 1054–59, 1081–85*t*, 1111–15, 1138–44. [for German translation, see same author, *Ceskoslovenska Parasitologie*, 6.9–56. 1959).

Kennedy, J. E. & Wise, G. N. (1971). Retinochoroidal vascular anastomosis in uveitis. *American Journal of Ophthalmology*, **71**, 1221–5.

Kijistra, A., Lugendijk, L., Baarsma, G. S., Rothova, A., Schweitzer, C. M. C., Tinamerman, Z., de Vries, J. & Briebaart, A. C. (1989). Aqueous humor analysis as a diagnostic tool in Toxoplasma uveitis. *International Ophthalmology*, **13**, 383–6.

Kijistra, A., Hoekzema, R., van der Lelij, A., Doekes, G. & Rothova, A. (1990). Humoral and cellular immune reactions against retinal antigens in clinical disease. *Current Eye Research*, **9** [Suppl.] 85–9.

Koch, F. L. P., Wolf, A., Cowen, D. & Paige, B. H. (1943). Toxoplasmic encephalomyelitis. Significance of ocular lesions in the diagnosis of infantile or congenital toxoplasmosis. *Archives of Ophthalmology*, **29**, 1–25.

Kramar, J. & Vrabec, F. (1960). The inoculation of parasites *Toxoplasma gondii* into the eyes of albino rats. *Ceskolovenska Parasitologie*, **7**, 245–50.

Lakhanpal, V., Schocket, S. S. & Nirankari, V. S. (1983). Clindamycin in the treatment of toxoplasmic retinochoroiditis. *American Journal of Ophthalmology*, **95**, 605–13.

Leopold, I. H. (1963). Drug therapy in uveitis. *American Journal of Ophthalmology*, **56**, 709–25.

Levaditi, C., Schoen, R. & Sanchis-Bayarri, V. (1928). Infection toxoplasmique experimentale d'oeil. *Compte Rendu de la Societe de Biologie (Paris)*, **98**, 1414–19.

Lou, P., Kazdan, J. & Basu, P. K. (1978). Ocular toxoplasmosis in three consecutive siblings. *Archives of Ophthalmology*, **96**, 613–14.

Malbrel, C. (1981). Complication hemorragique d'une choroidite toxoplasmique. *Bulletin des Societes d'Ophtalmologie de France*, **81**, 633–4.

Manners, R. M., O'Connell, S., Guy, E. C., Lanning, C. R., Etchells, D. E. & Joynson, D. H. M. (1994). Use of the polymerase chain reaction to detect *Toxoplasma gondii* in the vitreous of a patient with acquired ocular toxoplasmosis. *British Journal of Ophthalmology*, **78**, 483–4.

Matthews, J. D. & Weiter, J. J. (1988). Outer retinal toxoplasmosis. *Ophthalmology*, **95**, 941–6.

McMenamin, P. G., Dutton, G. D., Hay, J., & Cameron, S. (1986). The ultrastructural pathology of congenital murine toxoplasmic retinochoroiditis. I. The morphology of cysts within the retina. *Experimental Eye Research*, **43**, 529–43.

Miller, S. A. & Bresnick, G. (1978). Familial bilateral macular colobomata. *British Journal of Ophthalmology*, **62**, 261–4.

Mittelviefhaus (1992). Clindamycin – therapie bei Verdacht auf Toxoplasmose-Retinochoroiditis. *Klinische Monatsblatter Fur Angenheilkunde*, **200**, 123–7.

Montoya, J. G. & Remington, J. S. (1996). Toxoplasmic chorioretinitis in the setting of acute acquired toxoplasmosis. *Clinical Infectious Diseases*, **23**, 277–82.

Nicholson, D. H. & Wolchok, E. B. (1976). Ocular toxoplasmosis in an adult receiving long-term corticosteroid therapy. *Archives of Ophthalmology*, **94**, 248–54.

Nussenblatt, R. B., Gery, I., Ballintine, E. J. & Wacker, W. B. (1980a). Cellular immune responsiveness of uveitis patients to retinal S-antigen. *American Journal of Ophthalmology*, **89**, 173–9.

Nussenblatt, R. B., Gery, I. & Wacker, W. B. (1980b). Experimental autoimmune uveitis: cellular immune responsiveness. *Investigative Ophthalmology and Visual Science*, **19**, 686–90.

Nussenblatt, R. B., Mittal, K. K., Fuhrman, S., Sharma, S. D. & Palestine, A. G. (1989). Lymphocyte proliferative responses of patients with ocular toxoplasmosis to parasite and retinal antigens. *American Journal of Ophthalmology*, **107**, 632–41.

O'Connor, G. R. (1970). The influence of hypersensitivity on the pathogenesis of ocular toxoplasmosis. *Transactions of the American Ophthalmological Society*, **68**, 501–47.

O'Connor, G. R. (1982). Protozoal infections. In *Pathobiology of Ocular Disease. A Dynamic Approach*, ed. A. Garner. New York, NY: Marcel Dekker, pp. 346–58.

O'Connor, G. R. (1983). Factors relating to the initiation and recurrence of uveitis. XL Edward Jackson Memorial Lecture. *American Journal of Ophthalmology*, **96**, 577–99.

O'Connor, G. R. & Frenkel, J. K. (1976). Dangers of steroid treatment in toxoplasmosis. *Archives of Ophthalmology*, **94**, 213–16.

Ohno, S., O'Connor, G. R. & Kimura, S. J. (1977). HLA antigens and toxoplasmic retinochoroiditis. *Tohoku Journal of Experimental Medicine*, **123**, 91–4.

Oprerneak, E. M., Scales, D. K. & Sharpe, M. R. (1992). Trimethoprim–sulphamethoxazole therapy for ocular toxoplasmosis. *Ophthalmology*, **99**, 920–5.

Owens, P. L., Goldberg, M. F. & Busse, B. J. (1979). Prospective observation of vascular anastomoses between the retina and choroid in recurrent toxoplasmosis. *American Journal of Ophthalmology*, **88**, 402–5.

Pearson, P. A., Piracha, A. R., Sen, H. A. & Jaffe, G. J. (1999). Atovaquone for the treatment of toxoplasma retinochoroiditis. *Ophthalmology*, **106**, 148–53.

Perkins, E. S. (1961). *Uveitis and Toxoplasmosis*. London: Churchill.

Perkins, E. S. (1973). Ocular toxoplasmosis. *British Journal of Ophthalmology*, **57**, 1–17.

Perkins, E. S. (1981). Hereditary and congenital factors in inflammations of the uveal tract. *Transactions of the Ophthalmic Societies of the United Kingdom*, **101**, 304–7.

Piper, R. C., Cole, C. R. & Shadduck, J. A. (1970). Natural and experimental ocular toxoplasmosis in animals. *American Journal of Ophthalmology*, **69f**, 662–8.

Remington, J. S. & Desmonts, G. (1976). Toxoplasmosis. In *Infectious Diseases of the Fetus and Newborn Infant*, pp. 191–332. Philadelphia: WB Saunders.

Remington, J. S., Efron, B., Cavanaugh, E., Simon, H. J. & Trejos, S. (1970). Studies on toxoplasmosis in El Salvador. Prevalence and incidence of toxoplasmosis as measured by the

Sabin-Feldman dye test. *Transactions of The Royal Society of Tropical Medicine and Hygiene*, 64, 252–67.

Rieger, H. (1952). Uber uveitere auf toxoplasmosis adultorum acquisita verdachtige Falle von retinitis exsudativa externa centralis. *Klinische Monatablatter Fur Augenheilkunde*, 120, 33–50.

Rollins, D. F., Tabbara, K. F., Ghosheh, R. & Nozik, R. A. (1982). Minocycline in experimental ocular recurrent toxoplasmosis in the rabbit. *American Journal of Ophthalmology*, 93, 361–5.

Rothova, A., van Knapen, F., Baarsma, G. S., Kruit, P. J., Loewer-Sieger, D. H. & Kijistra, A. (1986). Serology in ocular toxoplasmosis. *British Journal of Ophthalmology*, 70, 615–22.

Rothova, A., Buitenhuis, H. J., Meenken, C., Baarsma, G. S., Boen-Tan, T. N., de Jong, P. T. V. M., Schweitzer, C. M. C., Timmerman, Z., de Vries, J., Zaal, M. J. W. & Kijistra, A. (1989). Therapy of ocular toxoplasmosis. *International Ophthalmology*, 13, 415–19.

Rothova, A., Bosch-Driessen, L. E., van Loon, N. H. & Treffers, W. F. (1998). Azithromycin for ocular toxoplasmosis. *British Journal of Ophthalmology*, 82, 1306–8.

Saari, K. M., Paivonsalo, T. & Partti, E. (1984). Argon laser coagulation in the treatment of recurrent active toxoplasmic retinochoroiditis. In *Uveitis Update*, ed. K. M. Saari. Amsterdam: Elsevier Science Publishers, pp. 529–38.

Sabates, R., Pruett, R. C. & Brockhurst, R. J. (1981). Fulminant ocular toxoplasmosis. *American Journal of Ophthalmology*, 92, 497–503.

Schlaegel, T. F. (1978). *Ocular Toxoplasmosis and Pars Planitis*. New York: Grune & Stratton.

Sidikaro, Y., Silver, L., Holland, G. N. & Kreiger, A. E. (1991). Rhegmatogenous retinal detachments in patients with AIDS and necrotizing retinal infections. *Ophthalmology*, 98, 129–35.

Siegel, S. E., Lunde, M. N., Gelderman, A. H., Halterman, R. H., Brown, J. A., Levine, A. S. & Graw, R. G. Jr. (1971). Transmission of toxoplasmosis by leukocyte transfusion. *Blood*, 37, 388–94.

Silveira, C., Belfort, R., Burnier, M. & Nussenblatt, R. (1988). Acquired toxoplasmic infection as the cause of toxoplasmic retinochoroiditis in families. *American Journal of Ophthalmology*, 106, 362–4.

Silveira, C., Belfort, R., Nussenblatt, R., Farah, M., Takahashi, W., Imarnura, P. & Burnier, M. (1989). Unilateral pigmentary retinopathy associated with ocular toxoplasmosis. *American Journal of Ophthalmology*, 107, 682–4.

Smith, R. E. & Ganley, J. P. (1972). Ophthalmic survey of a community. A. Abnormalities of the ocular fundus. *American Journal of Ophthalmology*, 74, 1126–30.

Sorsby, A. (1972). *Modern Ophthalmology; Topical Aspects*, Volume 4. London: Butterworths, pp. 1176–77.

Spalter, H. F., Campbell, C. J., Noyori, K. S., Rittler, C. M. & Koester, C. J. (1966). Prophylactic photocoagulation of recurrent toxoplasmic retinochoroiditis. A preliminary report. *Archives of Ophthalmology*, 75f, 21–31.

Stern, G. A. & Romano, P. E. (1978). Congenital ocular toxoplasmosis. Possible occurrence in siblings. *Archives of Ophthalmology*, 96, 615–17.

Swartzberg, J. E., Maresca, R. M. & Remington, J. S. (1977). Clinical study of gastrointestinal complications associated with clindamycin therapy. *Journal of Infectious Diseases*, 135 [Suppl.] S99–S103.

Tabbara, K. F. & O'Connor, G. R. (1975). Ocular tissue absorption of clindamycin phosphate. *Archives of Ophthalmology*, 93, 1180–5.

Tabbara, K. F. & O'Connor, G. R. (1980). Treatment of ocular toxoplasmosis with clindamycin and sulfadiazine. *Ophthalmology*, 87, 129–34.

Tabbara, K. F., Dy-Liacco, J., Nozik, R. A., O'Connor, G. R. & Blackman, J. (1979). Clindamycin in chronic toxoplasmosis. Effect of periocular injections on recoverability of organisms from healed lesions in the rabbit eye. *Archives of Ophthalmology*, 97, 542–4.

Tate, G. W. & Martin, R. G. (1977). Clindamycin in the treatment of human ocular toxoplasmosis. *Canadian Journal of Ophthalmology*, 12, 188–95.

Thompson, J. R., Du, L. & Rosenthal, A. R. (1989). Recent trends in the registration of blindness and partial sight in Leicestershire. *British Journal of Ophthalmology*, 73, 95–9.

Toussaint, D. & Wanderhaeghen, J. J. (1975). Ocular toxoplasmosis, trigeminal herpes zoster and pulmonary tuberculosis in a patient with Hodgkins disease. *Ophthalmologica* (*Basel*), 171, 237–43.

Vail, D., Strong, J. C. Jr. & Stephenson, W. V. (1943). Chorioretinitis associated with positive serologic tests for Toxoplasma in older children and adults. *American Journal of Ophthalmology*, 26, 133–41.

Vainisi, S. I. & Campbell, L. H. (1969). Ocular toxoplasmosis in cats. *Journal of the American Veterinary Medical Association*, 154, 141–52.

Wallace, G. D. (1969). Serologic and epidemiologic observations on toxoplasmosis on three Pacific atolls. *American Journal of Epidemiology*, 90, 103–11.

Werry, H. & Honegger, H. (1987). Pars-plana Vitrektomie bei chronischer Uveitis. *Klinische Monatsblatter Fur Augenheilkunde*, 191, 9–12.

Willerson, D., Aaberg, T. M., Reeser, F. & Meredith, T. A. (1977). Unusual ocular presentation of acute toxoplasmosis. *British Journal of Ophthalmology*, 61, 693–8.

Wyler, D. J., Blackman, H. J. & Lunde, M. N. (1980). Cellular hypersensitivity to toxoplasmal and retinal antigens in patients with toxoplasmal retinochoroiditis. *American Journal of Tropical Medicine and Hygiene*, 29, 1181–6.

Yeo, J. H., Jakobiec, F. A., Iwamato, T., Richard, G. & Kreissig, L. (1983). Opportunistic toxoplasmic retinochoroiditis following chemotherapy for systemic lymphoma. A light and electron microscopic study. *Ophthalmology*, 90, 885–98.

Yoshizumi, M. O. (1976). Experimental Toxoplasma retinitis. A light and electron microscopical study. *Archives of Pathology and Laboratory Medicine*, 100, 487–90.

Zscheile, F. P. (1964). Recurrent toxoplasmic retinitis with weakly positive methylene blue dye test. *Archives of Ophthalmology*, 71, 645–8.

12

Laboratory diagnosis of toxoplasma infection

D. H. M. Joynson and E. C. Guy

Toxoplasma Reference Unit, Public Health Laboratory, Singleton Hospital, Swansea, Wales

The laboratory diagnosis of infection with *Toxoplasma gondii* often plays a key role in determining optimal clinical management. In the immunocompetent, where toxoplasmosis usually poses no significant clinical threat, confirmation of acute infection can exclude other potentially more serious aetiologies. In other clinical scenarios where toxoplasma infection can result in severe sequelae, interpretation of laboratory findings poses significant challenges. A major complication is that the parasite can present in an acute, chronic, latent or reactivated form, and discrimination of these is often crucial in understanding clinical relevance. Further, an accurate diagnosis may be made substantially more difficult if certain organs are involved (eye, brain) or by the presence of an underlying disease (HIV infection) or medical procedures (cardiac transplant). Ironically, perhaps, it is in such clinical groups that the most severe sequelae of toxoplasma infection occur.

As with many other diseases, the diagnosis of *T. gondii* infection rests upon conclusions drawn from clinical, radiological and laboratory investigations. However, due to the often nonspecific symptoms and signs, or frequently asymptomatic nature of this infection, diagnosis in most cases relies primarily upon laboratory testing. In addition to confirming infection, such tests can aid in determining prognosis, influence management, and assist in monitoring response to treatment. Further, from an epidemiological perspective, laboratory testing (serological and parasitological) is an integral component of case definitions and classification systems that have been constructed for *T. gondii* infections in immunocompetent women and their congenitally infected offspring (Lebech et al. 1996) (see Appendices).

The prime objective of this chapter is to assist the clinical investigation and management of *T. gondii* infection by providing an overview of principal laboratory methods used by specialist or reference centres. Nonspecialist centres may prefer to use other tests, e.g. latex agglutination, IgG enzyme immunoassay, etc. as their primary test before determining whether or not to refer the serum for further testing. Practical strategies for investigation and interpretation of results will be presented for each of the key clinical groups.

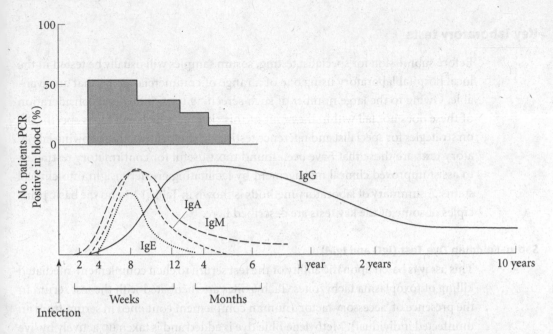

Figure 12.1 Schematic time course of immunoglobulin response to toxoplasma infection and persistence of apparent parasitemia

The laboratory tests that are used most commonly for initial investigation are serological, targeting detection of IgG, IgM and, in some circumstances, IgA specific for *T. gondii*. A range of kit formats is available commercially and results are usually produced in a quantitative or semi-quantitative form. Where confirmation of initial serology is required, or in clinical scenarios where such methods are potentially unhelpful (e.g. immunodeficiency, neonatal investigation) or additional information is required to support management, a range of secondary tests is available. In addition to enhanced serological methods, these secondary tests include a series of assays based on direct detection of the parasite or its subcellular components (microscopy, parasite culture and nucleic acid detection).

The immunological response to *T. gondii* infection is summarized in Figure 12.1. Typically, IgM appears first about 1–2 weeks after infection closely followed by IgA and IgE. Generally, these acute-phase immunoglobulins peak at about 2 months. The time at which they can no longer be detected is highly variable depending upon the sensitivity of the assay employed, but is usually about 6–9 months (12–18 months or longer where tests with enhanced sensitivity are used). In a small minority of cases IgM can persist for several years (to date, the maximum in the authors' experience is 14 years). IgG appears after IgM, typically reaching maximal levels at about 4 months, then declines to a lower level over the next 12–24 months. IgG persists for decades.

Key laboratory tests

Before submission for specialist testing, serum samples will usually be tested in the local hospital laboratory using one of a range of commercial assays that are available. Owing to the large number of such screening tests, individual consideration of these does not fall within the remit of this chapter, which will focus specifically on strategies for specialist and reference testing. In this context, the following laboratory tests are those that have been found most useful for confirmatory testing or to assist improved clinical management by facilitating greater insight into clinical status. A summary of laboratory methods is shown in Table 12.1 and the basic principles of some of the key tests are described here.

Sabin–Feldman Dye Test (IgG and IgM)

This assay is based upon the ability of the test serum to elicit complement-mediated killing of toxoplasma tachyzoites. Tachyzoites are incubated with the test serum in the presence of 'accessory factor' (human complement contained in serum from an uninfected individual). Methylene Blue dye is added and is taken up actively by live tachyzoites, while cells killed by complement (activated by the test serum) appear as 'ghosts'.

The Dye Test (DT) (Sabin & Feldman 1948) is usually carried out in a microtitre plate format with the test serum being diluted across the plate. The end-point of this titration is taken as the dilution of serum required to elicit killing of 50% of the tachyzoites.

Enzyme immunoassay (EIA)

A wide range of EIA-based assays are available for the detection of toxoplasma-specific immunoglobulins, in particular, IgG, IgM and IgA classes, although assays detecting IgE are also used successfully by some laboratories. In some immunoglobulin class-specific assays, the patient's antibody is captured onto the well of a microtitre plate, usually by a class-specific monoclonal antibody (e.g. antihuman IgG, -A, or -M) that has been previously attached chemically to the well. Toxoplasma antigen that has been suitably labelled (e.g. with horseradish peroxidase, alkaline phosphatase, biotin, etc.) is added to the well and is bound by any toxoplasma-specific antibody in the patient's serum. After washing to remove unbound antigen, bound antigen is detected colorimetrically by addition of the appropriate enzyme substrate or biotin-detection system. Measurement of the amount of coloured product formed permits quantification of the amount of toxoplasma-specific antibody in the patient's serum.

In addition to the 'capture' EIA system described, a wide range of alternative formats can be adopted. For example, toxoplasma antigen can be attached directly

Table 12.1. Laboratory investigations in toxoplasma infection

	Assay	Type	Diagnostic information provided	Notes
Primary (screening) assays	IgG	Serology	Infected?	+ve finding does not confirm active/acute infection
	IgM	Serology	Recent infection?	+ve finding suggests acute infection −ve finding on repeat testing (2–3 weeks) excludes T. gondii infection in the immunocompetent
	IgM + IgG	Serology	Infected?	
Secondary (confirmatory & reference) assays	Sabin-Feldman Dye Test (IgM + IgG)	Serology	Confirmation of infection status	'gold standard' assay for confirmation of T. gondii infection
	IgM EIA	Serology	Recent infection?	+ve finding suggests acute infection.
	IgA EIA	Serology	Recent infection?	+ve finding suggests acute infection.
	ISAGA-M	Serology	Recent infection?	More sensitive than standard assays
	ISAGA-A	Serology	Recent infection?	More sensitive than standard assays
	IgG Avidity	Serology	Estimate duration of infection	Primarily used to determine whether infection has occurred prior to, or during, pregnancy. Avidity results should not be interpreted in absence of other serology
	PCR	Direct detection	Confirm presence of T. gondii DNA in a range of clinical specimens	Provides no insight into cell viability. Cannot discriminate tachyzoite (active) from bradyzoite (quiescent)
	Culture	Direct detection	Confirm presence of T. gondii in a range of clinical specimens	Confirms parasite viability. Cannot discriminate tachyzoite (active) from bradyzoite (quiescent)
	Microscopy	Direct detection	Identify organism	Can discriminate tachyzoite (active) from bradyzoite (quiescent) form
	Histopathology	Indirect detection	Detect characteristic changes in host cell morphology	Can imply but not confirm T.gondii infection

to the microplate well and incubated with patient's serum. Bound antibody is then detected using a class-specific monoclonal antibody that is enzyme-labelled.

Immunosorbent agglutination assay (ISAGA)

This is a commercial assay (bioMerièux) for the detection of toxoplasma-specific IgM (ISAGA-M) and IgA (ISAGA-A) that is typically significantly more sensitive than standard EIA methods. This increased sensitivity can be a major advantage in clinical scenarios where low levels of antibody might be expected, e.g. HIV infection, immunosuppression, in neonates, etc. However, despite its greater sensitivity, our experience at the Toxoplasma Reference Unit, Swansea (UK) is that ISAGA-M is less useful than standard IgM EIA in assessing the risk of maternal toxoplasma infection in pregnancy. This is because unlike in standard IgM EIAs, which typically detect IgM for 6–9 months after infection, ISAGA-M can remain positive often greater than 12–15 months after infection. Thus, use of the latter would generate a significant number of additional IgM-positive cases where there is clearly no risk to the pregnancy but that would still require further laboratory investigation (and might possibly result in the local clinician considering amniocentesis).

IgG avidity

As the immune response to an invading pathogen matures, successive generations of antibody are produced that typically have progressively higher affinity for target epitopes. The overall effect of this process is that the avidity of binding of immunoglobulin molecules increases with time. An avidity index is the ratio of antibody bound to the antigen (usually measured by EIA) in the presence and absence of an appropriate disrupting agent such as urea.

Avidity cannot give a precise measure of the duration of infection but can discriminate with a degree of certainty (circa 90%) early (<3 months) and later (>6 months) infections (Joynson et al. 1990). Thus, avidity is of most use when employed in support of other assays such as DT and IgM EIA.

Polymerase chain reaction (PCR)

The presence of T. gondii in a given specimen can be confirmed by direct detection of specific regions of the parasite genome. PCR and other gene amplification techniques can be designed to target specific regions of the T. gondii genome and, by repeated DNA synthesis at such regions, can produce, for example, up to one billion DNA copies within 2–3 hours. Such quantities of PCR product can be readily visualized using gel electrophoresis.

Although exquisitely sensitive and rapid, PCR presents a number of technical challenges. In particular is the potential for obtaining false-positive results due to contamination of specimens with trace amounts of toxoplasma DNA (originating either from other infected samples or in the form of the amplified DNA produced within the laboratory during previous testing). To date, two major multicentre evaluations and comparisons of PCR methods have taken place within Europe (Guy et al. 1996; Pelloux et al. 1998). Both studies confirmed a wide range in level of performance and diagnostic accuracy among participating laboratories.

A significant finding of these studies was that not only did the majority of laboratories employ PCR methods targeting the *B1* gene *of T. gondii*, but PCR methods targeting the *P30* gene appeared to be inferior in performance. Other factors that may complicate clinical interpretation of PCR positive findings are the inability of the assay to discriminate between the active (tachyzoite) and quiescent (bradyzoite) forms of the parasite, and the inability to discriminate between viable and attenuated parasites.

Other laboratory tests: present and future

A range of additional tests for the investigation of toxoplasma infection are available but are used less widely, each of which is reported to provide helpful additional information in determining optimal clinical management. One such method is the HS/AC assay, an agglutination-based method employing two distinct antigen preparations (methanol-treated [AC]/formalin-treated [HS]) that react differentially with IgG produced early and later in infection (Thulliez et al. 1986). The HS/AC assay addresses the same question of duration of infection as IgG avidity and, although used less widely than the latter, has shown potential as an alternative confirmatory assay.

The enzyme-linked immunofiltration assay (ELIFA) is a method that, potentially, can provide invaluable information in the diagnosis and management of congenital toxoplasma infection in the neonate (Pinon & Gruson 1982). Major problems are that IgM and IgA may not be detectable in the congenitally infected infant for up to several weeks or more after birth with current assays. ELIFA offers an alternative strategy for early serodiagnosis by permitting the detection of neonatal IgG by resolution from passively acquired maternal IgG. Any IgG isotypes that react specifically with toxoplasma antigen and are unique to the neonate will indicate a neonatal immune response and hence serologically confirm congenital infection. An alternative strategy for discrimination between maternal and neonatal IgG is the use of immunoblot (Western blot) (Remington et al. 1985). By this method the range of toxoplasma antigens reactive with any given serum sample can be identified. Identification of any toxoplasma antigen reactive with the neonatal serum but not with the matched maternal serum would, again, indicate a specific neonatal immune response. The relative performances of ELIFA and immunoblot remain to be elucidated, but both address a clinical circumstance where early diagnosis can either expedite commencement of appropriate antitoxoplasma therapy or can prevent unnecessary treatment and reduce parental concern when congenital infection is excluded.

Clinical groups

Immunocompetent patients

Even though acute toxoplasma infection is usually a trivial clinical event in otherwise healthy individuals, diagnosis of toxoplasma in this group is often important for excluding a range of other possible aetiologies, e.g. lymphoproliferative disorders, which may require further, invasive, investigation and may result in unnecessary anxiety for the patient. Histopathological examination of a lymph node biopsy sample reveals a distorted architecture with large, irregular follicles with reactive hyperplasia and clusters of pale epithelioid histiocytes blurring the follicular outline. There is no caseation but germinal centres contain numerous mitoses of regular pattern and focal distension of sinuses with monocytoid cells (Stansfeld 1961; Dorfman & Remington 1973). These appearances, which are typical of toxoplasmic lymphadenopathy but not pathognomonic, usually result in a request for serology. The protozoon is infrequently seen in such biopsy samples and is also infrequently cultured successfully from lymph nodes. In acute infection, apparent parasitaemia as indicated by positive PCR, can persist for some 12–16 weeks (Guy & Joynson 1995). However, as with lymph node biopsy, culture from the blood of immunocompetent individuals is difficult. A range of serological screening tests is available commercially that can demonstrate the presence of toxoplasma antibodies. However, the most useful reference serological tests for confirmation of acute infection are the gold standard DT used in combination with IgM EIA. The DT will determine whether or not the patient has been infected at any time with *T. gondii* while the IgM EIA will indicate if this infection has been acquired within the previous 6–9 months. Probably due to the incubation period of infection and the nonspecific and often mild early sequelae, initial samples are often already *T. gondii* antibody-positive and, hence, seroconversion is rarely demonstrated. However, repeat sampling in early infection may demonstrate a significant rise in specific immunoglobulin levels.

Chronic active toxoplasmosis

In a very small clinical subset of immunocompetent patients, toxoplasma infection can present as a chronic active form where symptoms persist for many years usually with periods of remission (O'Connell et al. 1993). In addition to the anticipated IgG, specific antitoxoplasma IgM can usually be continually demonstrated by EIA and toxoplasma nucleic acid detected by PCR. Treatment reduces symptoms and may result in the disappearance of IgM and nucleic acid but these may be redetected when treatment ceases. In addition to repeated testing for IgM over a period of months or years, IgG avidity, which can provide an estimate of the duration of infection, is often helpful in confirming chronic infection.

Ocular infection

The diagnosis of toxoplasmic retinochoroiditis is primarily clinical, being based upon the visual examination of the retina. The only significant serological result is a negative finding, as this would essentially exclude *T. gondii* as the causative agent though very rarely a patient may have toxoplasma antibody demonstrable in aqueous humour but not in serum (Desmonts 1966). The detection of antitoxoplasma IgG alone in serum does not confirm a clinical diagnosis of toxoplasma ocular disease and is thus limited to adding a degree of support to the clinical diagnosis. The additional detection of antitoxoplasma IgM adds stronger support since retinochoroiditis can sometimes occur as a consequence of an acute toxoplasma infection (Manners et al. 1994; Montoya & Remington 1996).

A definitive laboratory diagnosis of acute toxoplasmic retinochoroiditis requires investigation of aqueous or vitreous humour. Diagnosis is achieved by confirming the presence of the parasite by culture or nucleic acid detection (Aouizerate et al. 1993) or by confirmation of intraocular antibody production. The levels of ocular and serum antitoxoplasma antibodies are compared to determine the Goldmann–Witmer Coefficient (Witmer 1978). A coefficient ratio of 3 or above is reported to be indicative of acute toxoplasmic retinochoroiditis. However, when the eye infection is quiescent, it is possible that none of the above methods will aid diagnosis.

A very important caveat in the use of serology to confirm acute ocular toxoplasmosis is that this condition can also occur without any change in serum antibody levels. In our experience, a rise in antitoxoplasma IgG levels or the reappearance of antitoxoplasma IgM is relatively rare. For example, antitoxoplasma IgM has been detected only in about 4% of sera submitted to the Swansea Toxoplasma Reference Unit from cases with a clinical diagnosis of ocular toxoplasmosis and the presence of IgG.

If toxoplasmic retinochoroiditis is diagnosed in children there are, at present, no laboratory investigations available to determine unequivocally if the infection was acquired *in utero*. Of course, negative toxoplasma serology in the mother would very strongly suggest that the child's infection was acquired postnatally.

Preconception screening

Many women who feel that they are at risk or are otherwise anxious to avoid infection request testing before they conceive.

The reference serological tests employed are the DT and IgM EIA. If toxoplasma antibodies are absent then the foetus will be at risk if the mother acquires toxoplasma during pregnancy and she can be advised of precautions to avoid infection. A positive DT and the absence of IgM indicates infection some time in the past and the proposed pregnancy should not be at risk from toxoplasma unless the mother is, or becomes, immunocompromised.

If serology confirms an acute infection, then our current practice is to suggest delaying conception for at least 6 months after the onset of infection (if asymptomatic) or 6 months after resolution of signs and symptoms. We recommend retesting after that time to confirm that the acute infection has resolved or is resolving, and, if this is the case, then the women can conceive even if low levels of antitoxoplasma IgM can still be detected. In this circumstance, antitoxoplasma chemotherapy is not required.

Potentially useful reference diagnostic tests for immunocompetent patients and ocular disease are summarized in Table 12.2.

Immunosuppressed patients

Patients whose immune system is suppressed either as a consequence of other disease, e.g. haematological malignancies, or treatment, e.g. corticosteroids, are at risk from either newly acquired toxoplasma infection or by reactivation of previously acquired latent infection. The clinical diagnosis of toxoplasmosis in such patients is difficult since the signs and symptoms of the underlying disease can mimic those of active toxoplasma infection.

Determination of baseline toxoplasma antibody level in serum collected at the presentation of the underlying disorder or before commencement of immunosuppressive therapy is essential. Patients without antibody are susceptible to infection and should be given advice on precautions required to avoid exposure to toxoplasma (see Appendices).

Reactivation of infection is often, but not always, associated with a rise in IgG antibody level. (Sera should always be tested in parallel with the baseline serum to confirm a significant rise.) The ISAGA for IgM should also be performed as this is a more sensitive test than EIA.

Where serology alone is unable to provide a definitive answer, the demonstration of the parasite by culture or nucleic acid detection in blood or cerebrospinal fluid (CSF) may be helpful. In this particular clinical context, however, these techniques are inappropriate for samples containing brain or heart tissue since they cannot distinguish between tissue cysts that may already be present in these organs during latent/quiescent infection and the tachyzoite form of the parasite associated with an acute infection. In such cases, histopathological examination of tissues

Table 12.2. Potentially helpful reference diagnostic tests for the investigation of toxoplasma infection in immunocompetent patients

	Dye Test	EIA IgM	ISAGA	IgG avidity	Culture	PCR	Histopathology
Acute toxoplasma infection							
Blood	+	+	−		+	+	−
Lymph node	+	+	+		+	+	+
Chronic active toxoplasmosis							
Blood	+	−	−	+			−
Preconception							
Blood	+	+	+				
Ocular toxoplasmosis							
Blood	+	−	−				
Aqueous/Vitreous humour	+	+	−		+	+	−

stained with an immunoperoxidase stain may reveal evidence of an acute or reactivated infection.

Transplant patients

This clinical group is not only at risk from acute or reactivated infection as a consequence of immunosuppression, but infection may be acquired in the form of tissue cysts present in the donated tissues, principally the heart but also the liver (Speirs et al. 1988). In bone marrow or kidney transplantation, transfer of toxoplasma is less likely.

Prior to transplantation, donor and recipient serum samples should be tested using the DT and IgM EIA. If a mismatch is identified, i.e. the donor is *T. gondii*-antibody-positive while the recipient is *T. gondii*-antibody-negative, prophylaxis should be considered (especially in heart and liver transplant patients) as an acute toxoplasma infection in such patients carries a risk of considerable morbidity and mortality. However, such a 'toxoplasma mismatch' does not exclude transplantation of tissues to the recipient (see Chapter 6).

The susceptible recipient of an organ from a *T. gondii*-antibody-positive donor that potentially contains tissue cysts should be carefully monitored for evidence of acute infection. This is very important in heart transplant recipients and especially so in those not receiving prophylactic antibiotics. Serial serum samples from such patients should be tested for *T. gondii* antibodies especially in recipients with symptoms consistent with toxoplasmosis. The DT and IgM EIA should be used to demonstrate seroconversion, rising titres and thus an acute infection. The detection of nucleic acid by gene amplification may also be helpful. Because of the unavoidable time delay associated with culture, this technique is of little use in the immediate management of seriously ill patients. If the diagnosis remains unconfirmed after these investigations, histopathological examination of biopsy samples of transplanted organs may need to be considered.

Reactivation of latent toxoplasma infection may be demonstrated by the DT (rising titres compared to pretransplant samples) and ISAGA for IgM. PCR of blood may also be helpful. If cerebral toxoplasmosis is suspected, examination of the CSF for nucleic acid with PCR and antibody levels should be performed.

The potential severity and rapidity with which sequelae can develop underlines the need both for prospective clinical assessment of risk and careful monitoring for signs and symptoms including repeated serological testing. However, the patient's condition may warrant commencing treatment on clinical suspicion alone before laboratory results are available. An important caveat in interpreting serological findings in such patients who have received significant blood transfusions is that the serological profile can be confused by the passive transfer of antibody from donated blood.

If both organ donor and recipient are shown to have no toxoplasma antibodies present then there is no risk from the donated organ. However, the recipient is susceptible to infection via natural routes and should be advised of precautions required to avoid infection (see Appendices).

Immunocompromised (HIV-infected) patients

Toxoplasmic encephalitis is the most common opportunistic infection of the CNS in HIV-infected patients occurring in up to 40% of patients with acquired immunodeficiency syndrome (AIDS). Unless treated, this can result in severe morbidity and often death (see Chapter 5).

These severe sequelae underline the importance of appropriate laboratory investigations in potential cases of acute/reactivated toxoplasma infection. Nevertheless, an unequivocal diagnosis can still be difficult and the significance, interpretation and prognostic value of some laboratory tests remain uncertain or controversial. For example, one study found that approximately 20% of HIV-infected patients with histopathologically-confirmed toxoplasmic encephalitis had undetectable levels of specific antitoxoplasma IgG (Porter & Sande 1992). However, other studies suggest that the majority of patients with toxoplasmic encephalitis will have detectable IgG; Subauste et al. (1997) estimated that the false-negative rate in such patients is about 3%.

As in other immunosuppressed patients, determination of baseline toxoplasma antibody levels is essential in sera collected at the time the diagnosis of HIV infection is made. *Toxoplasma gondii*-antibody-negative patients are susceptible to infection and should be given advice on precautions to avoid exposure to toxoplasma. It is prudent to retest *T. gondii*-antibody-negative patients particularly if immunodeficiency is profound.

Nearly all active toxoplasma infections in these patients are due to reactivation, the risk of which is increased as the patient becomes more immunocompromised – especially when the CD4 T-cell count is less than $100/mm^3$ and often accompanied by corresponding reduction in CD8 T-cells (Israelski & Remington 1992).

If reactivation manifests itself as a disseminated toxoplasma infection, the DT may, but not always, show an increase in titre and the ISAGA test may demonstrate the presence of IgM. It is pertinent to note that a significant rise in titre, i.e. 'serological reactivation', can occur without any clinical signs or symptoms. The use of PCR for testing blood for the diagnosis of an apparent toxoplasma parasitaemia may help in this particular situation.

Toxoplasmic encephalitis can occur without any change in DT or presence of IgM, and PCR of blood is not particularly helpful. However, high antibody levels are often found in patients with toxoplasmic encephalitis and PCR of CSF can be of help in making the diagnosis. A PCR-positive result confirms toxoplasmic encephalitis but a negative PCR finding does not necessarily exclude it since, depending on the location of the lesion, tachyzoites may not have passed into the ventricles. Occasionally, serological and radiological techniques fail to provide an answer and brain biopsy may be performed. Needle biopsy samples have been reported as being frequently negative (Wanke et al. 1987). PCR of brain tissue is unhelpful in the diagnosis of toxoplasmic encephalitis, as the current technology cannot distinguish between quiescent cysts and active infection. Histopathological examination utilizing stains, e.g. Giemsa and the immunoperoxidase technique (Conley et al. 1981), is much more likely to demonstrate an active infective process. For a detailed description of the pathology of cerebral toxoplasmosis see Chapter 5. The organism can also be detected by microscopy and PCR of broncho-alveolar lavage samples and ocular fluids in patients with toxoplasmic pneumonitis and retinochoroiditis respectively.

The predictive role of IgG antibody levels in identifying the early development of toxoplasmic encephalitis has been studied and conflicting reports have been published. Some workers have concluded that IgG levels are not useful in predicting the development of toxoplasmic encephalitis (Danneman et al. 1991), while others have found that the incidence of toxoplasmic encephalitis was increased in patients with high IgG antibody levels and that IgG levels were significantly associated with the recurrence of toxoplasmic encephalitis (Derouin et al. 1996; Belanger et al. 1999).

The occurrence of low CD4 T-cell counts (less than 150–200/mm^3) and the presence of *T. gondii* IgG antibody is generally accepted as being a good predictor of the development of toxoplasma reactivation, especially toxoplasmic encephalitis.

Potentially useful reference diagnostic tests for immunosuppressed/compromised patients are summarized in Table 12.3.

Pregnant women

When an acute toxoplasma infection occurs in an immunocompetent pregnant woman, the impact on the mother's health is minimal. Regretfully, this is not the case for the foetus as the infection can be fatal or result in gross abnormality. The investigation of such an event is a complex process that, in effect, involves three 'patients' (the mother, foetus and neonate) who are inextricably linked within one evolving clinical episode. Each requires a different diagnostic approach (Table 12.4)

The most crucial decision is whether or not an acute toxoplasma infection has impacted adversely on the pregnancy. The decision is often not clear-cut and a clinical judgement has to be made on the basis of clinical, ultrasonographic and laboratory findings. This decision is crucial because the future management of the pregnancy will be significantly altered, investigations are invasive and carry a small but definite risk of foetal death and current treatment carries the potential risk of toxicity.

Table 12.3. Potentially helpful reference diagnostic tests for the investigation of toxoplasma infection in immunosuppressed/compromised patients

	Dye Test	EIA IgM	ISAGA IgM	PCR blood	PCR CSF	Histopathology
Disseminated toxoplasma infection	+	±	+	+	NA	−
Toxoplasmic encephalitis	+	±	+	−	+	+

Table 12.4. Reference laboratory protocol for the investigation of toxoplasma infection in pregnancy. Key tests are shown in parentheses

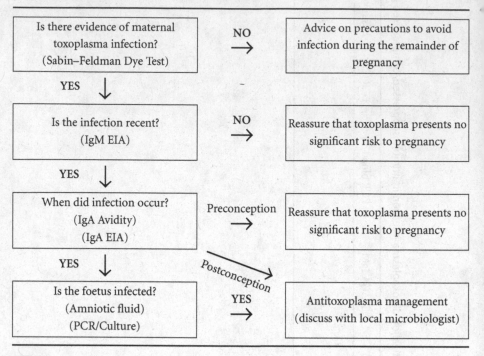

Is there evidence of maternal toxoplasma infection? (Sabin–Feldman Dye Test)	NO →	Advice on precautions to avoid infection during the remainder of pregnancy
↓ YES		
Is the infection recent? (IgM EIA)	NO →	Reassure that toxoplasma presents no significant risk to pregnancy
↓ YES		
When did infection occur? (IgA Avidity) (IgA EIA)	Preconception →	Reassure that toxoplasma presents no significant risk to pregnancy
↓ YES	Postconception ↘ YES →	
Is the foetus infected? (Amniotic fluid) (PCR/Culture)		Antitoxoplasma management (discuss with local microbiologist)

Maternal infection

There have been very few reports of congenital infection occurring where an immunocompetent women has acquired toxoplasma 3 or more months before conception. This, therefore, appears to be an extremely rare occurrence and it is generally accepted that when infection occurs several weeks prior to conception there is no significant risk to the foetus of congenital infection.

In order, therefore, to determine whether or not a pregnancy is at risk from toxoplasma infection, the following questions must be considered:

- Is there evidence of maternal toxoplasma infection?
- Is the infection recent?
- When did infection occur in relation to conception?

Unless monthly prenatal screening is performed, seroconversion (i.e. definitive evidence of an acute infection occurring during pregnancy) is infrequently demonstrated. However, the usual scenario is that the reference laboratory receives a single maternal serum sample, which was collected at some time during the first or second trimester and was found to be *T. gondii*-antibody-positive in a screening test carried out in the local hospital laboratory, or was antibody-negative but reference testing was requested for clinical or other reasons.

This sample should be investigated in the reference laboratory initially using the DT and IgM EIA. The DT can confirm whether or not the pregnant woman has become infected at any time previously with toxoplasma while the detection of IgM can identify infections probably (but not invariably) acquired up to 6–9 months earlier. The more sensitive IgM immunosorbent agglutination assay (ISAGA, bioMerièux) is not helpful in this particular investigation as it can detect IgM persisting for longer than 1 year after infection has been acquired (and thus unnecessarily include additional women for whom toxoplasma infection presents no risk to their pregnancy).

If the DT is negative, the patient should be advised on precautions required to avoid infection for the remainder of the pregnancy. When the DT is positive and IgM is not detected the patient can be reassured that the pregnancy should not be at risk where the duration of pregnancy is 6 months or less unless the mother is immunocompromised or a foetal abnormality has been detected. If gestation is 6 months or more it is advisable to test an earlier serum sample if available.

However, when both the DT and IgM are positive, further laboratory testing is required in order to provide a more precise estimate of the duration of infection. Measurement of IgG avidity can be particularly helpful for this purpose since, at present, this method can discriminate infections of less than 3 months from those of greater than 6 months duration (Joynson et al. 1990; Lappalainen et al. 1993). In addition, detailed questioning of the pregnant woman can be helpful in revealing clinical features which may help in timing the onset of infection.

Very importantly, a second serum should be requested immediately in order to both confirm the original result and to allow comparison for possible changes in titre. When an acute toxoplasma infection is confirmed in a pregnant woman, it is essential that the parents should be counselled regarding the risk to the foetus and management options discussed.

Foetal infection

The rate of transmission to the foetus in the first trimester is about 14%, rising to 29% in the second and 59% in the third, the average rate of transmission being about 30–40%. Recent data (see Table 7.1) suggest lower transmission rates but comparison with previous studies may not be valid. Infection of the foetus is not an inevitable outcome of maternal toxoplasmosis and thus an accurate and timely diagnosis of foetal infection is crucial. Perhaps it is even more important to demonstrate that the foetus is not infected, therefore avoiding an unnecessary termination.

The diagnosis of foetal infection is based upon the detection of the parasite and/or specific antibody responses in the foetus. Ultrasound alone can support, but not confirm, the diagnosis. Typical abnormalities found in an infected foetus by this technique are cerebral ventricular dilation and intracranial densities.

Cordocentesis affords the opportunity to demonstrate nonspecific biochemical and haematological abnormalities, and detection of both the parasite and specific antitoxoplasma IgM/IgA. However, these specific antibodies may be absent in confirmed foetal infections; one study found positive IgM results in only 12% of infected foetuses aged 22–24 weeks, 39% at 25–30 weeks and 59% after 30 weeks. No positive results were reported prior to 22 weeks of gestation (Hohlfeld et al. 1994). The presence of IgA also confirms congenital infection but, like IgM, is frequently not found. However, because the risk of contamination of foetal blood by maternal blood is difficult to exclude, the diagnostic significance of these tests is reduced. Culture of the parasite from foetal blood or amniotic fluid provides unequivocal evidence of infection. Unfortunately, isolation from mice can take 3–6 weeks and tissue culture though faster may be less sensitive when fewer parasites are present in the inoculum.

The finding that PCR for the detection of toxoplasma nucleic acid in amniotic fluid was as good if not better than previous diagnostic methods involving cordocentesis (Hohlfeld et al. 1994; Forestier et al. 1998) was a significant step forward for the following reasons:

- Rapid diagnosis – in ideal circumstances a result can be available within 24 hours.
- Amniocentesis is safer and less likely than cordocentesis to cause a miscarriage.
- Unlike cordocentesis, which is performed in a few specialist centres, amniocentesis is available in most obstetric departments.
- Amniocentesis can be performed much earlier in pregnancy (at about 16–18 weeks) than cordocentesis (about 22 weeks).

Thus amniocentesis, together with PCR, opens a window of opportunity allowing the earlier institution of therapy to prevent transmission of infection and avoiding an unnecessary termination. Alternatively, if congenital infection has occurred, it may facilitate earlier termination (if that is desired by the parents) or commencement of specific antitoxoplasma chemotherapy to halt or limit foetal damage at an earlier stage than would have been possible with previous techniques.

However, although PCR is a highly specific and sensitive technique it still has potential limitations and PCR results should not be interpreted in isolation from other tests. Thus, it is still the practice of the Toxoplasma Reference Unit, Swansea (UK) to culture amniotic fluid or foetal blood/tissues in addition to using molecular diagnostic techniques (Table 12.4).

Neonatal infection

The classic triad of congenital infection (hydrocephalus, cerebral calcification and retinochoroiditis) is infrequently seen and perhaps up to 85% of congenitally infected babies are born apparently normal. Occasionally clinical features present in the first weeks or months of life but if congenitally infected children are followed for a sufficiently long time – up to 20 years of age – it appears that most will develop some stigmata of the disease. It has been reported that early treatment of congenital toxoplasmosis will limit the frequency of retinochoroiditis and cause the disappearance of cerebral opacities.

If clinical benefit as a consequence of appropriate treatment can be achieved then the diagnosis of neonatal infection becomes crucial. It can be relatively straightforward in a baby with characteristic clinical and serological findings which are confirmed by parasite detection. Unfortunately, diagnosis is less straightforward in the majority of cases. It is essential that thorough clinical and ophthalmological examinations of the neonate be performed together with ultrasound of the brain. However, frequently no abnormalities can be detected and the diagnosis rests solely upon laboratory investigations.

Direct detection of the parasite is attempted by culture and PCR of the placenta, amniotic fluid and cord blood. Multisite sampling of the placenta is recommended as the distribution of parasite does not appear to be uniform (unpublished observation). Detection of parasite in the placenta alone, while providing strong evidence, cannot be considered as unequivocal confirmation of foetal infection.

Cord blood and a matched maternal sample should be subjected to serological testing. Since maternal IgG is transferred passively to the foetus *in utero*, a positive DT result in the neonate is of limited value unless levels are significantly elevated compared to maternal titres. Detection of neonatal IgM and IgA by EIA and/or ISAGA are regarded as being diagnostic of neonatal infection but the risk of contamination by maternal blood should be excluded. If specific antitoxoplasma IgM or IgA are found in cord blood, then it is recommended that neonatal serum is collected 2–3 weeks later and retested to confirm the original findings.

It is salutary to note that IgM and IgA may not be demonstrable in perhaps 20–30% of congenitally infected neonates (Remington et al. 1995). Thus, the only way at present to confirm or refute the diagnosis of congenital infection in such cases is to monitor serologically the baby ideally at monthly intervals for the first year of life. Maternal IgG antibodies will decline and disappear, the final negative serology demonstrating that congenital infection has not occurred. The persistence of positive DT antibody after 12 months confirms infection. Treatment of an infected neonate may initially result in reduction of DT levels but these usually increase again when therapy is stopped.

Potentially helpful reference diagnostic tests currently available for the investigation of toxoplasma infection in the pregnant woman and neonate are summarized in Table 12.5. However, new methods to distinguish between maternal and neonatal antitoxoplasma IgG are urgently required to assist clinical management when crucial decisions relating to treatment need to be made. Methods currently under evaluation in European multicentre trials include immunoblot and ELIFA (Pinon et al. 2001).

Table 12.5. Potentially helpful reference diagnostic tests for the investigation of toxoplasma infection in pregnancy.

	Pregnant woman	Foetus		Neonate		
		Amniotic fluid	Blood	Cord blood	Placenta	Amniotic fluid
Dye Test	+	–	+	+	–	–
IgM/IgA EIA	+	–	+	+	–	–
IgM/IgA ISAGA	–	–	+	+	–	–
IgG avidity	+	–	–	–	–	–
PCR	–	+	+	+	+	+
Culture	–	+	+	+	+	+

Immunocompromised pregnant woman

Reactivation of latent infection and consequent transmission to the foetus has been reported in women with a cell-mediated immune deficiency. This includes patients with systemic lupus erythematosus, Hodgkin's lymphoma and HIV infections. The frequency of congenital toxoplasmosis in the offspring of HIV-infected mothers has been reported to be very low – 0.1% (European Collaborative Study and Research Network on Congenital Toxoplasmosis 1997). However, in another study, mothers who were HIV infected and developed acute toxoplasmosis during pregnancy passed both infections to 75% of their offspring (Mitchell et al. 1990).

It is essential, therefore, that the baseline toxoplasma antibody status should be determined as soon as the diagnosis of HIV infection is made in women irrespective of whether they are pregnant or not. If the DT is negative, they should be advised of precautions to avoid infection.

If the DT is positive but no IgM is detected, then a pregnancy in an HIV-positive woman will probably only be at risk if she becomes severely immunocompromised (CD4$^+$ T cell count <100 cells/mm^3). Reactivation of toxoplasma infection can occur with or without a change in DT titres or the reappearance of specific IgM. PCR of blood may demonstrate an apparent parasitaemia, occurring as a result of reactivation.

If an acute maternal infection occurs in an HIV-positive patient, then the investigations and management mirror those of the immunocompetent pregnant woman. However, amniocentesis may not be advisable because of the risk of transmitting HIV infection to the foetus. Pregnant women in this category require careful monitoring of both their immune status and their toxoplasma infection.

Statistical characteristics of diagnostic/screening laboratory tests

In a diagnostic laboratory, the ideal test would both identify all patients with a particular disease while excluding all those without that same disease. To find how close to

Table 12.6. Predictive values for a laboratory test in hypothetical diseases with differing prevalences

Prevalence of hypothetical disease per 1000 population	Diagnostic test	
	Sensitivity 98%	Specificity 98%
	PPV (%)	NPV (%)
200	92.4	99.5
20	49.5	99.9
2	8.9	99.9

this ideal an individual test comes, basic statistical characteristics of diagnostic tests can be determined. These will not be considered in detail here, but briefly these are:

Sensitivity – this indicates the percentage of patients with a specific disease who will have a positive test result. This enables the true-positive rate and false-negative rate of the test to be determined.

Specificity – this indicates the percentage of patients without a given disease who will have a negative test result. This enables the true-negative rate and false-positive rate of the test to be determined.

It is pertinent to note at this stage that the above statistical terms may be confused by the same words having a different meaning when used in the context of laboratory testing. In the latter, sensitivity is defined as the ability of a test to detect the lowest concentration of a particular substance while specificity means the ability of a test to only detect a single specific substance.

Positive predictive value (PPV) – The PPV of a test indicates the probability (expressed as a percentage) that a positive result correctly identifies the presence of disease.

Negative predictive value (NPV) – The NPV of a test indicates the probability (expressed as a percentage) that a negative result correctly identifies the absence of disease.

It is important to realize that the PPV and NPV depend not only upon the sensitivity and specificity of the test but, crucially, also upon the prevalence of disease in the population in question. Variations in prevalence will result in very substantial differences in the PPV whereas the NPV usually remains relatively unaltered. This is illustrated in the following theoretical example (Table 12.6).

The example presented in Table 12.6 demonstrates that if antenatal screening for toxoplasma infection in pregnancy was introduced in the UK, where the prevalence is approximately 2/1000, there could be a substantial number of false-positive results. Thus, if clinical action were to be instituted on the basis of a single screening test then, at best, parents' worries and anxieties could be heightened and, at worst, healthy, normal foetuses could be put at risk.

However, in the context of congenital toxoplasmosis, this would be an incorrect application of the result of a screening test. Here, the screening test should be regarded as no more than the process by which a group of sera are selected which then rapidly undergo further extensive diagnostic investigation to make a definitive diagnosis. Only then would the parents be informed of their results and counselled accordingly. Since further clinical action would only be required in the eventually small number of cases with a definitive diagnosis, the potential problems associated with false-positive results in the screening test are obviated.

Summary

This chapter has considered a wide range of laboratory methods for the investigation of toxoplasma infection in a number of differing clinical scenarios. Central to the adoption of particular tests by a diagnostic laboratory and the combinations in which they may be applied helpfully is that selection of these must be determined by the clinical questions being asked and the answers that are required to influence clinical decisions. A test that is appropriate in one clinical situation may be inappropriate in another. Further, since the vast majority of laboratory investigations do not achieve the ideal of 100% sensitivity and specificity, an understanding of the characteristics of the diagnostic tests available is crucial to their application and interpretation in differing clinical scenarios.

The strategies for laboratory investigation presented here have been developed and are used routinely within the Public Health Laboratory Service Toxoplasma Reference Unit that serves England and Wales (approximately 20,000 specimens received in 1999). While it is recognized that the investigation strategies described here may be imperfect or may otherwise be unsuitable for some laboratories, it is hoped that they will, at least, provide helpful additional insight into some of the key issues and may provide a useful starting point for laboratories wishing to extend or expand their range of diagnostic services to include more specialized testing for toxoplasma infection.

REFERENCES

Aouizerate, F., Cazenave, J., Poiret, L., Verin, Ph., Cheryrou, A., Begueret, J. & Lagoutte, F. (1993). Detection of *Toxoplasma gondii* in aqueous humor by polymerase chain reaction. *British Journal of Ophthalmology*, 77, 107–9.

Belanger, F., Derouin, F., Grangeot-Keroski, L. & Mayer, L. (1999). Incidence and risk factors of toxoplasmosis in a cohort of human immunodeficiency virus-infected patients: 1988–1995. *Clinical Infectious Diseases*, 28, 575–81.

Conley, F. K., Jenkins, K. A. & Remington, J. S. (1981). *Toxoplasma gondii* infection of the central nervous system. Use of the peroxidase-antiperoxidase method to demonstrate toxoplasma in formalin fixed, paraffin embedded tissue sections. *Human Pathology*, 12, 690–8.

Danneman, B. R., Israelski, D. M., Leoung, G. S., McGraw, T., Mills, J. & Remington, J. S. (1991). Toxoplasma serology, parasitemia and antigenemia in patients at risk for toxoplasma encephalitis. *AIDS*, 5, 1363–5.

Derouin, F., Deport, C., Pueyos, S., Morland, P., Letrillart, B., Chêneg, G., Ecohichon, J.-L., Luft, B., Aubertin, J., Hafner, R., Vildé, J. L. & Salamon, R. (1996). Predictive value of *Toxoplasma gondii* antibodies on the occurrence of toxoplasmic encephalitis in HIV-infected patients. *AIDS*, 10, 1521–7.

Desmonts, G. (1966). Definitive serological diagnosis of ocular toxoplasmosis. *Archives of Ophthalmology*, 76, 839–51.

Dorfman, R. F. & Remington, J. S. (1973). Value of lymph node biopsy in the diagnosis of acute acquired toxoplasmosis. *New England Journal of Medicine*, 289, 878–81.

European Collaborative Study and Research Network on Congenital Toxoplasmosis (1997). Low incidence of congenital toxoplasmosis in children born to women infected with human immunodeficiency virus. *European Journal of Obstetrics and Gynaecology*, 176, 555–9.

Forestier, F., Hohlfeld, P., Sole, Y. & Daffos, F. (1998). Prenatal diagnosis of congenital toxoplasmosis by PCR extended experience. *Prenatal Diagnosis*, 18, 407–9.

Guy, E. C. & Joynson, D. H. M. (1995). Potential of the polymerase chain reaction in the diagnosis of active toxoplasma infection by the detection of parasite in blood. *Journal of Infectious Diseases*, 172, 319–22.

Guy, E. C., Pelloux, H., Lappalainen, M., Aspöck, H. A., Melby, K. K., Holberg-Pettersen, M., Petersen, E., Simon, J. & Ambroise-Thomas, P. (1996). Interlaboratory comparison of polymerase chain reaction for the detection of *Toxoplasma gondii* DNA added to samples of amniotic fluid. *European Journal of Clinical Microbiology and Infectious Disease*, 15, 836–9.

Hohlfeld, P., Daffos, F., Costa, J. M., Thulliez, P., Forestier, F. & Vidand, M. (1994). Prenatal diagnosis of congenital toxoplasmosis with a polymerase chain reaction test on amniotic fluid. *New England Journal of Medicine*, 331, 695–9.

Israelski, D. M. & Remington, J. S. (1992). AIDS associated toxoplasmosis. In *The Medical Management of AIDS*, 3rd edn., ed. M. A. Sande, P. A. Volderding, pp. 319–45. Philadelphia: WB Saunders.

Joynson, D. H. M., Payne, R. A. & Rawal, B. K. (1990). Potential role of IgG avidity for diagnosing toxoplasmosis. *Journal of Clinical Pathology*, 43, 1032–3.

Lappalainen, M., Koskela, P., Koskiniemi, M., Ammala, P., Hiilesmaa, V., Teramo, K., Raivio, K. O., Remington, J. S. & Hedman, K. (1993). Toxoplasmosis acquired during pregnancy improved serodiagnosis based on avidity of IgG. *Journal of Infectious Diseases*, 167, 691–7.

Lebech, M., Joynson, D. H. M., Seitz, H. M., Thulliez, R., Gilbert, R. E., Dutton, G. N., Øulisen, B. & Petersen, E. (1996). Classification system and case definitions of *Toxoplasma gondii* infection in immunocompetent women and their congenitally infected offspring. *European Journal Clinical Microbiology and Infectious Diseases*, 15, 799–805.

Manners, R. M., O'Connell, S., Guy, E. C., Joynson, D. H. M., Lanning, C. R. & Etchells, D. E. (1994). Use of polymerase chain reaction to detect *Toxoplasma gondii* in the vitreous of a patient with acquired ocular toxoplasmosis. *British Journal of Ophthalmology*, 78, 483–4.

Mitchell, C. D., Erlich, S. S., Mastrucci, M. T., Hutto, S. C., Parks, W. P. & Scott, G. B. (1990). Congenital toxoplasmosis occurring in infants perinatally infected with human immunodeficiency virus. *Paediatric Infectious Disease Journal*, 9, 129–32.

Montoya, J. G. & Remington, J. S. (1996). Toxoplasmic chorioretinitis in the setting of acute acquired toxoplasmosis. *Clinical Infectious Diseases*, 23, 277–82.

O'Connell, S., Guy, E. C., Dawson, S. J., Francis, J. M. & Joynson, D. H. M. (1993). Chronic active toxoplasmosis in an immunocompetent patient. *Journal of Infection*, 27, 305–10.

Pelloux, H., Guy, E., Angelici, M. C., Horst, A., Bessières, M.-H., Blatz, R., Pesso, M. D., Girault, V., Gratzl, R., Holberg Peterson, M., Johnson, J., Krüger, D., Lappalainen, M., Naessens, A. & Olsson, M. (1998). A second European collaborative study on polymerase chain reaction for *Toxoplasma gondii*, involving 15 teams. *FEMS Microbiology Letters*, 165, 231–7.

Pinon, J. M., Dumon, H., Chemla, C., Franck, J., Petersen, E., Lebech, M., Zufferey, J., Bessieres, M-H., Marty, P., Holliman, R., Johnson, J., Luyasu, V., Lecolier, B., Guy, E., Joynson, D. H. M., Decoster, A., Enders, G., Pelloux, E. & Candolfi, G. (2001). Strategy for diagnosis of congenital toxoplasmosis: evaluation of methods comparing mothers and newborns and standard methods for postnatal detection of immunoglobulin G, M, and A antibodies. *Journal of Clinical Microbiology*, 39, 2267–71.

Pinon, J. M. & Gruson, N. (1982). Interet des profils immunologiques compares ELIFA dans le diagnostic precoce de la toxoplasmose congenitale. *Lyon Medical*, 248, 27–30.

Porter, S. B. & Sande, M. A. (1992). Toxoplasmosis of the central nervous system in the acquired immunodeficiency syndrome. *New England Journal of Medicine*, 327, 1643–8.

Remington, J. S., Araujo, F. G. & Desmonts, G. (1985). Recognition of different Toxoplasma antigens by IgM and IgG antibodies in mothers and their congenitally infected newborns. *Journal of Infectious Diseases*, 152, 1020–4.

Remington, J. S., McLeod, R. & Desmont, G. (1995). Toxoplasmosis. In *Infectious Diseases of the Foetus and Newborn*, 4th edn., ed. J. S. Remington & J. O. Klein, pp. 140–267. Philadelphia: WB Saunders.

Sabin, A. B. & Feldman, H. A. (1948). Dyes as microchemical indicators of a new immunity phenomenon affecting a protozoon parasite (Toxoplasma). *Science*, 108, 660–3.

Spiers, G. E., Hakim, M., Calne, R. Y. & Wreghitt, T. G. (1988). Relative risk of donor-transmitted *Toxoplasma gondii* infection in heart, liver and kidney transplant recipients. *Clinical Transplantation*, 2, 257–60.

Stansfeld, A. G. (1961). The histological diagnosis of toxoplasmic lymphadenitis. *Journal of Clinical Pathology*, 14, 565–73.

Subauste, C. S., Wong, S. Y. & Remington, J. S. (1977). AIDS-associated toxoplasmosis. In *The Medical Management of AIDS*, ed. H. A. Sande & P. A. Volberding, pp. 343–62. Philadelphia: WB Saunders.

Thulliez, P., Remington, J. S., Santoro, F., Ovlaque, G., Sharma, S. & Desmonts, G. (1986). A new agglutination reaction for the diagnosis of the developmental stage of acquired toxoplasmosis *Pathologie Biologie Paris*, 34, 173–7.

Wanke, C., Tuazon, C. U., Kovacs, A., Dina, T., Davis, B. O., Barton, N., Katz, D., Lande, M., Levy, C. & Conley, F. K. (1987). Toxoplasma encephalitis in patients with acquired immune deficiency syndrome diagnosis and response to therapy. *American Journal of Tropical Medicine and Hygiene*, 36, 509–616.

Witmer, R. (1978). Clinical implications of aqueous humor studies in uveitis. *American Journal of Ophthalmology*, 86, 39–45.

13

Antitoxoplasma chemotherapy

R. E. McCabe

School of Medicine, University of California, California, USA

Introduction

Toxoplasma gondii is an obligate intracellular protozoon that was discovered in the gondi in 1908. In the1930s and 1940s toxoplasma was discovered to cause congenital disease in neonates (Sabin 1941) and severe disseminated disease in adults (Pinkerton & Henderson 1941). Subsequently toxoplasma was found to cause transient, nonsuppurative lymphadenopathy, usually in the head and neck regions, in immunocompetent patients (Remington et al. 1995). In the 1970s toxoplasma became appreciated as a cause of disease in iatrogenically immunosuppressed patients, primarily solid-organ transplant recipients. In the 1980s toxoplasma attained notoriety as the most common cause of encephalitis/brain abscess in acquired immunodeficiency syndrome (AIDS) patients.

Toxoplasma includes varied strains of differing virulence. Different animal species differ markedly in their resistance to toxoplasma infection, e.g. rats are highly resistant but mice are very susceptible, and some inbred strains of mice are more susceptible than others (Suzuki et al. 1989*b*). Cell-mediated immunity, activated macrophages, antibody and cytokines participate in host defence against toxoplasma, most frequently and extensively studied in murine models. Both CD8+ lymphocytes and CD4+ lymphocytes appear important for murine defence (Gazzinelli et al. 1991; Nagasawa et al. 1991; Subauste et al. 1991). CD8+ cells are cytotoxic for toxoplasma-infected cells and secrete interferon gamma. CD4+ cells are needed to effect drug cures in experimentally infected mice (Araujo 1992). Of the cytokines, interferon gamma has been studied most extensively. Interferon gamma activates macrophages and other cells to kill toxoplasma, is effective when administered *in vivo*, and neutralization of interferon gamma with a monoclonal antibody exacerbates toxoplasmic encephalitis (McCabe et al. 1984; Suzuki et al. 1989*b*). Interleukin-6 (IL-6) impairs host defence perhaps by antagonizing the macrophage-activating effect of interferon gamma (Beaman et al. 1992), IL-10 deactivates macrophages activated to kill toxoplasma *in vitro* (Gazzinelli et al. 1992), and IL-12 enhances the survival of toxoplasma-infected mice (Gazzinelli et al. 1993). Tumour necrosis factor triggers antitoxoplasma activity of interferon-gamma-primed macrophages (Sibley et al. 1991). In 'unactivated cells', toxoplasma reside in parasitophorous vacuoles that do not fuse with lysosomes and so are protected from cellular cidal mechanisms (Sibley et al. 1985). Experimentally, toxoplasma can be killed by reactive oxygen and nitrogen intermediates, tryptophan depletion and phagosome acidification.

IgG, IgM and IgA antibodies are produced in response to toxoplasma infection, and their detection is very useful diagnostically. However, antibody appears to play only a modest role in host defence.

Clinical scope

The acute acquired infection is without clinical signs or symptoms in up to 90% of immunocompetent patients. Transient head and neck lymphadenopathy is the most common sign (McCabe et al. 1987), and the acute acquired infection in the nonpregnant, immunocompetent host is usually not treated. Adenopathy persists or recurs rarely, and clinically significant organ system involvement (e.g. encephalitis, myocarditis, hepatitis, pneumonitis) does not occur very often.

Foetal infection only occurs when a woman acquires infection during pregnancy or immediately before conception. Immunocompromised women, especially if infected with human immunodeficiency virus (HIV), who were infected previously with toxoplasma may rarely experience reactivation of the infection during pregnancy, resulting in foetal infection. If the immunocompetent mother is not treated for toxoplasma infection, about 40% of foetuses will become infected (Wong & Remington 1994; Remington et al. 1995). The likelihood of foetal infection is greatest, about 60%, when maternal infection is acquired in the third trimester, but in most cases an apparently healthy baby is delivered.

Antitoxoplasma chemotherapy administered to the mother appears to prevent foetal infection in about 60% of cases (Wong & Remington 1994; Remington et al. 1995) and, if the foetus becomes infected, treatment of the mother limits the signs and symptoms of the infection in the child (Wong & Remington 1994). In addition, several recent studies have demonstrated sensitive and specific detection of foetal infection *in utero* (Grover et al. 1990; Stepick-Biek et al. 1990; Cazenave et al. 1992; Lappalainen et al. 1993; Wong & Remington 1994; Remington et al. 1995). Since infection in the mother is usually clinically silent, effective chemotherapeutic prevention of congenital toxoplasma infection and/or *in utero* diagnosis requires a systematic and accurate screening programme, as done in France (Remington et al. 1995). Acting upon incomplete or unreliable data will probably result in unindicated abortions and untreated infections.

The congenitally infected infant can be severely affected, but most appear normal at the time of birth, although this figure is influenced by the care given to examination of the infant (McAuley et al. 1994). Retinochoroiditis, hydrocephalus and cerebral calcifications detected in the neonate usually indicate first or early second trimester infection. The most common laboratory abnormalities involve the cerebrospinal fluid (CSF), e.g. pleocytosis and elevated protein concentration. Apparently severe damage in neonates due to toxoplasma infection does not necessarily preclude successful therapy and relatively normal development.

The majority of infants who are infected with toxoplasma and appear normal in the neonatal period will develop sequelae that become apparent later in life, e.g. retinochoroiditis in most, and seizures, hearing loss, lower than expected scores on intelligence tests, neuroendocrine abnormalities and developmental delay in smaller proportions. Antitoxoplasma chemotherapy during the first year of life can limit progressive tissue destruction while adequate immunity develops and might prevent the development of sequelae that become apparent only later in childhood (Wilson et al. 1980).

Although the peak incidence of toxoplasmic retinochoroiditis is in the second and third decades of life, most cases are thought to be caused by the recrudenscence of congenital infection rather than by newly acquired infection. When the retinochoroiditis is judged to be active by ophthalmological examination, then specific antitoxoplasma treatment is recommended.

Toxoplasma gondii-antibody-negative recipients of transplant organs (especially heart) from *T. gondii*-antibody-positive donors (i. e. toxoplasma mismatches) can develop toxoplasma infection and disease shortly after transplantation (Luft et al. 1983; McGregor et al. 1984; Hakim et al. 1986; Wreghitt et al. 1989). Toxoplasmosis, in heart transplant recipients, frequently mimics rejection. Antitoxoplasma chemotherapyapy is usually successful. 'Prophylactic' treatment of *T. gondii*-mismatched recipients with pyrimethamine for 6 weeks in the post-transplantation period can prevent the development of clinically overt infection (Wreghitt et al. 1989). Data concerning toxoplasma infection in other transplant recipients are discussed in Chapter 6.

Toxoplasmosis in AIDS patients may present as disease in any organ, but most commonly presents as brain abscess(es) and represents reactivation of infection acquired in the remote past. Toxoplasmic encephalitis occurs in approximately 10% of all patients with AIDS. It is estimated that 30–40% of *T. gondii*-antibody-positive patients with AIDS in the United States will develop toxoplasmic encephalitis if they do not receive prophylaxis (Beaman & Remington 1992; Luft & Remington 1992). In AIDS populations that have high prevalences of toxoplasma infection, e.g. in France, the total number of patients who develop toxoplasmic encephalitis will be significantly greater. Treatment of clinically overt toxoplasma infection is usually successful in patients with AIDS. Treatment is directed initially at controlling the signs and symptoms of acute disease, which is then followed by suppressive treatment for the remainder of the patient's life to prevent recrudescence of disease (Haverkos 1987; Leport et al. 1988). Studies indicate that prophylaxis (e.g. with trimethoprim–sulphamethoxazole) can prevent toxoplasmic encephalitis in AIDS patients (Beaman & Remington 1992).

Chemotherapeutic agents

Pyrimethamine

Pyrimethamine, an antimalarial substituted phenylpyrimidine, cures animals experimentally infected with toxoplasma (Eyles & Coleman 1953, 1955; Cook & Jacobs 1958). Pyrimethamine is a folic acid antagonist that is usually used in combination with other folic acid antagonists, sulphadiazine or trisulphapyrimidines (sulphamethazine, sulphamerazine, sulphadiazine), thereby synergistically inhibiting toxoplasma both *in vitro* and *in vivo*. Dihydropteroate synthase converts *para*-aminobenzoic acid to dihydrofolic acid, which then is converted to tetrahydrofolic acid by dihydrofolic acid reductase, and subsequently used for purine synthesis (Kucers & Bennett 1979; Allegra et al. 1987). Sulphonamides inhibit the first conversion mediated by dihydrofolic acid synthetase, and pyrimethamine inhibits the second step mediated by dihydrofolic acid reductase. Administered tetrahydrofolate (folinic acid, leucovorin) is taken up by mammalian cells and can achieve rescue from these folic acid antagonists. Toxoplasma cannot take in folinic acid, but can absorb folic acid, thereby partially bypassing the synergistic activity of pyrimethamine and sulphonamide. Hence folinic acid should be used to prevent toxicity, but folic acid should not be used since it might thwart the therapeutic effect.

The plasma half-life of pyrimethamine in adults, which is cleared by hepatic metabolism, is approximately 100 hours but with a wide range (35–139 hours), possibly due to genetic metabolic differences (Weiss et al. 1988; Jacobson et al. 1996). Approximately 10–25% penetrates the CSF in patients with AIDS and toxoplasmic encephalitis (Weiss et al. 1988) or those with meningeal leukemia (Geils et al. 1971). In patients with AIDS, doses correlate poorly with serum and CSF levels (Weiss et al. 1988), and studies do not agree as to whether pyrimethamine's pharmacokinetics differ between HIV-infected and -uninfected patients (Jacobson et al. 1996) and the extent of interpatient pharmacokinetic variation (Winstanley et al. 1995). Limited data suggest that serum levels of >0.75 μg/ml when pyrimethamine is used in combination with sulphonamide and >3.0 μg/ml when used singly may be desirable in the treatment of toxoplasmic encephalitis (Geils et al. 1971; Weiss et al. 1988). Pyrimethamine has been administered in markedly differing schedules, varying from daily to once every 3 or 4 days. Serum pyrimethamine levels are not routinely available to clinicians.

The major determinants of dose and dosing interval in clinical practice are severity of disease and toxicity. The usual loading dose in adults is 200 mg for the first day in two divided doses. The standard loading regimen may be inadequate for producing therapeutic serum concentrations quickly, and a single loading dose of 500 mg, which might prove difficult to tolerate, or 200 mg per day in two divided doses for 3 days have both been proposed as alternatives (Jacobson et al. 1996). Dosages then vary from 25 to 100 mg/day, with the lower dosages indicated for pregnant women, immunocompetent patients, and for suppressive maintenance therapy in patients with AIDS. In acute disease, dosages of 50–75 mg per day are used commonly. The prolonged half-life of pyrimethamine indicates that serum and tissue accumulation will occur, and so toxic levels might occur if relatively high doses are used (Jacobson et al. 1996). Doses are not adjusted for renal impairment.

The folic acid antagonism of pyrimethamine may cause reversible thrombocytopaenia, granulocytopaenia and megaloblastic anaemia (Kaufman & Geisler 1960; Winstanley et al. 1995). These effects may be compounded by the concomitant administration of sulphonamide drugs. To counteract or prevent bone marrow suppression, folinic acid (calcium leucovorin) is administered intramuscularly or orally at a dose of 5–10 mg per day (but occasionally up to 50 mg per day in two divided doses, especially in patients with AIDS). Therefore, patients on this therapy should have determinations of haemoglobulin concentrations, white blood cell count and platelet count twice a week if possible. Folic acid cannot be substituted for folinic acid since folic acid will antagonize the effect of pyrimethamine on *T. gondii* (Frenkel & Hitchings 1957).

Pyrimethamine at very high doses has been shown to be teratogenic in animals (Remington et al. 1995) and should not be used in the first trimester of pregnancy. Other side-effects attributed to pyrimethamine include nausea, headache and dysgeusia. Rash has been a particular problem in patients with AIDS (see below). Pyrimethamine is available only in tablet form.

Sulphonamides

Sulphadiazine or trisulphapyrimidines (sulphamethazine, sulphamerazine and sulphadiazine) are combined with pyrimethamine to synergistically inhibit toxoplasma multiplication. Sulphonamides and pyrimethamine inhibit sequential steps in folic acid metabolism: sulphonamides inhibit dihydrofolic acid synthetase and pyrimethamine inhibits dihydrofolic acid reductase. Sulphapyrazine, sulphamerazine, sulphamethazine and sulphadiazine are about equally effective but superior to other tested sulphonamides (Eyles & Coleman 1953, 1955). Others, such as sulphisoxazole (but see trimethoprim–sulphamethoxazole below), are often used to treat bacterial infections (Feldman 1973), but should not be used in the treatment of toxoplasma infection.

The loading dose of sulphadiazine or trisulphapyrimidines is 75 mg/kg up to 4 g, followed by 50–100 mg/kg per day up to 8 g/day in two to four divided doses. Parenteral forms of sulphadiazine or trisulphapyrimidines are not available in the United States. The sulphonamide drugs are well absorbed from the gastrointestinal tract, penetrate well into CSF and are excreted in the urine. The serum half-life of sulphadiazine is 10–12 hours in patients with normal kidney function, and the serum half-life doubles when the creatinine clearance is less than 10 ml/min, requiring dose adjustments.

Adverse reactions to sulphonamides are common and include Stevens–Johnson syndrome (Carroll et al. 1966), hepatitis, bone marrow suppression (especially when combined with pyrimethamine), nausea and diarrhoea. The last two effects are more characteristics of the sulphonamides with a long serum half-life, such as sulphadiazine and trisulphapyrimidine.

Crystalluria, nephrolithiasis and acute reversible renal failure are relatively common with the poorly soluble drugs such as sulphadiazine but are not common with the more soluble sulphasoxazole and sulphamethoxazole (Nissen et al. 1950; Goadsby et al. 1987; Carbone et al. 1988; Sahai et al. 1988; Oster et al. 1990). Cystalluria can be detected by light microscopy of urine sediment while ultrasonography may demonstrate stones or sludge due to crystals. Renal failure can be reversed with hydration and alkalinization of the urine. Trisulphapyrimidines may be less nephrotoxic than sulphadiazine, since the solubility characteristics of the different sulphonamides are independent of each other and each component of the trisulphapyrimidines is administered at a relatively low dose (Lehr 1957).

Trimethoprim–sulphamethoxazole

This combination is less effective than the combination of pyrimethamine and sulphonamide *in vitro* and *in vivo*. However, limited observations of patients with AIDS and toxoplasmic encephalitis have indicated response rates of approximately 75% to trimethoprim–sulphamethoxazole, and it has been shown to offer effective prophylaxis against toxoplasmic encephalitis in patients with AIDS (Grossman & Remington 1979; Richards et al. 1995). Furthermore, trimethoprim–sulphamethoxazole is known to be effective for such central nervous infections as cerebral nocardiosis and Gram-negative bacillary meningitis (Smego et al. 1983; Levitz & Quintiliani 1984).

Trimethoprim–sulphamethoxazole is 85–90% absorbed after oral ingestion, and an intravenous formulation is available. Penetration into the CSF is about 40% in patients with uninflamed meninges. The serum half-lives for the trimethoprim and sulphamethoxazole components are similar, 8–15 hours and 7–12 hours respectively in patients with normal renal functions; dosages need to be adjusted in patients with renal failure. Trimethoprim–sulphamethoxazole is given at 5 mg/kg (trimethoprim component) for patients with toxoplasmic encephalitis and normal renal function.

Macrolides/azalides

Spiramycin has long been used to treat toxoplasma infection, particularly in primary maternal infection in pregnancy. Recently introduced macrolides, e.g. clarithromycin, azithromycin and roxithromycin, appear to have promise for treating toxoplasmosis. The mechanism of anti- *T. gondii* activity is unknown. Spiramycin is not marketed in the United States but is available from the Food and Drug Administration in Washington DC.

Spiramycin is supplied in a syrup and tablets, and the usual dosage in adults is 2–4 g/day in divided doses. Spiramycin is usually very well tolerated but nausea, vomiting, diarrhoea and dysaesthesias are common side-effects at higher doses, as often happens with macrolides. Otherwise spiramycin is very safe which is perhaps its major attraction, especially when compared with pyrimethamine and sulphonamides. Spiramycin has no known adverse effects on the foetus. Spiramycin persists in tissues for a long time (Hudson et al. 1956; Sutherland 1962) which may account for the greater activity of spiramycin against toxoplasma compared with erythromycin. Most of an orally ingested dose is inactivated in the body with biliary excretion predominating over urinary excretion (Kucers & Bennett 1979).

When spiramycin was administered at 2 g/day, placenta drug levels were found to be more than twofold higher than in maternal serum, but cord blood levels were approximately half that in maternal serum (Hudson et al. 1956; Remington et al. 1995). Increasing the dose by 50% to 3 g/day doubled the concentration of spiramycin in the placenta, with smaller increases in cord blood and maternal serum. These data suggest that spiramycin would prevent transmission of toxoplasma across the placenta to the foetus, but, because of the relatively low cord blood levels, spiramycin might not be very effective for treating established foetal infection (Wong & Remington 1994). Patients with AIDS have developed toxoplasmic encephalitis while receiving spiramycin (Leport et al. 1986). This casts doubt on the suitability of spiramycin for the treatment of central nervous system toxoplasmic encephalitis. Individuals appear to differ significantly with respect to spiramycin pharmacokinetics (Remington et al. 1995), but serum levels are not commonly available to clinicians.

Macrolides

The new macrolides, clarithromycin and roxithromycin, and the azalide azithromycin are more stable to acid degradation in the gastrointestinal tract and are administered only once or twice daily. Azithromycin appears more active against toxoplasma than the other macrolides (Araujo et al. 1988). Azithromycin penetrates tissues very well and is concentrated to a remarkable extent in phagocytes, including macrophages, and levels within phagocytes can exceed those in serum by 10- to 1000-fold (Foulds et al. 1990; Piscitelli et al. 1992). Hence azithromycin may be particularly effective for treating intracellular pathogens such as toxoplasma. Azithromycin is active against the cyst form as well as intracellular tachyzoites, a property shared with atovaquone but not with other antitoxoplasma therepeutic agents. In one study, azithromycin at 200 mg/kg per day completely protected mice in experiments of both systemic toxoplasmosis and toxoplasmic encephalitis (Araujo et al. 1988). Food decreases absorption by 50%. The serum half-life is approximately 11–14 hours when sampled during the first 24 hours, with a terminal half-life of 68 hours. The tissue half-life has been estimated to be between 2 and 4 days (Schentag & Ballow 1991). These pharmacokinetic properties may reflect tissue redistribution (Araujo et al. 1988). Cerebrospinal fluid levels are very low. Elimination appears to be primarily biliary and transintestinal into the faeces. For treatment of toxoplasmic encephalitis, a dose of 1200–1500 mg every 24 hours has been recommended (Subauste et al. 1997).

The pharmacokinetics of clarithromycin are dose dependent, with disproportionate increases in peak concentration and serum half-life (2.3–6 hours) as the dose is increased (Fraschini et al. 1991; Hardy et al. 1992). Approximately 20–30% is excreted unchanged in the urine, and the dose needs to be decreased with severe renal impairment. The remainder is metabolized extensively by oxidation and hydrolysis in the liver, with the production of a 14-hydroxy metabolite with antimicrobial activity. Clarithromyin penetrates tissues very well and is concentrated in phagocytes, although not to so great an extent as azithromycin. Clarithromcyin has been shown to be effective against toxoplasmic infection in a murine model (Chang et al. 1988), but only limited clinical experience with clarithromycin for the treatment of toxoplasmic encephalitis in AIDS has been reported. In one study, clarithromycin was administered at a dose of 1 gram orally twice per day (twice the usual dose for common bacterial infection) in combination with pyrimethamine, with some success (Fernandez-Martin et al. 1992). Adverse events were common and included nausea and vomiting, hearing loss, liver toxicity, rash and severe thrombocytopaenia. The contribution of pyrimethamine could not be separated from that of clarithromycin. Of note, clarithromycin at a dose of 1 gram orally twice per day was associated with greater mortality when compared with a dose of 500 mg orally twice per day when used for disseminated *Mycobacterium avium-intracellulare* infection in patients with AIDS (Chaisson et al. 1994).

Roxithromycin, an ether oxime derivative of erythromycin, has proved to be effective in a murine model of toxoplasmosis (Chan & Luft 1986; Chang & Pechere 1987). Roxithromycin at a dosage of 300 mg three times a week was beneficial compared to an untreated control in a small European study (Durant et al. 1992) when used as prophylaxis for toxoplasmic encephalitis and disseminated M. avium-intra-cellulare. Adverse effects, e.g. digestive intolerance and hepatitis, were more common in patients who received roxithromycin.

Clindamycin

Clindamycin is less effective than pyrimethamine and sulphonamide in murine tox-oplasmosis (Araujo & Remington 1974), and its effectiveness can be difficult to dem-onstrate *in vitro* (Harriset al. 1988; Fichera et al. 1995). However, clindamycin has been used routinely in the treatment of toxoplasmic retinochoroiditis due to good clinical results, effectiveness in a rabbit model, and penetration into the choroid (Tabbara & O'Connor 1975, 1980; Lakhanpul et al. 1983). Clindamycin is rarely used to treat the primary maternal infection in pregnancy or congenital infection.

Although clindamycin penetrates the CSF poorly, considerable clinical experi-ence has been gained with the combination of pyrimethamine and clindamycin in the treatment of toxoplasmic encephalitis in patients with AIDS. This is because significant side-effects were associated with pyrimethamine and sulphonamide drug treatment of toxoplasmic encephalitis in patients with AIDS. Pyrimethamine and clindamycin in combination appear to be about as effective as pyrimethamine and sulphadiazine for the treatment of toxoplasmic encephalitis (Danneman et al. 1992). Clindamycin has been used at widely differing dosages, e.g. 2400–4800 mg i. v./day and 1200–2400 mg orally/day in divided doses orally and parenterally. One study (Gatti et al. 1993) reported that the bioavailability and peak concentrations of clindamycin were approximately 40% greater in patients with AIDS than in healthy volunteers; the authors speculated that this was possibly due to decreased gut metabolism of clindamycin because of AIDS enteropathy. Clindamycin is 90% absorbed when administered orally, is concentrated in macrophages and poly-morphonuclear leukocytes (Prokesch & Hand 1982) and attains relatively high concentrations in experimental abscesses (Joiner et al. 1981), perhaps accounting for its efficacy in toxoplasmic encephalitis. Clindamycin enters foetal blood and tissues when administered to pregnant women (Panzeret al. 1972). The half-life of clindamycin is 2.4 hours and it is extensively metabolized by the liver; the half-life doubles when there is severe renal impairment.

Atovaquone

Atovaquone (previously known as BW566C80) is an orally administered hydroxy-naphthoquinone originally developed as an antimalarial agent (Spencer & Goa 1995). Atovaquone is effective for treating mild to moderate *Pneumocystis carinii* pneumonia and is effective against *T. gondii in vivo* and *in vitro*. Atovaquone appears to inhibit mitochondrial electron transport in plasmodium species and ultimately inhibits pyrimidine synthesis. Atovaquone and azithromycin differ from other antitoxoplasma agents and combinations in that they kill tissue cysts, including brain cysts, *in vitro* and *in vivo* as well as tachyzoites (Araujo et al. 1992); other antitoxoplasma agents do not affect tissue cysts (Huskinson-Mark et al. 1991). Other hydroxynaphthoquinones have been shown to be active against *T. gondii in vitro* and *in vivo* (Khan et al. 1998).

The absorption of atovaquone is increased about threefold when ingested as a tablet with food compared with the fasted state. Serum levels correlate linearly with dose up to 450–750 mg, but relatively decreased absorption was observed at higher doses (Huskinson-Mark et al. 1991; Khan et al. 1998). Absorption may be increased and be more reliable with a suspension formulation. Atovaquone is highly lipophilic and more than 99% is bound to plasma proteins. The mean elimination half-life is between 45 and 77 hours. Enterohepatic circulation is likely and most of the drug is excreted unmetabolized in the faeces. Penetration of CSF is less than 1% in volunteers (Spencer & Goa 1995).

In clinical trials, rashes including erythema multiforme occurred in 12–41% (Kovacs and the NIAID Clinical Centre Intramural AIDS Program 1992; Torres et al. 1997). Other adverse effects include gastrointestinal distress, headache, insomnia, fever and liver function test abnormalities. Atovaquone has been used at dosages of 750 mg orally four times per day to treat toxoplasmic encephalitis in patients with AIDS (Kovacs and the NIAID Clinical Centre Intramural AIDS Program 1992) and ocular toxoplasmosis in patient with AIDS (Lopez et al. 1992).

Trimetrexate

Trimetrexate is used for salvage therapy for *Pneumocystis carinii* pneumonia. Trimetrexate inhibits dihydrofolate reductase to a much greater extent than either pyrimethamine or trimethoprim (Allegra et al. 1987; Kovacs et al. 1987). Trimetrexate is active in a murine model of toxoplasmosis, and exhibits additive or synergistic activity with sulphadiazine (Kovacs et al. 1987). In limited studies of patients with AIDS and toxoplasmic encephalitis, trimetrexate appeared effective but relapses occurred while patients were receiving the drug (Polla et al. 1989; Masuret al. 1993), indicating that it is effective transiently as a chemotherapeutic agent but ultimately will fail. The recommended dose is 45 mg/m^2 i.v. 6 hourly, administered with leucovorin 20 mg/m^2 6 hourly to counteract trimexate's antifolate activity. The intravenous preparation can be ingested orally (Masur et al. 1993). The serum half-life is 11 hours and 10–30% is excreted by the kidneys.

Dapsone

Dapsone, which inhibits *T. gondii* dihydropteroate synthase, is potentially promising because it is well absorbed orally, has been used extensively for other indications, has a long serum half-life, is inexpensive and is synergistic *in vitro* and *in vivo* with pyrimethamine. However, dapsone administered as a single agent was relatively ineffective in a murine model of toxoplasmosis, but in the same model appeared effective when administered with pyrimethamine (Derouin et al. 1991; Gatti et al. 1997). Clinical experience with dapsone for the treatment or prevention of toxoplasmosis is very limited, but dapsone may eventually have a role in suppressive treatment or prophylaxis. Dapsone is well absorbed after oral administration, distributes widely into host tissues, has a half-life of about 25 hours, is 70–80% protein bound and is excreted into the urine as glucuronide or sulphate conjugates. Data from patients with AIDS show that dapsone enters the CSF but with a high interpatient variability (Gatti et al. 1997). Data are not available to guide dose adjustments in renally impaired patients. Side-effects include bone marrow suppression, haemolytic anaemia (contraindicated in patients with glucose 6-phosphate dehydrogenase deficiency) and methaemoglobinaemia. Dapsone is available in 25-mg and 100-mg tablets, and has been used at 100 mg orally per day for treatment of toxoplasmic encephalitis, 100 mg twice weekly for the maintenance treatment for toxoplasmic encephalitis, and 50 mg per day, 100 mg twice weekly, and 200 mg weekly for primary prophylaxis of toxoplasmic encephalitis.

Tetracyclines

The investigation of tetracyclines has produced contradictory results in animal models (Chang et al. 1990). Doxycycline is effective *in vitro* at concentrations attainable in serum and is also effective in murine toxoplasmosis. Doxycycline is well absorbed after oral ingestion, an intravenous formulation is available and the dose is not adjusted in renal impairment. Clinical experience with doxycycline for toxoplasmosis is very limited, but at least one patient with AIDS and toxoplasmic encephalitis was treated with doxycycline at 100 mg orally twice per day in combination with pyrimethamine to suppress the infection (Morris & Kelly 1992). Minocycline has been shown to be active against *T. gondii* in mice (Chang et al. 1991), but human data are few regarding therapy of toxoplasmosis.

Trovafloxacin

A new fluoroquinolone approved for use in the United States, trovafloxacin, was found to be active against *T. gondii in vitro* and in a murine model, both singly and in combination with clarithromycin, pyrimethamine or sulphadiazine (Khan et al. 1996, 1997). There are no data for the treatment of humans with toxoplasmosis. Trovafloxacin is well absorbed after oral ingestion, an intravenous preparation is available, it becomes concentrated in phagocytes and the dose is not adjusted for renal impairment (Dalvie et al. 1997; Teng et al. 1997).

Other drugs
Rifabutin

Rifabutin is a rifamycin derivative used commonly to treat *M. avium-intracellulare* and *Mycobacterium tuberculosis* infection in patients with AIDS. It is active against *T. gondii in vitro* and *in vivo* both singly and in combination with trovafloxacin (Olliaro et al. 1994; Romand et al. 1996). Rifabutin's mechanism of activity against *T. gondii* is not known. Rifapentine, another rifamycin derivative, in a murine model appeared to be as active as atovaquone and superior to rifabutin (Araujo et al. 1996). Rifapentine is not avilable in the United States but has been used elsewhere to treat tuberculosis (Chan et al. 1994).

Ketolide antibiotics

Ketolide antibiotics are relatively acid-stable derivatives of erythromycin, and similarly have been shown to be active *in vitro* and in a murine model of toxoplasmosis (Araujo et al. 1997).

Pentamidine

Pentamidine is used parenterally to treat *Pneumocystic carinii* pneumonia and by aerosol administration to prevent *Pneumocystis carinii* pneumonia. It is active *in vitro* against *T. gondii,* as are nine pentamidine analogues (Lindsay et al. 1991).

Artemisinin (quinghaosu)

Artemisinin (quinghaosu) is an antimalarial agent used in humans that is derived from a Chinese herb. It is also active against *T. gondii in vitro,* as are derivatives of artemisinin (O-Yang et al. 1990). Mutants of *T. gondii* resistant to artemisinin have been selected in cultures that contain permissive concentrations of artemisinin (Berens et al. 1998).

Piritrexim

Piritrexim is a lipid-soluble inhibitor of dihydrofolate reductase, similar to trimitrexate, that was developed to treat malignancies. Piritrexim is not as effective as pyrimethamine in a murine model of systemic toxoplasmosis, but does have synergistic activity in combination with sulphadiazine (Araujo et al. 1987). Unlike pyrimethamine, piritrexim does not inhibit histamine *N*-methyltransferase and thus histamine-related adverse effects such as nausea and headache may be less frequent. Piritrexim has been used in humans in investigations of its potential for treating malignancies (Bleehen et al. 1995; Feun et al. 1995).

Arprinocid

Arprinocid is an anticoccidial purine analogue used in veterinary medicine that is a specific competitor of hypoxanthine transport across membranes (Wang et al.

1979*b*), and additionally has been found to inhibit dihydrofolate reductase in *Eimeria tenella* (Wang et al. 1979*a*). *Toxoplasma gondii*, which is incapable of *de novo* purine synethesis, salvages hypoxanthines to produce purines (Pfefferkorn & Pfefferkorn 1977). Arprinocid was found to be active in a murine model of toxoplasmosis (Luft 1986).

Poloxamers

Poloxamers are nonionic block copolymers that consist of a single chain of hydrophobic polyoxypropylene between two hydrophilic chains of polyoxyethylene. They are effective *in vitro* and in a murine model (Krahenbuhl et al. 1993). Poloxamers have been used in the pharmaceutical industry and can function as immunological adjuvants and upregulators of macrophage afferent effector function. Diclazuril is a benzene-acetonitrile derivative available commercially in many European and South American countries to prevent coccidiosis in poultry. It was found to be effective *in vitro* and in a murine model of toxoplasmosis (Lindsay & Blagburn 1993).

Of note is that 2′,3′-dideoxyinosine, which is commonly known as DDI and is an HIV nucleoside reverse transcriptase inhibitor used commonly to treat HIV, appears to kill *T. gondii* brain cysts in a murine model of chronic infection (Sarciron et al. 1997). There are no available human data regarding the anti-*T. gondii* activity of DDI.

5-Fluorouracil

5-Fluorouracil has *in vitro* activity against *T. gondii* (Harris et al. 1988) and anecdotally has been used to treat toxoplasmic encephalitis in a patient with AIDS (Dhiver et al. 1993).

Immunomodulators

Although immunomodulators such as IL-2 and interferon gamma are available, they have no established clinical role in the treatment of toxoplasmosis (Subauste et al. 1997). The use of immunomodulators is very attractive conceptually, since the immune response effectively stops multipliation of *T. gondii*, prevents or limits disease during the active infection and prevents the reactivation of latent infection in immunocompetent patients and in many severely immunocompromised patients. Augmentation or 'reconstitution' of the immune response, therefore, may be effective for prophylaxis or treatment. Immunomodulators that have demonstrated anti-*T. gondii* activity *in vivo* or *in vitro* include interferons gamma and beta, IL-2, IL-7 and IL-12, tumour necrosis factor and granulocyte-macrophage colony stimulating factor. Neutralization of IL-6 with monoclonal antibody reduces foci of acute inflammation in a murine model of cerebral toxoplasmosis (Suzuki et al. 1994). The use of highly active anti-HIV treatment regimens, often including protease inhibitors, will probably produce data concerning the effectiveness of this relatively nonspecific method of immune reconstitution on risk of acute toxoplasmosis and the necessity and nature of maintenance and primary prophylactic regimens.

Treatment regimens

Acute acquired infection in the immunocompetent patient

Up to 90% of newly acquired infections in the immunocompetent host either do not produce symptoms or are not severe enough to warrant medical attention or the pursuit of a specific diagnosis. The most common finding is cervical lymphadenopathy which is almost always self-limiting (McCabe et al. 1987). Treatment of the primary infection in an immunocompetent patient is not recommended unless the patient is pregnant, has severe or prolonged systemic symptoms, suffers significant organ dysfunction, such as myocarditis or encephalitis, or rarely if infection is acquired by blood transfusion or laboratory accident (anecdotally the latter infections tend to be severe). If treatment is indicated, the combination of pyrimethamine (25–50 mg/day) and sulphadiazine or trisulphapyrimidines (6–8 gm/day) with folinic acid is recommended for 2–4 months, at which time the need for additional therapy is determined. Other drugs and regimens are likely to be effective, but there are no controlled trials comparing one regimen with another to help guide the clinician in caring for immunocompetent hosts.

Toxoplasma infection in the immunodeficient patient

Toxoplasma infection in these patients can result either from either primary infection or by reactivation of latent infection. The newly acquired primary infection should always be treated even when signs or symptoms are absent. When the reactivation of infection is diagnosed, treatment should be started. Quiescent latent infection without signs or symptoms is usually not treated in the immunodeficient patient. Prophylaxis against the reactivation of latent infection is indicated in patients with AIDS who are positive for toxoplasma antibody because of their extremely high risk for reactivation of infection.

The treatment of toxoplasmosis in the immunodeficient patient is divided into three phases: primary prevention (e.g. a patient with AIDS positive for toxoplasma antibody, but who has never had active toxoplasmosis), acute phase (i. e. acute signs and symptoms of infection) and the maintenance or suppressive phase (for patients who have suffered an episode of toxoplasmosis). Treatment recommendations are summarized in Tables 13.1, 13.2 and 13.3 respectively.

For the acute phase, the standard regimen is a combination of pyrimethamine and sulphonamide, although studies have shown that the combination of pyri-

Table 13.1. Treatment of acute toxoplasmic encephalitis in patients with AIDS[1]

Regimen[2]	Dose
I. Pyrimethamine	200 mg oral load, then 75–100 mg orally four times per day
+ sulphadiazine (triple sulphas)	1–2 gm orally four times per day
II. Pyrimethamine	see above
+ clindamycin	60 mg orally/i.v. 6 hourly
III. Pyrimethamine	see above
+ clarithromycin	1 gm orally twice per day
IV. Pyrimethamine	see above
+ azithromycin	1200–1500 mg orally four times per day
V. Pyrimethamine	see above
+ dapsone	100 mg orally four times per day

[1]Treatment of acute encephalitis is for at least 6–8 weeks, until signs and symptoms controlled, followed by life-long maintenance therapy.
[2]Regimens I and II are preferred. Two agents should be used, including pyrimethamine if possible. When pyrimethamine is used, folinic acid, usually 10–15 mg orally four times per day, should be added. Other agents are discussed in the text and include trimethoprim–sulphamethoxazole, atovaquone, 5-fluorouracil, trimetrexate, and doxycycline.

methamine and clindamycin will produce similar clinical results for toxoplasmic encephalitis in patients with AIDS (Danneman et al. 1992; Katlama et al. 1992). Pyrimethamine can be loaded at 100 mg orally twice a day, on the first day followed by 50–75 mg orally per day. Sulphadiazine or trisulphapyrimidines are administered at 4–8 g orally per day in four divided doses. Folinic acid at 10 mg orally four times a day, but up to 50 mg per day, is usually added to counteract the antifolate activities in host cells of the pyrimethamine–sulphonamide combination. Folic acid cannot be used since it will counteract the anti-*T. gondii* activity of pyrimethamine. Treatment is continued for at least 3–6 weeks when acute signs and symptoms of infection should be controlled.

In patients without AIDS the course of treatment is frequently continued for 6 months or longer but is usually terminated when the disease is controlled and the immune system is stable, with little risk of relapse of toxoplasmosis (Carey et al. 1973; Ruskin & Remington 1976; Hakes & Armstrong 1983). For patients with AIDS, whose immune system deteriorates steadily, treatment is life-long to prevent relapse. A common regimen for patients with AIDS, toxoplasmic encephalitis and a response to highly active anti-HIV regimens, it is not known whether suppressive treatment can be discontinued, but prudence dictates continuing the suppressive treatment until good clinical data indicate that treatment

Table 13.2. Maintenance treatment of toxoplasmic encephalitis

Regimen	Dose
I. Pyrimethamine	25–50 mg orally four times per day
+ sulphadiazine	0.5–1.0 g orally four times per day
II. Pyrimethamine	see above
+ clindamycin	300–450 mg orally three times per day, four times per day
III. Pyrimethamine	25 mg orally twice weekly
+ sulphadiazine	0.5 g orally four times per day twice weekly

Treatment is continued for life. Folinic acid is used with pyrimethamine, usually 10 mg orally four times per day. In regimen III, folinic acid was used at 15 mg twice weekly. Regimens I and III are effective at preventing *Pneumocystis carinii* pneumonia. Regimen III is less effective than regimen I and probably regimen II.

Table 13.3. Prophylaxis to prevent a first episode of toxoplasmic encephalitis in patients with AIDS

Regimen	Dose
I. Trimethoprim–sulphamethoxazole	One double strength tablet orally four times per day
II. Pyrimethamine	50 mg orally four times per day
+ dapsone	60 mg orally four times per day
III. Pyrimethamine	25 mg orally twice weekly
+ dapsone	100 mg orally once or twice weekly

Folinic acid is used with pyrimethamine, usually 10 mg orally four times per day when pyrimethamine is used daily, and 15 mg orally with each dose of pyrimethamine when the latter is administered once or twice weekly.

can be stopped or modified. A common regimen for maintenance therapy is pyrimethamine at 25–50 mg per day in combination with sulphadiazine at 2 g orally per day, with use of folinic acid.

Use of pyrimethamine and sulphadiazine in patients with AIDS has proved effective as 80–90% of patients respond. However, this regimen is toxic for up to 40% of patients and that has necessitated the evaluation of other agents, most notably clindamycin. A randomized but un-blinded study (Danneman et al. 1992) of 56 patients compared pyrimethamine in combination with either sulphadiazine or clindamycin for the treatment of acute but clinically diagnosed cases of toxoplasmic encephalitis for 6 weeks. The respective doses were pyrimethamine, 200 mg loading dose then 75 mg/day; sulphadiazine, 100 mg/kg up to 8 g/day; clindamycin, 1200 mg i. v. every 6 hours for 3 weeks, followed by oral clindamycin at 300 mg every 6 hours or 450 mg every 8 hours. The two treatment arms yielded very similar results, but patients treated with pyrimethamine and sulphadiazine exhibited trends toward greater survival but slower defervescence and less complete radiological responses. Toxicity was more common in patients treated with sulphadiazine, especially thrombocytopenia (Haverkos 1987; Danneman et al. 1992).

A much larger European study (Katlama et al. 1992) of 299 patients compared patients treated with either pyrimethamine (50 mg/day) combined with sulphadiazine (4 g/day) or with pyrimethamine (50 mg/day) and clindamycin (2.4 g/day orally). The treatment results were similar between the two arms, but more than half of the crossovers from the pyrimethamine and clindamycin arm were for 'clinical worsening', suggesting that pyrimethamine and clindamycin might be less effective than pyrimethamine and sulphadiazine. The relatively slow clinical response and observed mortality raise the issue of whether superior results could be achieved with all three agents, pyrimethamine, sulphadiazine and clindamycin in combination, but this problem has not been studied.

There are few data that rigorously examine other agents in the treatment of toxoplasmosis in the immunocompetent patient. Anecdotal data indicate that available single agents are not likely to be reliable for treatment of acute toxoplasmosis in the immunodeficient. In general, if regimens other than pyrimethamine with sulphonamide or clindamycin are used, a combination should be used that includes pyrimethamine whenever possible.

The combination of pyrimethamine with dapsone (100 mg/day) has been used in patients who are either intolerant of, or failed to respond to, pyrimethamine and sulphadiazine (Subauste et al. 1997). Azithromycin is being evaluated for the treatment, suppression and prophylaxis of toxoplasmic encephalitis. Doses of 900 mg, 1200 mg and 1500 mg per day orally are being used in combination with pyrimethamine for acute toxoplasmic encephalitis. Azithromycin in one report (Lane et al. 1994) was disappointing at a dose of 1200 mg daily, since two patients exhibited progressive disease after 2 weeks of treatment, thus raising doubts as to its efficacy as a single agent and suggesting that the dose of 1500 mg per day might be prudent to treat acute disease. In another report, azithromycin at a dose of 500 mg per day failed in two patients (Wynn et al. 1993).

Clarithromycin at 1 g orally twice per day was used in combination with pyrimethamine (75 mg/day) for 6 weeks with some success in an uncontrolled study of 13 patients with acute toxoplasmic encephalitis (Fernandez-Martin et al. 1992). Eight patients responded, as shown radiographically and clinically, two withdrew from the study voluntarily and three due to toxicity. Adverse events were common and included severe thrombocytopaenia, liver toxicity, hearing loss, rash, nausea and vomiting.

Trimethoprim–sulphamethoxazole, widely used for the prophylaxis and treatment of *Pneumocystis carinii* pneumonia especially in patients with AIDS, anecdotally has been used successfully to treat acute toxoplasmic encephalitis (Subauste et al. 1997) at a dose of 20 mg/kg per day (trimethoprim component). The adverse effects of trimethoprim–sulphamethoxazole are well known and include hepatitis, rashes including Stevens–Johnson syndrome, hyponatraemia and bone marrow suppression.

Atovaquone (BW566C80) is a hydroxynapthoquinone that appears to be cidal to toxoplasma cysts (Huskinson-Mark et al. 1991; Araujo et al. 1992) and is used to treat and prevent *Pneumocystis carinii* pneumonia. A European group (Clumeck et al. 1992) treated 28 patients with mild cerebral toxoplasmic encephalitis using atovaquone at 750 mg orally four times per day for 6 weeks. The disease progressed in four (14%) patients, as shown radiologically or clinically, and they subsequently responded to pyrimethamine and sulphadiazine. Adverse effects were common, including liver toxicity, rash and gastrointestinal disturbance. In a United States study (Kovacs and the NIAID Clinical Centre Intramural AIDS Program 1992), eight patients with toxoplasmic encephalitis who were either intolerant or had failed standard therapies were treated with atovaquone at 750 mg orally four times per day indefinitely. Evaluation at week 6 found that seven patients had improved radiographically and one remained stable. Five patients died at weeks 16–60 without evidence of toxoplasmosis. The same dose of atovaquone was used as salvage therapy, due to either intolerance to other agents or clinical failure, for 93 patients with toxoplasmic encephalitis (Torres et al. 1997). Clinical and radiological improvements at week 6 were 52% and 37% respectively, and at week 18 the respective improvements were 26% and 15%. The patients who had large trough plasma atovaquone concentrations ($\geq$18.5 µg/ml) responded much better than patients with small trough concentrations ($\leq$8.6 µg/ml).

Trimetrexate, related to methotrexate, inhibits toxoplasma dihydrofolate reductase much more potently than trimethoprim, and is used to treat *Pneumocystis carinii* pneumonia. Trimetrexate initially appeared effective for toxoplasmic encephalitis, but patients suffered relapses while receiving the drug (Gluckstein & Ruskin 1995). Folinic acid must be used with trimetrexate.

A small series of 16 patients with 19 episodes of toxoplasmic encephalitis, reported in a letter (Dhiver et al. 1993), examined the use of 5-flourouracil at a dose of 1.5 mg/kg per day and clindamycin at 1.8–4.8 g/day for the treatment of cerebral toxoplasmosis, both as initial treatment and as secondary treatment prompted by the adverse consequences of pyrimethamine and sulphadiazine therapy. 5-Flourourcil has activity *in vitro* against toxoplasma (Harris et al. 1988). Success was reported for all but one patient with few adverse effects (rash in three patients and haematological toxicity in one patient). Forty-eight days was the longest reported treatment course.

Drug-induced toxicity is a common management problem. The combinations of pyrimethamine–sulphonamide or pyrimethamine–clindamycin are strongly preferred to other regimens unless toxicity is intolerable. Folinic acid should be used routinely, at doses up to 50 mg/day to prevent bone marrow depression. The role of recombinant colony stimulating factors is unknown. Gastrointestinal intolerance can be addressed symptomatically or by evaluation for coexisting infection or pathology, e.g. *Helicobacter pylori, Mycobacterium avium-intracellulare,* peptic ulcer disease and pancreatitis. In a European trial (Katlama et al. 1992) comparing pyrimethamine and sulphadiazine with pyrimethamine and clindamycin, two patients treated with clindamycin died of *Clostridium difficile* pseudomembranous colitis.

Rash is very common in patients receiving pyrimethamine–sulphonamide; and in the aforementioned un-blinded European trial (Katlama et al. 1992) two patients treated with pyrimethamine–sulphonamide died of acute epidermolysis. Rash is not necessarily due to the sulphonamide. In this trial, 29% of patients receiving pyrimethamine and clindamycins suffered a rash compared with 39% of those receiving pyrimethamine and sulphadiazine. Whether to continue treatment in the presence of a rash is a matter of clinical judgement. In this same trial, most patients treated with pyrimethamine and clindamycin who suffered a rash did not have their treatment with these agents discontinued. Several desensitization protocols for trimethoprim–sulphamethoxazole have been published (Bell 1985; Smith et al. 1987; Gluckstein & Ruskin 1995; Piketty et al. 1995; Sande et al. 1998), the protocols vary in length from several hours to several days.

Crystalluria is a well-recognized complication of sulphonamide therapy, especially with sulphadiazine, and can cause haematuria and acute renal failure (Nissen et al. 1950; Goadsby et al. 1987; Carbone et al. 1988; Sahai et al. 1988; Oster et al. 1990). Typical crystals can be seen by microscopic examination of urine. Treatment is primarily hydration and urine alkalinization. The sulphonamide can be continued despite crystalluria, although hydration needs to be assured. Triple sulphonamides are less likely to cause crystalluria than sulphadiazine, since the solubility of each sulphonamide is independent of that of the others.

The role of corticosteroids has not been defined precisely but they are frequently used to control intracranial hypertension and oedema due to encephalitis. Corticosteroids do not appear to affect survival significantly, or affect proportion of survival significantly (Luft et al. 1984). Corticosteroids may hinder the evaluation of response to treatment, since clinical and radiographical responses may be observed with corticosteroids alone, and may also hinder the detection of toxoplasma lesions on computed tomography (CT) scan even when contrast is used. Seizures are common in toxoplasmic encephalitis and anticonvulsants are commonly used to prevent them. Because of the adverse effects including rashes and problems with drug interactions common to anticonvulsants, it may be wiser to use anticonvulsants only to treat established seizure disorders (Cohn et al. 1989).

A vexing issue is whether and/or when to perform a brain biopsy when a patient possibly has toxoplasmic encephalitis. Brain biopsies are morbid, expensive, require special expertise/equipment, can present an enormous burden to a system that serves many patients with AIDS and may not provide treatment-altering information. The differential diagnosis of space-occupying lesions in patients with AIDS is broad and includes infections with toxoplasma, mycobacteria, bacteria, viruses and fungi, as well as neoplasms, especially lymphomas and Kaposi's sarcoma. The relative likelihood of each disease depends on the patient population served, e.g. the population-based infection rate with *M. tuberculosis* or toxoplasma, as well as medical care strategies and execution, e.g. screening and prophylaxis practices. Thus, each medical system needs to develop an approach to treat space-occupying lesions in the brain in patients with AIDS.

A detailed flow diagram, appropriate for medical centres in the United States, has been proposed by Luft and Remington (1992). In brief, immediate brain biopsy is warranted for patients with *T. gondii* antibody with CD4 counts less than 200/μl and single lesions on magnetic resonance imaging (MRI) scan (which is a more sensitive technique than the CT scan for detecting toxoplasmic brain abcesses). At the initial evaluation of a patient with AIDS, especially if they have a very low CD4 count, factors to consider are whether the patient's serum has toxoplasma antibody and whether the radiological studies (CT or MRI) are typical of toxoplasmic encephalitis. If the serum is negative for toxoplasma antibody, then toxoplasmic encephalitis is unlikely but not completely eliminated. If no other diagnosis is considered reasonable, then a biopsy should be performed if technically feasible. On CT scanning, toxoplasmic encephalitis typically presents as multiple ring-enhancing hypodense lesions at the corticomedullary interface and in the basal ganglia. A patient positive for toxoplasma antibody and with such a scan is usually considered to have toxoplasmic encephalitis and an empirical treatment trial is reasonable. If the CT scan is not typical of toxoplasmic encephalitis, then a MRI scan is recommended. The MRI scan can demonstrate masses not demonstrated on CT scan (Levy et al. 1985; Kupfer et al. 1987), and if multiple enhancing lesions are demonstrated then empirical treatment is reasonable. If only a single lesion is demonstrated, especially by MRI, then a diagnosis other than toxoplasmic encephalitis needs to be considered and biopsy should be considered.

If empirical treatment is undertaken, quick clinical improvement, as assessed by neurological examination in a study of patients treated with pyrimethamine and clindamycin, is expected (Luft et al. 1993). Of 47 patients, 18 improved by day 3 of treatment, 30 by day 7, and 32 by day 14. Hence the large majority of patients who were to respond did so by day 7. Twelve patients did not respond clinically; two were biopsied and found to have lymphoma. Four of the remaining ten patients were considered 'treatment failures', one proved by biopsy, and two by response to pyrimethamine and sulphadiazine. Hence if the patient has a neurological examination that allows the assessment of improvement, and if no improvement is observed by day 7, biopsy should be considered. In the same study, radiological improvement appeared to lag clinical improvement, but the majority responded by week 3 of treatment.

Differentiation of toxoplasmic encephalitis from neoplasia may be aided by new imaging techniques. Positron emission tomographic (PET) brain scanning with 2-fluorodeoxyglucose in patients with AIDS and contrast enhancing lesions on CT or MRI scans can accurately differentiate between toxoplasmic encephalitis (hypometabolic lesions) and lymphoma (hypermetabolic) (Pierce et al. 1995; Villringer et al. 1995). Progressive multifocal leukoencephalopathy (PML) presented hypermetabolic lesions with PET scanning in this study. Another study (Lorberboym et al. 1996) yielded similar results with thallium-201 SPECT scanning.

Toxoplasma primarily causes encephalitis in patients with AIDS, but it has been recovered from many other organs, especially the lungs (usually with symmetrical lung infiltrates on chest radiographs), blood, pancreas, gastrointestinal tract, eye, heart, lymph nodes, testes and liver (Rabaud et al. 1996). Lung involvement and the detection of toxoplasma organism in the blood portends a poor prognosis. Treatment regimens for extra-CNS toxoplasmosis have not been evaluated critically, but pyrimethamine combined with sulphonamide is recommended.

A relapse of toxoplasmic encephalitis occurs in at least 50% of patients when there is no maintenance or suppressive chemotherapy, and the relapse is often demonstrable radiographically at the side of previous lesions (Haverkos 1987). Maintenance therapy is plagued by patient intolerance and noncompliance, and poorly controlled studies regarding efficacy and tolerability. The combination of pyrimethamine (25–50 mg/day) and sulphonamide (2–4 g/day) appears to be the most effective and is the current standard for maintenance therapy. Limited data suggest that pyrimethamine (25 mg) and sulphadiazine (75 mg/kg or 4–8 g/day) administered twice weekly might be effective compared with historical controls, but were less effective than when pyrimethamine and sulphadiazine were administered daily (Pedrol et al. 1990). In this study, by 12 months, relapse had occurred in 6% and 30% of patients, respectively, receiving daily compared with biweekly pyrimethamine and sulphadiazine. Of considerable practical importance is that the combination of pyrimethamine and sulphonamide also effectively prevents *Pneumocystis carinii* pneumonia.

Clindamycin can be substituted for sulphonamide at 300–450 mg 6 hourly to 8 hourly in the daily regimen if sulphonamide is not tolerated (Israelski & Remington 1988; Remington et al. 1991; Luft et al. 1993). Pyrimethamine combined with clindamycin does not prevent *Pneumocystis carinii* pneumonia. Pyrimethamine has been used as a single agent without reliable success, and doses as high as 100 mg/day may be needed if that option is chosen (Maslo et al. 1992). Fansidar™, a pyrimethamine and sulphadoxine combination that has a long serum half-life, might be effective when administered biweekly for suppression. However, relapses (Israelski & Remington 1988) and severe side-effects, including Stevens–Johnson syndrome and toxic epidermal necrolysis, have occurred with this regimen. Pyrimethamine (50 mg per week) combined with dapsone (50 mg per day) appeared effective as primary prophylaxis (see below) but more data are needed with this regimen for maintenance therapy (Girard et al. 1993).

The usefulness of the newer macrolides for maintenance therapy remains to be determined but the use of only a single agent, in the absence of strong data, is discouraged. If used, the macrolide should probably be used in combination with pyrimethamine until data supporting other regimens are available. The macrolides have the advantage of providing prophylaxis, and they are also a component of the treatment regimen for *Mycobacterium avium-intracellulare* infection.

The management of patients who suffer relapses of toxoplasmic encephalitis has not been examined critically. Options include the use of high doses of the standard combination of pyrimethamine and sulphonamide, or the use of agents not previously used, but which, given limited available data, are considered less potent than the combination of pyrimethamine and sulphonamide. The antimicrobial resistance of toxoplasma has not been discovered clinically, although the primary resistance of toxoplasma and the development of resistance during therapy have been largely unexplored. Developing appropriate *in vitro* systems has been difficult. Agents that are effective *in vivo* are ineffective in some *in vitro* systems (Harris et al. 1988). Mutants resistant to antitoxoplasma agents can be selected *in vitro* (Ricketts & Pfefferkorn 1993; Pfefferkorn & Borotz 1994), but the development of resistance clinically has not been documented or frequently sought (Cazenave et al. 1992). Strains of *T. gondii* differ regarding their tropism, virulence and susceptibility to antimicrobial agents (Suzuki et al. 1989*a*). These properties are not measured in the clinical setting and are not used in patient management.

Prophylaxis to prevent toxoplasmic encephalitis is commonly used for high-risk groups, especially patients with AIDS and heart transplant recipients. Prophylaxis has been used successfully for mismatched heart transplant recipients, i.e. those who are antibody-negative receiving a heart from an antibody-positive donor (Hakim et al. 1986; Wreghitt et al. 1989). Although toxoplasmic encephalitis afflicts 25–50% of *T. gondii*-antibody-positive patients with AIDS, few well-designed comparative trials have been conducted to determine the efficacy and tolerability of prophylactic regimens. Prophylaxis to prevent an initial episode of toxoplasmosis differs from suppressing toxoplasmosis that has been evident clinically; the latter situation is variably termed suppressive, secondary prophylactic, or maintenance therapy. Toxicity, intolerance and inconvenience are less likely to be acceptable to the patient and physician for primary prophylaxis. Beaman and Remington (1992) summarized the situation by stating that most prophylactic regimens have been shown to have some efficacy, but it is doubtful that monotherapy with existing agents will be reliably effective. Prophylaxis is reviewed by Richards et al. (1995).

A double-blind, placebo-controlled trial compared pyrimethamine at 25 mg orally three times a week with clindamycin at 300 mg orally twice per day (Jacobson et al. 1992, 1994) for patients with toxoplasma antibody and CD4 lymphocyte counts less than 200/μl. The clindamycin arm of the trial was stopped prematurely due to unacceptable toxicity, primarily diarrhoea in 31% and rash in 21% of 52 treated patients. Toxicity in the pyrimethamine and placebo arms was minimal. Mortality was significantly higher among patients receiving pyrimethamine compared with placebo in this study, but increased mortality was not observed in another study of prophylactic pyrimethamine. Toxoplasmic encephalitis was rare in both the pyrimethamine and placebo arms, probably due to common use of trimethoprim–sulphamethoxazole for *Pneumocystis carinii* pneumonia prophylaxis. Thus available data suggest that pyrimethamine at 25 mg per week and three times a week appears ineffective (Leport et al. 1993; Mallolas et al. 1993; Jacobson et al. 1994), especially if patients are receiving trimethoprim–sulphamethoxazole. This is possibly due, at least in part, to the confounding prophylactic effect of trimethoprim–sulphamethoxazole against *T. gondii*.

Several studies have indicated that trimethoprim–sulphamethoxazole is effective prophylaxis for toxoplasmic encephalitis. Trimethoprim–sulphamethoxazole is a very attractive prophylactic agent since it is inexpensive, convenient and very effective prophylaxis for *Pneumocystis carinii* pneumonia as well as that caused by other pathogens, e.g. *Streptococcus pneumoniae*, *Staphylococcus aureus*, *Nocardia* spp., *Listeria monocytogenes*. An Australian study (Carr et al. 1992) retrospectively compared trimethoprim–sulphamethoxazole at 160 mg trimethoprim/800 mg sulphamethoxazole twice a day twice a week with aerosolized pentamidine for prophylaxis of pneumocystis pneumonia. None of 22 *T. gondii*-positive patients who received trimethoprim–sulphamethoxazole developed toxoplasmic encephalitis compared with 14 (39%) of 36 seropositive patients in the aerosolized pentamidine group. Studies of similar design support these results (Carr et al. 1992; Leport et al. 1993), and doses used for prophylaxis of *Pneumocystis carinii* pneumonia appear effective for the prophylaxis of toxoplasmic encephalitis.

Hypersensitivity, especially rash attributed to trimethoprim–sulphamethoxazole, is its major drawback. Continuation of treatment despite the rash, possibly with concomitant steroids or desensitization of the patient to sulphonamides, has been successful. Desensitization protocols range from quick (less than 1 day) to very slow (about 1 month) (Bell et al. 1985; Smith et al. 1987). Oral trimethoprim–sulphamethoxazole has been used safely in patients who appeared to suffer hypersensitivity reactions when given intravenous trimethoprim–sulphamethoxazole (Shafer et al. 1989).

Dapsone and pyrimethamine act synergistically against *T. gondii* (Derouin et al. 1991; Gatti et al. 1997) and the combination is effective prophylaxis for *Pneumocystis carinii* pneumonia. Several studies have examined this combination for toxoplasmic encephalitis. A combination of dapsone at 100 mg and pyrimethamine at 25 mg, each administered weekly, is about as effective as trimethoprim–sulphamethoxazole, three times a week (Dunn et al. 1997). Dapsone and pyrimethamine, administered twice weekly at 100 mg and 25 mg respectively, completely prevented toxoplasmic encephalitis in a group of 109 patients, 50% of whom were positive for toxoplasma antibody (Clotet et al. 1991). However, another trial (Girard et al. 1993) suggested incomplete efficacy. Dapsone prescribed at 50 mg daily and pyrimethamine at 50 mg weekly resulted in 11% of patients developing toxoplasmic encephalitis, significantly better results than achieved by the aerosolized pentamidine control group. Trimethoprim–sulphamethoxazole (one double strength tablet twice a day three times a week) appears to be about as effective as pyrimethamine (25 mg/week) combined with dapsone (100 mg/week), but in this study trimethoprim–sulphamethoxazole was better at preventing *Pneumocystis carinii* pneumonia (Podzamczer et al. 1993). Administering pyrimethamine at 25 mg twice weekly and dapsone at 100 mg twice weekly might be more effective than once weekly administration (Clotet et al. 1991; Richards et al. 1995).

Fansidar™ (pyrimethamine–sulphadoxine) has been used at regimens of three tablets every 2 weeks and one tablet biweekly (Subauste et al. 1997). As noted above, severe hypersensitivity reactions plague the use of Fansidar™.

The macrolides have been little studied. Roxithromycin at 300 mg three times a week was significantly more effective than control (aerosolized pentamidine) in the prevention of toxoplasmic encephalitis and mycobacterial infections (Durant et al. 1992). Drug-related adverse effects, especially hepatitis and gastrointestinal disturbances, were more common with roxithromycin.

Clarithromycin, when used singly, appeared ineffective at preventing toxoplasmic encephalitis. Ten patients, including eight positive for toxoplasma antibody, were treated for *M. avium-intracellulare* infection with clarithromycin (2 g/day) and other agents. Three patients developed toxoplasmic encephalitis after 6, 9 and 69 days of clarithromycin treatment. The 30% (or 38% using toxoplasma positives as the at-risk group) incidence of toxoplasmic encephalitis is high and perhaps no different than the incidence expected in untreated controls. In another study (Raffi et al. 1995), toxoplasmic encephalitis occurred despite the use of clarithromycin for *M. avium-intracellulare.*

Toxoplasmic encephalitis, in common with most opportunistic infections in patients with AIDS, strikes when the CD4 count is less than 200/μl, with the risk increasing as the CD4 count decreases. The exact CD4 count at which to start prophylaxis for toxoplasmic encephalitis is not clear, but counts of 100 cells/μl have been proposed as reasonable (Jacobson et al. 1994; USPHS/IDSA 1997) for patients who are toxoplasma antibody positive. Clinical data regarding prophylaxis in patients who have had low CD4 counts that have risen to levels greater than the aforementioned cut-offs with use of highly active antiretroviral therapy remain to be gathered and reported.

Treatment of infection in organ transplant recipients is reviewed more extensively in Chapter 6. Toxoplasmosis frequently mimics transplant rejection and/or the signs or symptoms may be attributed to other disease processes, and so clinical suspicion must be stimulated for diagnosis. All biopsy specimens should be examined for toxoplasma and serum obtained to detect seroconversion. Therapy with pyrimethamine and sulphadiazine is effective when started early, and it might be prudent to start therapy when seroconversion is detected. Signs and symptoms may not appear until months after seroconversion (Luft et al. 1983).

For heart transplants, a high-risk group for toxoplasmosis can be identified and, since intense immunosuppression is relatively short, prophylaxis for toxoplasmosis is conceptually attractive. At Papworth Hospital, UK, 21 *T. gondii*-antibody-positive patients received transplants from *T. gondii*-antibody-positive donors (Wreghitt et al. 1989). Four (57%) of the first seven patients developed toxoplasmosis within 20–32 days after transplantation. Pyrimethamine then was administered at 25 mg/day for 6 weeks after transplantation to the subsequent 14 high-risk patients, and only 2 (14%) developed toxoplasmosis.

Primary maternal toxoplasma infection in pregnancy

Treatment of pregnant woman with primary toxoplasma infection has two goals: to prevent infection of the foetus by blocking transmission of toxoplasma across the placenta, and to treat the infected foetus when such infection is diagnosed. Although data are not definitive (Wong & Remington 1994; Remington et al. 1995), spiramycin appears to prevent transmission across the placenta, which occurs after a clinically significant lag period that allows diagnosis and initiation of treatment, but is ineffective treatment for the infected foetus. Pyrimethamine combined with sulphadiazine appears to be an effective treatment for the infected foetus, but such treatment is much more toxic and inconvenient than spiramycin. Furthermore, pyrimethamine, due to concerns about teratogenicity, should not be used in the first trimester and there is concern about using pyrimethamine before 18 weeks of gestation.

Spiramycin (3 g/day in three divided doses) can be used throughout pregnancy if the foetus is judged not to be infected. Use of spiramycin has been associated with a 60% reduction in the incidence of congenital toxoplasmosis (Remington et al. 1995). If the foetus is determined to be infected, pyrimethamine (50 mg/day) combined with sulphadiazine (4 g/day) is recommended, with folinic acid at 10–20 mg/day. Since pyrimethamine is potentially teratogenic in the first trimester, either spiramycin or sulphadiazine is used as a single agent during the first trimester. For foetal infection some French experts alternate 3-week courses of pyrimethamine and sulphonamide, with 3-week courses of spiramycin until term. Folinic acid is added to avert the toxicity of pyrimethamine and sulphonamide, and blood counts, including platelets, need to be monitored closely. Bone marrow suppression is usually easily reversed with increased dosages of folinic acid and/or interruption of treatment with pyrimethamine and sulphadiazine, with resumption when toxicity has abated (Boyer 1996).

An example of a successful approach to preventing congenital toxoplasmosis despite acute maternal infection was provided by a French group (Alger 1997), who combined drug treatment with prenatal *in utero* diagnosis in 746 pregnant women with primary infection. Spiramycin at 3 g/day was administered as soon as maternal infection was suspected or diagnosed, and treatment was continued throughout the pregnancy. If toxoplasma infection was diagnosed in the foetus, then pyrimethamine (50 mg/day), sulphadiazine (3 g/day), and folinic acid were administered to the mother for 3 weeks alternating with 3 weeks of spiramycin (3 g/day). With this approach, the percentage of infants severely damaged by toxoplasmosis was reduced from 21% (historical control) to 2%. Alternatively, a few women who had toxoplasmosis diagnosed in their foetus received daily spiramycin (3 g/day) and the combination of pyrimethamine (25 mg) and sulphadoxine (1500 mg) (Fansidar™) every 10 days until delivery.

Diagnosis of *in utero* infection has already been discussed. A foetus at risk is identified by diagnosing infection acquired during pregnancy. If maternal infection is diagnosed, then a sonogram can be obtained to detect microcephaly, calcifications, hydrops, or placental thickening. The sonogram will be suggestive of infection in approximately 30–40% of cases of congenital toxoplasmosis (Daffos et al. 1988; Hohlfeld et al. 1994). If normal or if diagnosis is uncertain, foetal blood can be obtained by cordocentesis to measure toxoplasma IgM, IgA and IgE, white blood cell and differential counts, platelet count and gamma-glutamyltransferase. Studies based on cordocentesis blood can detect 90% of infected foetuses. Amniocentesis is safer, more available, and polymerase chain reaction assays can be applied to amniotic fluid, quickly giving sensitive and specific results. However, quality control of polymerase chain reaction testing is a concern (Guy et al. 1996). Infection of the foetus can occur after the above tests have been done, probably due to the incompletely protective effect of the placenta. Serial ultrasounds can be done at 2- to 4-week intervals.

Data concerning concurrent HIV and latent toxoplasma infection in pregnant women are scant (Wong & Remington 1994). Toxoplasma infection can reactivate and be transmitted across the placenta but the risk appears to be low. Infected infants are also usually infected with HIV (Minkoff et al. 1997). It is not clear what treatment should be offered, if any, to a pregnant woman infected with both HIV and toxoplasma. Consideration should be given to spiramycin during the first trimester and the combination of pyrimethamine and sulphadiazine in the second and third trimesters, especially if there is evidence of advanced immunosuppression.

Congenital toxoplasmosis

All infants with congenital toxoplasmosis should be treated. The superiority of a particular regimen has not been established. The guidelines of Couvreur from Paris (Remington et al. 1995) have long served as a reasonable base for therapeutic decisions. Treatment is for 1 year, by which time the infant should have an immune system capable of controlling the infection. Treatment appears effective for the prevention of recurrent eye lesions, sensorineural hearing loss and neurodevelopmental handicaps.

Pyrimethamine combined with sulphadiazine is the cornerstone of therapy. For severe disease, Couvreur recommends pyrimethamine (2 mg/kg per day for 2 days, then 1 mg/kg per day) and sulphadiazine (100 mg/kg per day in two divided doses) for the first 6 months followed by monthly alternation with spiramycin (100 mg/kg per day). In subclinical infection, a combination of pyrimethamine and sulphadiazine is used for the first 6 weeks, followed by monthly alternation with spiramycin. Folinic acid at 5 mg 3 days per week is used with pyrimethamine plus sulphadiazine, and the dose is increased to 10 mg when the infant reaches 1 month of age, weighs 4.5 kg, or neutropaenia develops (750–900/mm^3). Pyrimethamine has been given at 1 mg/kg three times per week for the last 6–10 months of the course (McAuley et al. 1994).

Clinicians may decide to use pyrimethamine and sulphadiazine for the entire treatment course since spiramycin might not be as good at treating central nervous system disease. In the Chicago Collaborative Treatment Trial (McAuley et al. 1994), pyrimethamine was administered as a loading dose of 2mg/kg per day for 2 days, then 1 mg/kg per day each day for 2–6 months, then as 1mg/kg per day three times

Table 13.4. Treatment of congenital toxoplasmosis

Regimen	Dose
I. Pyrimethamine	2 mg/kg per day orally four times per day for 2 days, then 1 mg/kg per day for 6 months, then thrice weekly
+ sulphadiazine	100 mg/kg per day orally (two divided doses)
+ folinic acid	5–10 mg orally thrice weekly
II. Spiramycin	100 mg/kg per day orally (two divided doses)

Spiramycin is considered less effective than pyrimethamine and sulphadiazine for toxoplasma encephalitis and so regimen I is preferred for all overt cases of congenital toxoplasmosis. For subclinical cases, consideration can be given to starting streatment with regimen I for 6 weeks, then 6 weeks of spiramycin alternated with 4 weeks of regimen I. Treatment is until 12 months of age in all cases. Corticosteroids in high dosages (e.g. prednisolone 1–1.5 mg/kg per day orally in two divided doses are administered if retinochoroiditis, CSF protein >100 mg/dl, or severe disease is diagnosed, and then tapered over a 3-week period after disease is controlled.

per week. Sulphadiazine was administered at 100 mg/kg per day in two divided doses. Folinic acid was given at 5–10 mg three times per week, sometimes 5–20 mg daily due to neutropaenia. The dose was increased routinely to 10 mg three times per week when the infant reached 1 month of age or weighed more than 4.5 kg. The entire treatment regimen usually lasts 12 months but treatment for children with AIDS will probably need to be life-long. Treatment recommendations are summarized in Table 13.4.

The preparation and administration of pyrimethamine, sulphadiazine and folinic acid to infants can be difficult and a detailed programme has been published (McAuley et al. 1994). Pyrimethamine and sulphadiazine are available as suspensions and concentrations can be adjusted so that the volume ingested of each is one-half the infant's weight in kilograms. Folinic acid is administered as a crushed tablet given with formula, apple juice or cereal.

The major treatment-related toxicity is neutropaenia, and neutrophil counts should be measured twice weekly by heel-stick, with monthly measurements of platelet and haemoglobin levels. Blood counts should be followed frequently, e.g. twice weekly by heel-stick. Neutropaenia (less than 900/mm^3) occurred in 58% of infants in one series. Viral infections may promote neutropaenia. In the Chicago Collaborative Treatment Trial protocol (McAuley et al. 1994), when the absolute neutrophil count is less than 500/mm^3, pyrimethamine is withheld and folinic acid is increased to 10–20 mg/day until the neutrophil count is more than 1000/mm^3 for several weeks. Cell counts can be measured once per week. Significant anaemia or thrombocytopaenia occurred in 5.4% of patients (McAuley et al. 1994). It is recommended that folinic acid should be stopped 1 week after the discontinuation of pyrimethamine.

As for adults, adequate hydration is necessary to prevent crystalluria and renal failure due to sulphadiazine. No data are available to critically evaluate clindamycin, but it is expected to be efficacious if the combination of pyrimethamine and sulphadiazine cannot be tolerated.

CSF shunting procedures may be needed to relieve hydrocephalus. Prednisolone at a dose of 1mg/kg in two daily divided doses is recommended for infants with elevated CSF protein levels ($\geq$ 1 g/dl) or for active retinitis that threatens vision. The prednisolone is continued until the protein level is reduced to less than 1 g/dl or retinochoroiditis no longer threatens vision, at which time the dosage is tapered over a 3-week period.

Aggressive ophthalmological evaluation, sometimes requiring anaesthesia for adequate examination, is needed, and prednisolone is indicated as above when active retinochoroiditis threatens vision. Retinal detachment can occur. Patching and prismatic or corrective spectacles may be needed (Boyer 1996). Retinochoroiditis may recur later in life after apparently successful treatment. It is recommended that ophthalmological examination should be carried out once a month for 3 months after stopping treatment, then every 3–4 months until the child is mature enough to reliably report visual symptoms, and then every 6 months (McAuley et al. 1994). Toxoplasma serological test titres decline during therapy, but often increase (both IgG and IgM) when therapy is stopped, possibly reflecting renewed tachyzoite proliferation. The clinical significance of this observation is uncertain, but concern regarding the adverse effects of even modest tachyzoite replication on vision indicates compulsive and repeated ophthalmological evaluations.

With intensive therapy in the first year, focal neurological signs often resolve and normal development often occurs. Hydrocephalus, usually due to aqueductal obstruction, can occur during or after therapy. Ventricular enlargement should be sought by appropriate surveillance studies (e.g. head circumference measurements and radiological studies) with consideration given to CSF shunting if hydrocephalus is detected. Seizures can also occur during or after therapy. Phenobarbital may lower the serum concentrations of pyrimethamine in children, possibly by inducing hepatic enzymes that degrade pyrimethamine (McLeod et al. 1992; McAuley et al. 1994). The clinical significance of this observation is uncertain.

Empirical treatment in the neonatal period is frequent, often in anticipation of making a definitive diagnosis by serologically testing the infant. However, serological confirmation or rejection may require months. Hence one must balance the toxicity of the treatment against the likelihood of disease. If the infant appears well, and the diagnosis of congenital toxoplasmosis has not been established but is a realistic possibility (e.g. the mother is known to have acquired infection during pregnancy), then a course of pyrimethamine and sulphadiazine may be followed by spiramycin until the diagnosis is confirmed or refuted. If there is considerable doubt about the diagnosis of congenital toxoplasmosis (e.g. the infant appears well and it is unknown whether the mother acquired toxoplasma infection during pregnancy), spiramycin has been used until a diagnosis is established or refuted.

Ocular toxoplasmosis

Diagnosis is based on the ophthalmological demonstration of retinochoroiditis and the presence of toxoplasma IgG antibody in the serum. In the adult, toxoplasmic retinochoroiditis usually but not always represents the reactivation of previously acquired infection, and the toxoplasma IgM antibody titre is usually negative and the IgG antibody titre is small. Occasionally toxoplasma antibody can only be found in the aqueous humour. In difficult to diagnose cases, the aqueous humour can be studied with polymerase chain reaction to detect toxoplasma, herpes simplex virus, varicella-zoster virus and cytomegalovirus. Polymerase chain reaction studies appear more sensitive in patients with AIDS than in immunocompetent patients (Danise et al. 1997).

One regimen for active toxoplasmic retinochoroiditis is the combination of pyrimethamine and sulphadiazine (75 mg/day and 2 g/day, respectively, in one regimen) (Kaufman & Geisler 1960). Improvement usually occurs within 10 days of starting therapy, which is often administered for 1 month. If signs or symptoms of active infection persist, longer treatment or repeated courses are warranted, or consideration of alternative diagnoses. Treatment may be needed for months in some patients.

Ophthalmologists frequently use clindamycin to avoid the adverse effects attributed to pyrimethamine and sulphadiazine. Clindamycin concentrates highly in the rabbit choroid, iris and retina, and treats rabbit experimental toxoplasmic retinochoroiditis effectively (Tabbara & O'Connor 1975; Lakhanpul et al. 1983). Although the data obtained are essentially uncontrolled, clindamycin at 300 mg orally four times per day appears effective against human toxoplasmic retinochoroiditis, with results comparable to those obtained with pyrimethamine and sulphonamide (Tabbara & O'Connor 1980). Spiramycin is not usually recommended for the treatment of toxoplasmic retinochoroiditis because of high recurrence rates (Canamucio et al. 1963; Ghosh et al. 1965). Systemic corticosteroids are usually given when the macula is threatened.

Summary

Toxoplasma gondii was an under-appreciated cause of infection in both immunocompetent and immunocompromised patients until the AIDS epidemic struck, which thrust toxoplasmic encephalitis and toxoplasma infection into the main-stream of clinical practice. This increased interest in toxoplasma infection and disease (toxoplasmosis) has brought a focus to shortcomings in the diagnosis, treatment and prevention of infection and disease in all groups of patients. Apparently effective treatment regimens are available for each clinical entity of toxoplasma infection, but the lack of well-controlled trials, incomplete clinical efficacy, relatively poor drug potency, drug toxicity, unavailability of drugs, incomplete knowledge of pharmacokinetics and the almost completely unexplored issue of antimicrobial resistance continue to make the treatment of toxoplasmosis an art. Recommended treatment regimens are derived from *in vitro* and animal models and/or clinical practice at medical centres experienced in the treatment of toxoplasma infection. The onslaught of AIDS has allowed the relatively efficient diagnosis of large numbers of patients with toxoplasmic encephalitis, permitting some controlled trials that might benefit patients without AIDS as well. The mainstay of treatment, however, remains the relatively old anti-folate antibiotics, pyrimethamine and sulphadiazine supplemented by folinic acid to prevent marrow suppression. Newer and safer antibiotics, effective against both the tachyzoite and tissue cyst, are urgently required.

REFERENCES

Alger, L. S. (1997). Toxoplasmosis and parvovirus B19. *Infectious Disease Clinics of North America*, 11, 55–75.

Allegra, C. J., Kovacs, J. A., Drake, J. C. et al. (1987). Potent *in vitro* and *in vivo* antitoxoplasma activity of the lipid-soluble antifolate trimetrexate. *Journal of Clinical Investigation*, 79, 478–82.

Araujo, F. G. (1992). Depletion of CD4+ T cells but not inhibition of the protective activity of interferon gamma prevents cure of toxoplasmosis mediated by drug therapy in mice. *Journal of Immunology*, 149, 3003–7.

Araujo, F. G. & Remington, J. S. (1974). Effect of clindamycin on acute and chronic toxoplasmosis in mice. *Antimicrobial Agents and Chemotherapy*, 5, 647–51.

Araujo, F. G., Guptill, D. R. & Remington, J. S. (1987). *In vitro* activity of piritrexim against *Toxoplasma gondii*. *Journal of Infectious Diseases*, 156, 828–30.

Araujo, F. G., Guptill, D. R. & Remington, J. S. (1988). Azithromycin, a macrolide antibiotic with potent activity against *Toxoplasma gondii*. *Antimicrobial Agents and Chemotherapy*, 32, 755–7.

Araujo, F. G., Huskinson-Mark, J., Gutteridge, W. E. & Remington, J. S. (1992). *In vitro* and *in vivo* activities of the hydroxynaphthoquinone 566C80 against the cyst form of *Toxoplasma gondii*. *Antimicrobial Agents and Chemotherapy*, 36, 326–30.

Araujo, F. G., Khan, A. A. & Remington, J. S. (1996). Rifapentine is active *in vitro* and *in vivo* against *Toxoplasma gondii*. *Antimicrobial Agents and Chemotherapy*, 40, 1335–7.

Araujo, F. G., Khan, A. A., Slifer, T. L. et al. (1997). The ketolide antibiotics HMR 3647 and HMR 3004 are active against *Toxoplasma gondii in vitro* and in murine models of infection. *Antimicrobial Agents and Chemotherapy*, 41, 2137–40.

Beaman, M. H. & Remington, J. S. (1992). Prophylaxis for toxoplasmosis in AIDS. *Annals of Internal Medicine*, 117, 163–4.

Beaman, M., Wong, S. Y. & Remington, J. S. (1992). Cytokines, toxoplasma and intracellular parasitism. *Immunological Reviews*, 127, 97–117.

Bell, E. T., Tapper, M. L. & Pollock, A. A. (1985). Sulphadiazine desensitization in AIDS patients. *Lancet*, 1, 163.

Berens, R. L., Krug, E. C., Nash, P. B. & Curiel, T. J. (1998). Selection and characterization of *Toxoplasma gondii* mutants resistant to artemisinin. *Journal of Infectious Diseases*, 177, 1128–31.

Bleehen, N. M., Newman, H. V., Rampling, R. P. et al. (1995). A phase II study of oral piritrexim in recurrent high-grade (III, IV) glioma. *British Journal of Cancer*, 72, 766–8.

Boyer, K. M. (1996). Diagnosis and treatment of congenital toxoplasmosis. *Advances in Pediatric Infectious Diseases*, 11, 449–67.

Canamucio, C. J., Hallett, J. W. & Leopold, I. H. (1963). Recurrence of treated toxoplasmic uveitis. *American Journal of Ophthalmology*, 55, 1035–9.

Carbone, L., Bendixen, B. & Appel, G. (1988). Sulphadiazine-associated obstructive nephropathy occurring in a patient with the acquired immunodeficiency syndrome. *American Journal of Kidney Diseases*, 12, 72–5.

Carey, R. M., Kimball, A. C., Armstrong, D. & Lieberman, P. H. (1973). Toxoplasma: clinical experiences in a cancer hospital. *American Journal of Medicine*, 54, 30–8.

Carr, A., Tindall, B., Brew, B. J. et al. (1992). Low-dose trimethoprim-sulphamethoxazole prophylaxis for toxoplasma encephalitis in patients with AIDS. *Annals of Internal Medicine*, 117, 106–11.

Carroll, O. M., Bryan, P. A. & Robinson, R. J. (1966). Stevens–Johnson syndrome associated with long-acting sulphonamides. *Journal of American Medical Association*, 195, 691–3.

Cazenave, J., Forestier, F., Bessieres, M. et al. (1992). Contribution of a new PCR assay to the prenatal diagnosis of congenital toxoplasmosis. *Prenatal Diagnosis*, 12, 119–27.

Chaisson, R. E., Benson, C., Dub, M. et al. (1994). Clarithromycin therapy for bacteremic *Mycobacterium avium* complex disease. *Annals of Internal Medicine*, 121, 905–11.

Chan, J. & Luft, W. (1986). Activity of roxithromycin (RU 28965), a macrolide, against *Toxoplasma gondii* in mice. *Antimicrobial Agents and Chemotherapy*, 30, 323–4.

Chan, S. L., Yew, W. W., Porter, J. H. D. et al. (1994). Comparison of Chinese and Western rifapentines and improvement of bioavailability by prior taking of various meals. *International Journal of Antimicrobial Agents*, 3, 267–74.

Chang, H. R. & Pechere, J. C. (1987). Activity of Aroxithromycin against *Toxoplasma gondii* in murine models. *Journal of Antimicrobial Chemotherapy*, 20 [Suppl. B], 69–74.

Chang, H. R., Rudareanu, F. C. & Pechere, J. C. (1988). Activity of A-56268 (TE-031), a new macrolide, against *Toxoplasma gondii* in mice. *Journal of Antimicrobial Chemotherapy*, 22, 359–61.

Chang, H. R., Comte, R. & Pechere, J. C. (1990). *In vitro* and *in vivo* effects of doxycycline on *Toxoplasma gondii*. *Antimicrobial Agents and Chemotherapy*, 34, 775–80.

Chang, H. R., Comte, R., Piguet, P. F. et al. (1991). Activity of minocycline against *Toxoplasma gondii* infection in mice. *Journal of Antimicrobial Chemotherapy*, 27, 1855–9.

Clotet, B., Sirera, G., Romeu, J. et al. (1991). Twice-weekly dapsone-pyrimethamine for preventing PCP and cerebral toxoplasmosis [Letter]. *AIDS*, 5, 601–2.

Clumeck, N., Katlama, C., Ferrero, T. et al. (1992). Atovaquone (1,4-hydroxynaphthoquinone, 566C80) in the treatment of acute cerebral toxoplasmosis in AIDS patients. 32nd Interscience Conference on Antimicrobial Agents and Chemotherapy, October 11–14. Anaheim, CA 313.

Cohn, J., McMeeking, A., Cohen, W. et al. (1989). Evaluation of the policy of empiric treatment of suspected *Toxoplasma encephalitis* in patients with the acquired immunodeficiency syndrome. *American Journal of Medicine*, 86, 521–7.

Cook, M. K. & Jacobs, L. (1958). *In vitro* investigations on the action of pyrimethamine against *Toxoplasma gondii*. *Journal of Parasitology*, 44, 280–8.

Daffos, F., Forestier, F., Capella-Pavlovsky, M. et al. (1988). Prenatal management of 746 pregnancies at risk for congenital toxoplasmosis. *New England Journal of Medicine*, 318, 271–5.

Dalvie, D. K., Khosla & Vincent, J. (1997). Excretion and metabolism of trovafloxacin in humans. Drug metabolism and disposition. *The Biological Fate of Chemicals*, 25, 274–7.

Danise, A., Cinque, P., Vergani, S. et al. (1997). Use of polymerase chain reaction assays of aqueous humour in the differential diagnosis of retinitis in patients infected with human immunodeficiency virus. *Clinical Infectious Diseases*, 24, 110–16.

Danneman, B. R., McCutchan, J. A., Israelski, D. et al. (1992). Treatment of toxoplasma encephalitis in patients with AIDS. A randomized trial comparing pyrimethamine plus clindamycin to pyrimethamine plus sulphadiazine. *Annals of Internal Medicine*, 116, 33–43.

Derouin, F., Piketty, C., Chastang, C. et al. (1991). Anti-toxoplasma effects of dapsone alone and combined with pyrimethamine. *Antimicrobial Agents and Chemotherapy*, 35, 252–5.

Dhiver, C., Milandre, C., Poizot-Martin, I. et al. (1993). 5-Fluorouracil-clindamycin for treatment of cerebral toxoplasmosis. *AIDS*, 7, 143–4.

Dunn, D., Newell, M. L. & Gilbert, R. (1997). Low risk of congenital toxoplasmosis in children born to women infected with human immunodeficiency virus. *Pediatric Infectious Disease Journal*, 16, 84.

Durant, J., Hazime, F., Bernard, E. et al. (1992). An open randomized study of roxithromycin (RO) efficacy and tolerance in the primary prevention (PP) of pneumocystosis (PC) and cerebral toxoplasmosis (CT) in 52 HIV-positive patients. 32nd Interscience Conference on Antimicrobial Agents and Chemotherapy, October 11–14, Anaheim, CA, abstract #1216.

Eyles, D. E. & Coleman, N. (1953). Synergistic effect of sulphadiazine and Daraprim against experimental toxoplasmosis in the mouse. *Antibiotics and Chemotherapy*, 3, 483–90.

Eyles, D. E. & Coleman, N. (1955). An evaluation of the curative effects of pyrimethamine and sulphadiazine alone and in combination, on experimental mouse toxoplasmosis. *Antibiotics and Chemotherapy*, 5, 529–39.

Feldman, H. A. (1973). Effects of trimethoprim and sulphisoxazole alone and in combination on murine toxoplasmosis. *Journal of Infectious Diseases*, 128S, 774–7.

Fernandez-Martin, J., Leport, C., Morlat, P. et al. (1992). Pyrimethamine–clarithromycin combination for therapy of acute toxoplasma encephalitis in patients with AIDS. *Antimicrobial Agents and Chemotherapy*, 35, 2049–52.

Feun, L. G., Robsinon, W. A., Savaraj, N. et al. (1995). Phase II trial of piritrexim and DTIC using an alternating dose schedule in metastatic melanoma. *American Journal of Clinical Oncology*, 18, 488–90.

Fichera, M. E., Bhopale, M. K. & Roos, D. (1995). *In vitro* assays elucidate peculiar kinetics of clindamycin action against *Toxoplasma gondii*. *Journal of Infectious Diseases*, 157, 14–22.

Foulds, G., Shepard, R. M. & Johnson, R. B. (1990). The pharmacokinetics of azithromycin in human serum and tissues. *Journal of Antimicrobial Chemotherapy*, 25, [Suppl. A], 73–82.

Fraschini, F., Scaglione, G., Pintucci, G. et al. (1991). The diffusion of clarithromycin and roxithromycin into nasal mucosa, tonsils, and lung in humans. *Journal of Antimicrobial Chemotherapy*, 27, [Suppl. A], 61–6.

Gatti, G., Flaherty, J., Bubpp, J., White, J. et al. (1993). Comparative study of bioavailabilities and pharmacokinetics of clindamycin in healthy volunteers and patients with AIDS. *Antimicrobial Agents and Chemotherapy*, 37, 1137–43.

Gatti, G., Hossein, J., Malena, M. et al. (1997). Penetration of dapsone into cerebrospinal fluid of patients with AIDS. *Journal of Antimicrobial Chemotherapy*, 40, 113–15.

Gazzinelli, R. T., Hakim, F. T., Hieny, S. et al. (1991). Synergistic role of CD4+ and CD8+ T lymphocytes in interferon gamma production and protective immunity induced by an attenuated *Toxoplasma gondii* vaccine. *Journal of Immunology*, 146, 286–92.

Gazzinelli, R. T., Oswald, I., James, S. & Sher, A. (1992). IL-10 inhibits parasite killing and nitrogen oxide production by IFN-gamma activated macrophages. *Journal of Immunology*, 148, 1792–6.

Gazzinelli, R., Hieny, S., Wynn. et al. (1993). Interleukin-12 is required for the T-lymphocyte-independent induction of interferon-gamma by an intracellular parasite and induces resistance in T-cell-deficient hosts. *Proceedings of the National Academy of Sciences of the United States of America*, 90, 6115–19.

Geils, G. F., Scott, C. S. Jr., Baugh, C. M. & Butterworth, C. E. Jr. (1971). Treatment of meningeal leukemia with pyrimethamine. *Blood*, 38, 131–7.

Ghosh, M., Levy, P. M. & Leopold, I. H. (1965). Therapy of toxoplasmosis uveitis. *American Journal of Ophthalmology*, 59, 55–61.

Girard, P. M., Landman, R., Gaudebout, C. et al. (1993). Dapsone–pyrimethamine compared with aerosolized pentamidine as a primary prophylaxis against *Pneumocystis carinii* pneumonia and toxoplasmosis in HIV infection. *New England Journal of Medicine*, 328, 1514–20.

Gluckstein, D. & Ruskin, J. (1995). Rapid oral desensitization to trimethoprim–sulphamethoxazole (TMP–SMZ): use in prophylaxis for *Pneumocystis carinii* pneumonia in patients with AIDS who were previously intolerant to TMP–SMZ. *Clinical Infectious Diseases*, 20, 849–53.

Goadsby, P., Donaghy, A., Lloyd, A. & Wakefield, D. (1987). Acquired immunodeficiency syndrome (AIDS) and sulphadiazine-associated renal failure. *Annals of Internal Medicine*, 107, 783–4.

Grossman, P. L. & Remington, J. S. (1979). The effect of trimethoprim and sulphamethoxazole on *Toxoplasma gondii in vitro* and *in vivo*. *American Journal of Tropical Medicine and Hygiene*, **28**, 445–557.

Grover, C. M., Thulliez, P., Remington, J. S. & Boothroyd, J. D. (1990). Rapid prenatal diagnosis of congenital Toxoplasma infection by using polymerase chain reaction and amniotic fluid. *Journal of Clinical Microbiology*, **28**, 2297–301.

Guy, E. C., Pelloux, H., Lappalainen, M. et al. (1996). Interlaboratory comparison of polymerase chain reaction for the detection of *Toxoplasma gondii* DNA added to samples of amniotic fluid. *European Journal of Clinical Microbiology and Infectious Diseases*, **15**, 836–9.

Hakes, T. B. & Armstrong, D. (1983). Toxoplasmosis. Problems in diagnosis and treatment. *Cancer*, **52**, 1535–40.

Hakim, M., Esmore, D., Wallwork, J. et al. (1986). Toxoplasmosis in cardiac transplantation. *British Medical Journal*, **292**, 1108.

Hardy, D. J., Guary, D. R. P. & Jones, R. N. (1992). Clarithromycin, a unique macrolide. A pharmacokinetic, microbiological, and clinical overview. *Diagnostic Microbiology and Infectious Disease*, **15**, 39–53.

Harris, C., Salgo, M. P., Tanowitz, H. B. & Wittner, M. (1988). *In vitro* assessment of antimicrobial agents against *Toxoplasma gondii*. *Journal of Infectious Diseases*, **157**, 14–22.

Haverkos, H. W. (1987). Assessment of therapy for toxoplasma encephalitis. The TE study group. *American Journal of Medicine*, **82**, 907–14.

Hohlfeld, P., Daffos, F., Thulliez, P. et al. (1994). Prenatal diagnosis of congenital toxoplasmosis with a polymerase-chain-reaction test on amniotic fluid. *New England Journal of Medicine*, **331**, 695–9.

Hudson, D. G., Yoshihara, G. M. & Kirby, W. M. (1956). Spiramycin: clinical and laboratory studies. *Archives of Internal Medicine*, **97**, 57–61.

Huskinson-Mark, J., Araujo, F. G. & Remington, J. S. (1991). Evaluation of the effect of drugs on the cyst form of *Toxoplasma gondii*. *Journal of Infectious Diseases*, **164**, 170–7.

Israelski, D. & Remington, J. S. (1988). Toxoplasma encephalitis in patients with AIDS. *Infectious Disease Clinics of North America*, **2**, 429–45.

Jacobson, J. M., Davidian, M., Rainey, P. M. et al. (1996). Pyrimethamine pharmacokinetics in human immunodeficiency virus-positive patients seropositive for *Toxoplasma gondii*. *Antimicrobial Agents and Chemotherapy*, **40**, 1360–5.

Jacobson, M. A., Besch, C. L., Child, C. et al. (1992). Toxicity of clindamycin as prophylaxis for AIDS-associated toxoplasma encephalitis. *Lancet*, **339**, 333–4.

Jacobson, M. A., Besch, C. L., Child, C. et al. (1994). Primary prophylaxis for toxoplasma encephalitis in patients with advanced human immunodeficiency virus disease: results of a randomized trial. *Journal of Infectious Diseases*, **169**, 384–94.

Joiner, K. A., Lowe, B. R., Dzink, J. L. et al. (1981). Antibiotic levels in infected and sterile subcutaneous abscesses in mice. *Journal of Infectious Diseases*, **143**, 487–94.

Katlama, C., De Wit, S., Guichard, A. et al. (1992). A randomized European trial comprising pyrimethamine–clindamycin (P/C) to pyrimethamine–sulphadiazine(P/S) in AIDS toxoplasma encephalitis (TE). 32nd Interscience Conference on Antimicrobial Agents and Chemotherapy, October 11–14, Anaheim, CA, abstract #1215.

Kaufman, H. E. & Geisler, P. H. (1960). The haematologic toxicity of pyrimethamine (Daraprim) in man. *Archives of Ophthalmology*, 64, 140–6.

Khan, A. A., Slilfer, T., Araujo, F. G. & Remington, J. S. (1996). Provafloxacin is active against *Toxoplasma gondii*. *Antimicrobial Agents and Chemotherapy*, 40, 1855–9.

Khan, A. A., Slifer, T., Araujo, F. G. et al. (1997). Activity of trovafloxacin in combination with other drugs for treatment of acute murine toxoplasmosis. *Antimicrobial Agents and Chemotherapy*, 41, 893–97.

Khan, A. A., Nasr, M. & Araujo, F. G. (1998). Two 2-hydroxy-3-alkyl-1,4-naphthoquinones with *in vitro* and *in vivo* activities against *Toxoplasma gondii*. *Antimicrobiol Agents and Chemotherapy*, 42, 2284–9.

Kovacs, J. A., Allegra, W., Chabner, B. A. et al. (1987). Potent effect of trimetrexate, a lipid-soluble antifolate, on *Toxoplasma gondii*. *Journal of Infectious Diseases*, 155, 1027–32.

Kovacs, J. A. and the NIAID Clinical Centre Intramural AIDS Program. (1992). Efficacy of atovaquone in treatment of toxoplasmosis in patients with AIDS. *Lancet*, 340, 637–8.

Krahenbuhl, J. L. & Fukutomi, Y., Gu, L. (1993). Treatment of acute experimental toxoplasmosis with investigational poloxamers. *Antimicrobial Agents and Chemotherapy*, 37, 2265–9.

Kucers, A., Bennett, N. Mck. (eds). (1979). *The Use of Antibiotics*, 3rd edn. London: William Heinemann, pp. 517–21.

Kupfer, M., Zee, C. S., Colletti, P. M. et al. (1987). MRI evaluation of AIDS-related encephalopathy: toxoplasmosis vs. lymphoma. *MRI*, 8, 51–7.

Lakhanpul, V., Schocket, S. S. & Nirankari, V. S. (1983). Clindamycin in the treatment of toxoplasmic retinochoroiditis. *American Journal of Ophthalmology*, 95, 605–13.

Lane, H. C., Laughon, B. E., Falloon, J. et al. (1994). Recent advances in the management of AIDS-related opportunistic infections. *Annals of Internal Medicine*, 120, 945–55.

Lappalainen, M., Koskela, P., Koskiniemi, M. et al. (1993). Improved serodiagnosis based on avidity of IgG. *Journal of Infectious Diseases*, 167, 691–7.

Lehr, D. (1957). Clinical toxicity of sulphonamides. *Annals of the New York Academy of Science*, 69, 417–47.

Leport, C., Vilde, J. L., Katlama, C. et al. (1986). Failure of spiramycin to prevent neurotoxoplasmosis in immunosuppressed patients. *Journal of American Medical Association*, 255, 2290.

Leport, C., Raffi, F., Matheron, S. et al. (1988). Treatment of central nervous system toxoplasmosis with pyrimethamine/sulphadiazine combination in 35 patients with acquired immunodeficiency syndrome. Efficacy of long-term continuous therapy. *American Journal of Medicine*, 84, 94–100.

Leport, C., Morlat, P., Chene, G. et al. (1993). Pyrimethamine for primary prophylaxis of toxoplasmosis in HIV patients: a double-blind randomized trial. First National Conference on Human Retroviruses and Related Infections. Washington: American Society for Microbiology, abstract # 36.

Levitz, R. & Quintiliani, R. (1984). Trimethoprim–sulphamethoxazole for bacterial meningitis. *Annals of Internal Medicine*, 100, 881–90.

Levy, R. M., Rosenbloom, S. & Perrett, L. (1985). Neuroradiological findings in AIDS. A review of 200 cases. *American Journal of Neuroradiology*, 7, 833–9.

Lindsay, D. S. & Blagburn, B. L. (1993). Activity of diclazuril against *Toxoplasma gondii* in cultured cells and mice. *American Journal of Veterinary Medicine*, 55, 530–3.

Lindsay, D. S., Blagburn, B. L., Hall, J. E. & Tidwell, R. R. (1991). Activity of pentamidine and pentamidine analogs against *Toxoplasma gondii* in cell cultures. *Antimicrobial Agents and Chemotherapy*, 35, 1914–16.

Lopez, J. S., de Smet, M. D., Masur, H. et al. (1992). Orally administered 566C80 for treatment of ocular toxoplasmosis in a patient with the acquired immunodeficiency syndrome. *American Journal of Ophthalmology*, 113, 331–3.

Lorberboym, M., Estok, L., Machac, J. et al. (1996). Rapid differential diagnosis of cerebral toxoplasmosis and primary central nervous system lymphoma by thallium-201 SPECT. *Journal of Nuclear Medicine*, 37, 1150–4.

Luft, B. J. & Remington, J. S. (1992). Toxoplasma encephalitis in AIDS. *Clinical Infectious Diseases*, 15, 211–22.

Luft, B. J., Naot, Y., Araujo, F. G. et al. (1983). Primary and reactivated toxoplasma infection in patients with cardiac transplants: clinical spectrum and problems in diagnosis in a defined population. *Annals of Internal Medicine*, 99, 27–31.

Luft, B. J., Brooks, R. G., Conley, F. K., McCabe, R. E. & Remington, J. S. (1984). Toxoplasma encephalitis in patients with acquired immune deficiency syndrome. *Journal of American Medical Association*, 22, 913–6.

Luft, B. J., Hafner, R., Korzun, A. H. et al. (1993). Toxoplasma encephalitis in patients with the acquired immunodeficiency syndrome. *New England Journal of Medicine*, 329, 995–1000.

Luft, W. (1986). Potent *in vivo* activity of arprinocid, a purine analogue, against murine toxoplasmosis. *Journal of Infectious Diseases*, 154, 692–5.

Mallolas, J., Zamora, L., Gatell, M. et al. (1993). Primary prophylaxis for *Pneumocystis carinii* pneumonia: a randomized trial comparing cotrimoxazole, aerosolized pentamidine and dapsone, plus pyrimethamine. *AIDS*, 7, 59–64.

Maslo, C., Matheron, S. & Saimot, A. (1992). Cerebral toxoplasmosis: assessment of maintenance therapy. VIIIth International Conference on AIDS. Amsterdam, The Netherlands, abstract # PoB 123.

Masur, H., Polis, M. A., Tuazon, C. U. et al. (1993). Salvage trial of trimetrexate–leucovorin for the treatment of cerebral toxoplasmosis in patients with AIDS. *Journal of Infectious Diseases*, 167, 1422–6.

McAuley, J., Boyer, K. M., Patel, D. et al. (1994). Early and longitudinal evaluations of treated infants and children and untreated historical patients with congenital toxoplasmosis: the Chicago collaborative treatment trial. *Clinical Infectious Diseases*, 18, 38–72.

McCabe, R. E., Luft, B. J. & Remington, J. S. (1984). Effect of murine interferon gamma on murine toxoplasmosis. *Journal of Infectious Diseases*, 150, 961–2.

McCabe, R. E., Brooks, R. G., Dorfman, R. F. & Remington, J. S. (1987). Clinical spectrum in 107 cases of toxoplasmic lymphadenopathy. *Reviews in Infectious Disease*, 9, 754–74.

McGregor, C. G. A., Fleck, D. G., Nagington, J. et al. (1984). Disseminated toxoplasmosis in cardiac transplantation. *Journal of Clinical Pathology*, 37, 74–7.

McLeod, R., Rack, D., Foss, R. et al. (1992). Levels of pyrimethamine in sera and cerebrospinal and ventricular fluids from infants treated for congenital toxoplasmosis. *Antimicrobial Agents and Chemotherapy*, **36**, 1040–8.

Minkoff, H., Remington, J. S., Holman, S. et al. (1997). Vertical transmission of toxoplasma by human immunodeficiency virus-infected women. *American Journal of Obstetrics and Gynaecology*, **176**, 555–9.

Morris, J. T. & Kelly, J. W. (1992). Effective treatment of cerebral toxoplasmosis with doxycycline. *American Journal of Medicine*, **93**, 107–8.

Nagasawa, H., Manabe, T., Maekawa, Y. et al. (1991). Role of L3T4+ and Lyt-2+ T cell subsets in protective immune responses of mice against infection with a low or high virulent strain of *Toxoplasma gondii. Microbiology and Immunology*, **35**, 215–22.

Nissen, N., Aagaard, K. & Flindt-Hansen, E. (1950). Sulphonamide hematuria. *Acta Medica Scandinavica*, **138**, 301–14.

Olliaro, P., Gorini, G., Jabes, D. et al. (1994). *In vitro* and *in vivo* activity of rifabutin against *Toxoplasma gondii. Journal of Antimicrobial Chemotherapy*, **34**, 649–57.

Oster, S., Hutchison, F. & McCabe, R. (1990). Resolution of acute renal failure in toxoplasma encephalitis despite continuance of sulphadiazine. *Reviews in Infectious Disease*, **12**, 618–20.

O-Yang, K., Krug, E. C., Marr, J. J. & Berens, R. L. (1990). Inhibition of growth of *Toxoplasma gondii* by quinghaosu and derivatives. *Antimicrobial Agents and Chemotherapy*, **34**, 1961–5.

Panzer, J. D., Brown, D. C., Epstein, W. L. et al. (1972). Clindamycin levels in various body tissues and fluids. *Journal of Clinical Pharmacology*, **12**, 259–62.

Pedrol, E., Gonzalez-Clemente, J. M., Gatell, J. M. et al. (1990). Central nervous system toxoplasmosis in AIDS patients: efficacy of an intermittent maintenance therapy. *AIDS*, **4**, 511–17.

Pfefferkorn, E. R. & Borotz, S. E. (1994). Comparison of mutants of *Toxoplasma gondii* selected for resistance to azithromycin, spiramycin, or clindamycin. *Antimicrobial Agents and Chemotherapy*, **38**, 31–7.

Pfefferkorn, E. R. & Pfefferkorn, L. C. (1977). *Toxoplasma gondii*: specific labelling of nucleic acids of intracellular parasites in Lesch–Nyhan cells. *Experimental Parasitology*, **41**, 95–104.

Pierce, M. A., Johnson, M. D., Maciunas, R. J. et al. (1995). Evaluating contrast-enhancing brain lesions in patients with AIDS by using positron emission tomography. *Annals of Internal Medicine*, **123**, 594–8.

Piketty, C., Gilquin, J. & Kazatchkine, M. D. (1995). Efficacy and safety of desensitization to trimethoprim–sulphamethoxazole in human immunodeficiency virus-infected patients. *Journal of Infectious Diseases*, **172**, 611.

Pinkerton, H. & Henderson, R. G. (1941). Adult toxoplasmosis: a previously unrecognized disease entity simulating the typhus-spotted fever group. *Journal of American Medical Association*, **116**, 807–14.

Piscitelli, S. C., Danziger, L. H. & Rodvold, K. A. (1992). Clarithromycin and azithromycin: new macrolide antibiotics. *Clinical Pharmacy*, **11**, 137–52.

Podzamczer, D., Santin, M., Jimenez, J. et al. (1993). Thrice-weekly cotrimoxazole is better than weekly dapsone-pyrimethamine for the primary prevention of *Pneumocystis carinii* pneumonia in HIV-infected patients. *AIDS*, **7**, 501–6.

Polla, M. A., Masur, H., Tuazon, C. et al. (1989). Salvage trial of trimetrexate–leucovorin for treatment of cerebral toxoplasmosis in AIDS patients [Abstract]. *Clinical Research*, **37**, 437A.

Prokesch, R. C. & Hand, W. L. (1982). Antibiotic entry into human polymorphonuclear leukocytes. *Antimicrobial Agents Chemotherapy*, 23, 373–80.

Rabaud, C., May, T., Lucet, J. C. et al. (1996). Pulmonary toxoplasmosis in patients infected with human immunodeficiency virus. A French national survey. *Clinical Infectious Diseases*, 23, 1249–54.

Raffi, F., Struillou, L., Ninin, E. et al. (1995). Breakthrough cerebral toxoplasmosis in patients with AIDS who are being treated with clarithromycin. *Clinical Infectious Diseases*, 20, 1076–7.

Remington, J. S., Velde, J. L., Antunes, F. et al. (1991). Clindamycin for toxoplasma encephalitis in AIDS. *Lancet*, 338, 1142–3.

Remington, J. S., McLeod, R. & Desmonts, G. (1995). Toxoplasmosis. In *Infectious Diseases of the Foetus and Newborn Infant*, 4th edn., ed. J. S. Remington & J. O. Klein, pp. 140–267. Philadelphia: WB Saunders.

Richards, F. O., Kovacs, J. A. & Luft, B. J. (1995). Preventing toxoplasma encephalitis in persons infected with human immunodeficiency virus. *Clinical Infectious Diseases*, 21, [Suppl. 1], S49–56.

Ricketts, A. P. & Pfefferkorn, E. R. (1993). *Toxoplasma gondii*: susceptibility and development of resistance to anticoccidial drugs *in vitro*. *Antimicrobial Agents and Chemotherapy*, 37, 2358–63.

Romand, S., Bruna, C. D., Farinotti, F. & Derouin, F. (1996). *In vitro* and *in vivo* effects of ribabutin alone or combined with atovaquone against *Toxoplasma gondii*. *Antimicrobial Agents and Chemotherapy*, 40, 2015–20.

Ruskin, J. & Remington, J. S. (1976). Toxoplasmosis in the compromised host. *Annals of Internal Medicine*, 84, 193–9.

Sabin, A. B. (1941). Toxoplasma encephalitis in children. *Journal of American Medical Association*, 116, 801–7.

Sahai, J., Heimberger, T., Collins. et al. (1988). Sulphadiazine-induced crystalluria in a patient with the acquired immunodeficiency syndrome: a reminder. *American Journal of Medicine*, 84, 791–2.

Sande, M. A., Gilbert, D. N. & Moellering, R. C. (1998). *The Sanford Guide to HIV/AIDS Therapy*, 7th edn., pp. 1–108. Hye Park, VT.

Sarciron, M. E., Lawton, P., Saccharin, C. et al. (1997). Effects of 2′,3′-dideoxyinosine on *Toxoplasma gondii* cysts in mice. *Antimicrobial Agents and Chemotherapy*, 41, 1531–6.

Schentag, J. J. & Ballow, C. H. (1991). Tissue directed pharmacokinetics. *American Journal of Medicine*, 91, [Suppl. 3A], 5S–11S.

Shafer, R. W., Seitzman, P. A. & Tapper, M. L. (1989). Successful prophylaxis of *Pneumocystis carinii* pneumonia with trimethoprim-sulphamethoxazole in AIDS patients with previous allergic reactions. *Journal of Acquired Immune Deficiency Syndrome*, 2, 389–93.

Sibley, L. D., Weidner, E. & Krahenbuhl, J. L. (1985). Phagosome acidification blocked by intracellular *Toxoplasma gondii*. *Nature*, 315, 416–19.

Sibley, L. D., Adams, L. B., Fukutomi, Y. & Krahenbuhl, J. L. (1991). Tumor necrosis factor-alpha triggers anti-toxoplasma acitivity of IFN-gamma primed macrophages. *Journal of Immunology*, 147, 2340–5.

Smego, R., Moeller, M. S. & Gallis, H. A. (1983). Trimethoprim–sulphamethoxazole therapy for *Nocardia* infections. *Archives of Internal Medicine*, 143, 711–18.

Smith, R. M., Iwamoto, G. K., Richerson, H. B. & Flaherty, J. P. (1987). Trimethoprim–sulame-thoxazole desensitization in the acquired immunodeficiency syndrome. *Annals of Internal Medicine*, 10, 335.

Spencer, C. M. & Goa, K. L. (1995). Atovaquone. A review of its pharmacological properties and therapeutic efficacy in opportunistic infections. *Drugs*, 50, 176–96.

Subauste, C. S., Koniaris, A. H. & Remington, J. S. (1991). Murine CD8+ cytotoxic T lympho-cytes lyse *Toxoplasma gondi*-infected cells. *Journal of Immunology*, 147, 3955–9.

Subauste, C. S., Wong, S. Y. & Remington, J. S. (1997). AIDS-associated toxoplasmosis. In *The Medical Management of AIDS*, ed. M. A. Sande & P. A. Volberding, pp. 343–62. Philadelphia: WB Saunders.

Sutherland, R. (1962). Spiramycin: a reappraisal of its antibacterial activity. *British Journal of Pharmacology*, 19, 99–110.

Suzuki, Y., Conley, F. K. & Remington, J. S. (1989a). Differences in virulence and development of encephalitis during chronic infection vary with the strain of *Toxoplasma gondii*. *Journal of Infectious Diseases*, 159, 790–4.

Suzuki, Y., Conley, F. K. & Remington, J. S. (1989b). Importance of endogenous interferon gamma for prevention of toxoplasma encephalitis in mice. *Journal of Immunology*, 143, 2045–50.

Suzuki, Y., Yang, Q., Conley, F. K. et al. (1994). Antibody against interleukin-6 reduces inflammation and numbers of cysts in brains of mice with toxoplasma encephalitis. *Infection and Immunology*, 62, 2773–8.

Tabbara, K. F. & O'Connor, G. R. (1975). Ocular tissue absorption of clindamycin phosphate. *Archives of Ophthalmology*, 93, 1180–5.

Tabbara, K. F. & O'Connor, G. R. (1980). Treatment of ocular toxoplasmosis with clindamycin and sulphadiazine. *Ophthalmology*, 87, 129–35.

Teng, R., Dogolo, L. C., Willavize, S. A. et al. (1997). Oral bioavailability of trovafloxacin with and without food in healthy volunteers. *Journal of Antimicrobial Chemotherapy*, 39, [Suppl. B], S87–S92.

Torres, R. A., Weinberg, W. & Stansell, J. et al. (1997). Atovaquone for salvage treatment and sup-pression of toxoplasma encephalitis in patients with AIDS. *Clinical Infectious Diseases*, 24, 422–9.

USPHS/IDSA. (1997). Guidelines for the prevention of opportunistic infections in persons infected with human immunodeficiency virus. *Clinical Infectious Diseases*, 25, [Suppl. 3], S299.

Villringer, K., Jager, H., Dichgans, M. et al. (1995). Differential diagnosis of CNS lesions in AIDS patients by FDG-PET. *Journal of Computer Assisted Tomography*, 19, 532–6.

Wang, C. C., Simashkevich, P. M. & Stotish, R. L. (1979a). Mode of anticoccidial action of arpri-nocid. *Biochemical Pharmacology*, 28, 2241–8.

Wang, C. C., Tolman, R. L., Simashkevich, P. M. & Stotish, R. L. (1979b). Arprinocid, an inhibi-tor of hyoxanthine-guanine transport. *Biochemical Pharmacology*, 28, 2249–60.

Weiss, L. M., Harris, C., Berger, M., Tanowitz, H. B. & Wittner, M. (1988). Pyrimethamine concentrations in serum and cerebrospinal fluid during treatment of acute toxoplasma encephalitis in patients with AIDS. *Journal of Infectious Diseases*, 157, 580–3.

Wilson, C. B., Remington, J. S., Stagno, S. & Reynolds, D. W. (1980). Development of adverse sequelae in children born with subclinical congenital toxoplasma infection. *Pediatrics*, 66, 767–74.

Winstanley, P., Khoo, S., Szwandt, S. et al. (1995). Marked variation in pyrimethamine disposition in AIDS patients treated for cerebral toxoplasmosi. *Journal of Antimicrobial Chemotherapy*, 36, 435–9.

Wong, S. Y. & Remington, J. S. (1994). Toxoplasmosis in pregnancy. *Clinical Infectious Diseases*, 18, 853–62.

Wreghitt, T. G., Hakim, M., Gray, J. J. et al. (1989). Toxoplasmosis in heart and heart and lung transplant recipients. *Journal of Clinical Pathology*, 42, 194–9.

Wynn, R. F., Leen, C. L. S. & Brettle, R. P. (1993). Azithromycin for cerebral toxoplasmosis in AIDS. *Lancet*, 341, 2443–4.

14

Toxoplasma vaccines

J. L. Fishback[1] and J. K. Frenkel[2]

[1] School of Medicine, Department of Pathology & Oncology, The University of Kansas Medical Center, Kansas City, USA
[2] 1252 Vallecita Drive, Santa Fe, USA

Introduction

The rational design of vaccines should be considered within the context of the immunity that naturally develops against the targeted infection. It follows that each specific infection must be viewed in the context of the transmission cycle and epidemiology. The biological attributes of the microbe should be separated as much as possible from those of its hosts, and should be understood in terms of the evolution of the organism.

T. gondii has apparently evolved from a one-host intestinal coccidia of primitive cats. It has become a highly successful and stable two-host parasite. Its sexual cycle, which leads to oocyst production, occurs in the intestine of carnivorous cats, while extra-intestinal tissue cysts exist in the cats' prey. Prey animals that feed on the ground encounter the infectious oocyst stage from cat faeces. Evolution from the one-host primitive *T. gondii* to the two-host modern *T. gondii* was made possible by the evolution of the tissue cyst stage. Extension of infection into intermediate hosts with tissue cysts has enabled the transmission back to cats. Indeed, the *T. gondii* lifecycle has become so dependent upon tissue cysts that the transmission of infection to cats with tissue cysts is more efficient than the direct transmission from cat to cat via oocysts (Dubey & Frenkel 1976).

These facts are important for an understanding of immunity to *T. gondii* and the design of vaccines. The tissue cyst is an essential part of the evolved natural cycle. Although not essential for the maintenance of immunity, as will be discussed, all natural isolates of *T. gondii* have been selected for the persistence of tissue cysts, in spite of the immunity of intermediate hosts. It appears unlikely, therefore, that a vaccine can be produced that engenders immunity, suppressing tissue cysts and bradyzoites.

A second important observation is that the intestinal stages (leading to oocyst production only in cats) are under immunological control (Dubey & Frenkel 1974). Immune mechanisms in the intestinal compartment are distinct from those in the extra-intestinal compartment, and a separate vaccine is necessary to control intestinal infection in cats.

The majority of animals develop effective immunity against disease caused by *T. gondii*, protecting them from uncontrolled multiplication of the organism and the destruction of host cells. However, natural infection results in the immune state known as infection-immunity or premunition, because bradyzoites persist in tissue cysts. When animals recover from primary infection, they are protected against symptomatic disease if reexposed to *T. gondii*, yet they remain infected, probably for life, similar to infection with herpes simplex virus, cytomegalovirus or *Mycobacterium tuberculosis*. Reinfection probably occurs, but is clinically unimportant in the immunocompetent host. Tissue cysts may rupture from time to time throughout the lifetime of the host but, if normal immunity is maintained, the released bradyzoites are rapidly destroyed and no illness results.

It has been hypothesized that antigens secreted by the encysted bradyzoites serve to restimulate the host immune system over time, and thus are chiefly responsible for the excellent lifelong immunity of the premunition type (Capron & Dessaint 1988; Cesbron-Delauw & Capron 1993). These antigens have been called excreted-secreted antigens (ESA), and have been proposed as vaccine candidates. Natural reinfection may also serve to stimulate the immune system periodically. There is evidence from infection of Aotus monkeys and other animals that tissue cysts periodically rupture, which could also release antigens and restimulate cells of the immune system (Frenkel & Escajadillo 1987).

The development of chemically induced mutants of *T. gondii* by Pfefferkorn and Pfefferkorn (1976) has enabled the selection of a temperature-sensitive strain (ts-4) that does not persist (form cysts) in host tissues (Waldeland et al. 1983). Experiments with this strain proved for the first time that sterile immunity was possible in toxoplasmosis. The ts-4 strain protects mice from illness on challenge, with surprising efficacy against an oral challenge of 10^6 organisms, and 10^3 organisms 1 year later (Waldeland & Frenkel 1983). These results were later confirmed by others (Suzuki & Remington 1988; Hakim et al. 1991). These experiments demonstrate that concurrent infection is not necessary for the development and maintenance of good immunity to *T. gondii*, requiring a paradigm shift in thinking about immunity to intracellular infection.

In their test of the ts-4 strain as a vaccine for domestic pigs, Lindsay et al. (1993) outline five goals for future *T. gondii* vaccines. First, the vaccine must not cause disease in vaccinated animals. Second, it must not persist (i.e. form tissue cysts) in the tissues of animals. Third, it should protect against clinical disease. Fourth, it should protect against abortion and congenital infection caused by *T. gondii*. Fifth, it should prevent tissue cyst formation in challenged animals. Their test of the ts-4 live vaccine candidate in pigs fulfilled the first three requirements, was not evaluated against the fourth, and failed to fulfil their fifth requirement, in that (not surprisingly) tissue cysts were found after challenge.

Rather than considering the formation of tissue cysts after challenge to be a shortcoming of the ts-4 *T. gondii* vaccine, one should consider that sterile immunity to *T. gondii* does not occur in nature, and may be unachievable with natural strains. However, the mutant ts-4 strain demonstrates that immunization may eventually be a useful strategy to help prevent symptomatic disease, decrease the risk of congenital transmission, decrease the number of tissue cysts in meat animals and perhaps convey a higher degree of immunity against *T. gondii* to hosts that may become immunocompromised in later life. Newer immunization strategies may yet be able to improve upon naturally acquired immunity.

Epidemiological considerations

The role of prevention in controlling human toxoplasmosis has been stressed in the past (Frenkel 1981). It remains important, because good hand-washing techniques and the proper cooking of meat can do much to prevent the transmission of toxoplasmosis. Pregnant women and immunocompromised patients should be educated about the dangers of toxoplasmosis, and the means to prevent it. McCabe and Remington (1987) have proposed a serological screening programme for congenital toxoplasmosis, similar to the one currently in place in France (Daffos et al. 1987) but others have argued that preventive measures would be much more cost effective (Frenkel 1981; Thorpe et al. 1988; Leighty 1990). Such cost issues have become increasingly important in today's economic and regulatory environment, since medical practices once considered almost sacred, such as routine ultrasound scans during pregnancy, have been called into question (Berkowitz 1993). Vaccination programmes, which are themselves expensive, must only be considered if the usually cheaper prevention programmes fail to achieve an acceptable level of disease control. Cost-benefit analysis may show prevention to be effective in one geographical area, but not in another (Foulon 1992; Stray-Pederson & Jenum 1992). Where preventive measures fail, immunization may be practical.

Possible target species for a *T. gondii* vaccine, based on current knowledge of the lifecycle and epidemiology, would include:
1 humans, particularly women of child-bearing age,
2 domestic meat animals, and
3 the most prevalent definitive host, cats.
Human toxoplasmosis, in its acute form, is usually an asymptomatic disease, causing little morbidity and very low mortality. However, the foetus is at risk in acutely infected women, since it lacks a fully developed immune system. Later pregnancies are not at risk, since the woman has recovered from the acute illness and

has developed immunity. Thus, *T. gondii*-antibody-negative women of child-bearing age represent one group that can be targeted in any future immunization programmes designed to reduce the incidence of congenital toxoplasmosis.

In the setting of human immunodeficiency virus (HIV) infection, conferring primary immunity would be a useful goal, to prevent disease from primary infection and later recrudescence. However, it is speculation whether patients with a compromised immune system could be effectively immunized. Realistically, *T. gondii*-antibody-positive HIV patients would probably not benefit as much from a *T. gondii* vaccine as they would from the development of a cidal drug for encysted bradyzoites. If all encysted bradyzoites could be killed with chemotherapy, then a *T. gondii* vaccine for this subset of patients becomes unnecessary.

Domestic animals do not usually become symptomatic from *T. gondii* infection, but their infected meat can transmit the infection via the tissue cyst to unwary humans who prefer that their meat be served rare. Pork is one meat likely to transmit the infection. Using serological surveys, the United States Drug Administration (USDA) has estimated that 42% of pigs of breeding age and 23% of market-age pigs are infected (Dubey et al. 1991). Game animals such as deer are also known to have a high *T. gondii* antibody prevalence (Lindsay et al. 1991). Vaccination of domestic meat animals against toxoplasmosis may be a useful strategy for helping to prevent congenital infection and abortion, in terms of the number of tissue cysts formed in the meat of an immunized animal that may come in contact with *T. gondii* oocysts.

Domestic cats, the principal disseminators of *T. gondii* oocysts, could be vaccinated to prevent oocyst shedding. This strategy represents a departure from usual schemes, in that it attempts to control the epidemic at its source, the definitive host, rather than by vaccination of susceptible intermediate hosts, such as humans and domestic animals. The highest yield would probably be attained by immunizing the cats belonging to women of child-bearing age or to immunosuppressed patients, and cats on farms or ranches where abortions due to *T. gondii* occur in pigs and sheep. When the vaccination of cats is combined with that of humans and other animals, the risk of infection could decrease dramatically. Indeed, the combined vaccination of cats and intermediate hosts may be critical in locations harbouring cats with a high *T. gondii* antibody seroprevalence (such as Central America), where children become infected at a very young age. A vaccination programme in cats alone could be predicted to raise the average age of infection (as defined by Anderson & May 1982) by decreasing the concentration of infectious oocysts in the soil. The number of cases of congenital toxoplasmosis could therefore paradoxically increase in such areas, since young girls would acquire infection in their teens or early twenties, instead of age four or five years, due to the depletion of viable oocysts in the environment.

Experimental models

Several factors are important to consider when selecting an experimental model for testing a potential *T. gondii* vaccine. First, selection of the target species is critical when evaluating vaccine efficacy (Krahenbuhl et al. 1972). Mice and rabbits are rather susceptible to toxoplasmosis, with evidence of genetic predisposition now being recognized in mice (McLeod et al. 1989b). The lack of evolutionary selection by *T. gondii* of Australian marsupial species, which evolved in an environment free of cats, and of strictly arboreal neotropical monkeys who would not come into contact with *T. gondii* oocysts, probably explains the relative inability of these species to develop immunity against toxoplasmosis (Frenkel 1989). These particular species may lack the requisite histocompatibility antigens to develop a cellular immune response, and prevention of infection will be a more useful strategy than immunization.

Second, the *T. gondii* strain used for challenge is critical. For example, Krahenbuhl et al. (1972) used the C56 attenuated strain of *T. gondii* as the challenge organism in their killed vaccine study, and were able to show modest protection. In their study, a challenge with 5×10^4 tachyzoites of the C56 strain killed only about 50% of control mice after 14 days. When compared to the virtually 100% mortality that can be observed with one organism of the RH strain, the C56 strain can be seen as a poor test of immunity. Use of attenuated strains may be justified as a means to evaluate the immunogenicity of weak antigens. However, one should consider that by using low pathogenicity strains as a challenge, where controls die in 2 or 3 weeks (Bülow & Boothroyd 1991) the challenge may actually boost the immunity produced by the vaccine. For the most critical studies, controls should die in the first week.

Third, the route of infection and the stage of *T. gondii* used in the challenge may be important. It has been normal practice for workers to use the subcutaneous or intraperitoneal route for the challenge infection, usually with tachyzoites that have been serially passed in mouse peritoneum or cell culture. Although convenient, and the dose is more easily calculated, this practice may not be advisable. Since infections are acquired in nature by ingestion of tissue cysts or oocysts, this should be the preferred challenge route. Since oocysts and bradyzoites are not as easily counted as tachyzoites derived from mouse peritoneal macrophages, it is also preferable to titrate the challenge, so that a lethal dose 50 (LD_{50}) may be determined, as illustrated in Waldeland and Frenkel (1983). Some investigations have utilized oral challenges, including oocyst challenge by Lindsay et al. (1993) in their study of *T. gondii* vaccines in pigs and likewise Wilkins et al. (1988a, b) in a study of *T. gondii* vaccines in sheep. Darcy et al. (1992) and Khan et al. (1991) have also utilized oral bradyzoite challenges. The use of a vaccine capable of inducing immunity to the cyst stage has been suggested by Alexander et al. (1996).

Lastly, the choice of adjuvant has always been considered important when using killed vaccine preparations of any kind, including subunit preparations derived from cloned antigens. Several adjuvants have been explored, including liposome and immunostimulating complex (ISCOM) preparations. Waldeland and Frenkel (1983) studied several different adjuvants, including liposomes, but were able to show only a modest activity of 1.4 logs of protection with their killed preparation, as compared to the four or five logs of protection seen after immunization with a wild strain, attenuated by sulphadiazine prophylaxis. Uggla et al. (1988) first described an ISCOM preparation of killed *T. gondii* antigen, which protected mice against lethal challenge. Overnes et al. (1991) tested a killed vaccine with an ISCOM preparation in mice, and was able to improve overall survival time, but ultimately all of their study animals succumbed to toxoplasmosis after challenge. Buxton et al. (1989) also tested a similar ISCOM preparation in pregnant sheep as a means of preventing abortion, but was unable to show a significant difference in lamb mortality over controls. Another adjuvant tested is cholera toxin (Bourguin et al. 1993).

Prospective vaccines

Live vaccines suitable for intermediate hosts

Live vaccines have traditionally been used to generate the large antigenic mass sufficient to immunize a host. They require no adjuvants, and continue to proliferate within the host until immunity is achieved. Their principal disadvantage is that they cannot be used in an immunocompromised host, since the infection will not be controlled by the host immune response, and may cause death or severe morbidity. Live vaccines are also more subject to rapid environmental degradation than are killed preparations, and require refrigeration to ensure continued potency.

Wild strains of *T. gondii* can be successfully utilized as vaccines in intermediate hosts, under cover of static drugs such as sulphamerazine (Elwell & Frenkel 1984). Immunization by this method provides excellent immunity to challenge. However, tissue cysts are produced in the vaccinated animal, so immunity is of the premunition type. This would be undesirable in domestic meat animals, and would also be a problem in humans, since a vaccine recipient might later become immunosuppressed, either by HIV or iatrogenic immunosuppression for malignancy or transplantation.

The problem of residual tissue cysts was solved by using the mutant strains first developed by Pfefferkorn and Pfefferkorn (1976). A temperature-sensitive mutant, ts-4, was used to immunize mice and did not cause the formation of tissue cysts (Waldeland et al. 1983). The ts-4 strain protected mice against a challenge with the 106 organisms of the RH strain (Waldeland & Frenkel 1983; Suzuki & Remington

1988). Should the ts-4 strain be accidentally injected into an immunocomprom-ised host, its proliferation could be arrested by treatment with sulphamerazine. Still, commercial interest in ts-4 has been scant, since vaccine firms are unwilling to assume the legal risk entailed by a live vaccine.

A live vaccine (*T. gondii* tachyzoites of the S48 'incomplete strain') has been developed and marketed in New Zealand for sheep and goats (Wilkins et al. 1988*a*, *b*) and after further study (Buxton et al. 1991) was launched in the UK and Eire (Toxovax™). This strain is described as 'incomplete', in that it does not form oocysts in cats. It was derived from continuous passage twice weekly in mice, which leads to loss of *T. gondii* stages (Frenkel et al. 1976). This vaccine was able to prevent lamb losses, but was not able to prevent transmission of *T. gondii* to the offspring in approximately two-thirds of cases (Buxton et al. 1991). Studies have shown that this vaccine will induce a relatively long-lasting protection against toxoplasma challenge for up to 18 months (Buxton & Innes 1995). The S48 strain of *T. gondii* has not been shown to persist in ovine tissues but this does not necessarily mean that the vaccine strain will never produce tissue cysts. Vaccination of pigs with a similar strain has shown some degree of success (Dubey et al. 1994).

Live vaccines for the definitive feline host

A live vaccine for the definitive feline host presents a very different problem from that encountered in immunizing intermediate hosts. Cats rarely become ill from toxoplasmosis yet shed millions of oocysts in their faeces. Previously, it was shown that a complete strain (one that produced oocysts in cats) could be prevented from forming oocysts by chemoprophylaxis with sulphamerazine, monensin, or similar coccidiostatic ionophores (Frenkel & Smith 1982*a*, *b*). However, these methods were considered impractical commercially, since the drugs would have to be added to cat food, which might be consumed by humans. Therefore, a search was started for a mutant strain that did not complete the entire enteric cycle, using the techniques of Pfefferkorn and Pfefferkorn (1976). The mutants were screened in cats for lack of oocyst shedding (Frenkel et al. 1991).

The T-263 vaccine strain developed from these studies aims at interrupting the maturation of coccidian stages in the cat intestine, and provides a high degree of protection against oocyst shedding after challenge (Frenkel et al. 1991; Freyre et al. 1993). The mechanism by which the vaccine produces this effect has been studied. Recombination experiments suggest that the vaccine proliferates in the feline small intestine and eventually produces only one sexual gamete, which leads to reproductive failure and lack of oocyst production (Frenkel et al. 1991).

The nature of the gut immune response to *T. gondii* remains relatively unknown. However, toxoplasmosis in cats can be altered by immunosuppression with corticosteroids, producing disseminated lesions (Dubey & Frenkel 1974). Therefore, a live

Table 14.1. Immunity to oocyst shedding in kittens after oral vaccination*

| | Vaccination (T-263 bradyzoites) | | Challenge (T-265 bradyzoites) | |
| | Oocyst shedding determined by: | | Oocyst shedding determined by: | |
	Faecal flotation	Mouse inoculation	Faecal flotation	Mouse inoculation
T-263 vaccine	0/61	0/61	6/61	6/61
T-265 control	NA#	NA	22/22	22/22

*Combined data from Frenkel et al. (1991) and Freyre et al. (1993). In the latter experiments, two doses of the vaccine were given before challenge.
#Not applicable.

vaccine in cats suffers from some of the same problems as a live vaccine in humans: it should not be given to potentially immunosuppressed animals. Any cat receiving the vaccine should be serologically negative for feline immunodeficiency virus (FIV) and feline leukaemia virus (FeLV), both of which may cause immunosuppression.

Studies of an oral bradyzoite preparation of T-263 in 61 kittens show a cumulative efficacy of approximately 90% in preventing the shedding of *T. gondii* oocysts in the cats' faeces (Table 14.1). This is similar to the percentage of cats that would shed oocysts upon a second exposure to *T. gondii* after natural infection (Frenkel & Smith 1982*a, b*). The vaccine appears to be safe for most cats but deaths have been reported in cats that were infected with FeLV 11 months prior to vaccination (Choromanski et al. 1994). Interestingly, Mateus-Pinella et al. (1999) have demonstrated that vaccinating cats found around a piggery was associated with a consequent reduction in toxoplasma infections in the swine.

Killed vaccines

For the purposes of this chapter, we define a killed vaccine as one that is derived from killed, whole *T. gondii* organisms. Over the years, many research groups have attempted to immunize animals against toxoplasmosis by using killed preparations of *T. gondii* tachyzoites and bradyzoites. Success has been modest. Indeed, Krahenbuhl et al. (1972) resorted to challenge with an attenuated strain in an to attempt to show some immune effect with their killed preparation. The search for an effective adjuvant has dominated research for inert *T. gondii* vaccine preparations.

Two studies have compared the efficacy of killed vaccines and live preparations. The original paper utilizing ts-4 as a live vaccine (Waldeland & Frenkel 1983) also

Table 14.2. Survival* after challenge with *T. gondii* oocysts of mice vaccinated with live or killed tachyzoites of various strains#

Challenge dose (no. of oocysts)	Strains of *T. gondii* used in vaccines						
	Live RH	Live M-7741	Live ts-5	Live ts-4	Killed RH	Killed M-7741	Control (saline)
10^6	0/4	5/5		2/3			
10^5	2/5	6/6	2/5	5/6			
10^4	1/5	6/6	1/6	5/6	0/6	0/6	0/6
10^3	1/4	6/6	1/6	6/6	0/6	0/6	0/6
10^2			1/6	6/6	0/6	0/6	0/6
10^1			3/6	5/6	0/6	0/6	0/6
10^0					0/6	0/6	0/6

*Survival expressed as the number of mice that survived for more than 1 month after challenge, over total number challenged.

#Adapted from Table III, p. 63, Waldeland & Frenkel (1983).

examined chemoprophylaxis of wild strains and several killed preparations. The results are reproduced in Table 14.2. One can see that the ts-4 strain shows a similar level of immunity upon oral challenge with 10^6 oocysts to that of a wild strain infection (strain M-7741) attenuated by drug administration. No mice vaccinated with a killed preparation survived challenge, even with only one oocyst.

Killed preparations were also compared to the ts-4 vaccine by Bourgin et al. (1993). Combined with sonicated tachyzoite antigens, a preparation that contained cholera toxin was administered orally, and protected approximately 50% of mice from an oral challenge with strain 76K bradyzoites that killed 100% of controls. The number of brain cysts in vaccinated animals, as determined by counting aliquots of brain suspension by light microscopy, was significantly less than controls. The ts-4 vaccine, by contrast, protected 100% of mice.

Killed vaccines have also been examined in animals other than mice. Wilkins et al. (1987) examined a killed preparation, with Freund's incomplete antigen as an adjuvant, to see if it could prevent lambing losses in sheep. They found similar lambing losses between vaccinated and un-vaccinated sheep after intravenous tachyzoite challenge. They concluded that a killed preparation would not be effective, and went on to investigate live vaccines.

Although there are numerous other studies of killed preparations, the story is the same. Killed vaccines do not produce comparable immunity achieved by natural infection or vaccination with the ts-4 strain. The results of Bourgin et al. (1993) are interesting, since it has been suggested by McLeod et al. (1988) that oral immunization might be the best way to induce good immunity to toxoplasmosis.

Recombinant or subunit vaccines

Recombinant or subunit vaccines hold forth the possibility that, by precise selection of strong immunostimulating antigens and deletion of any immunosuppressive antigens, a vaccine could be formulated from the parts that are greater than the whole (killed preparations). In pursuit of such goals, there has been a great deal of activity in classifying and cloning the various protein antigens of T. gondii. Cesbron-Delauw and Capron (1993) have provided a useful summation chart of the proteins cloned utilizing the genetic nomenclature scheme suggested by Sibley et al. (1991). We shall focus our discussion of subunit or recombinant vaccines on the three classes of proteins that appear to be important in the immune response to T. gondii: the surface antigens (SAG), the rhoptry-associated proteins (ROP), and the dense granules (GRA). Both SAG and GRA appear to be included in the broad category of ESA, although GRA proteins are thought to constitute the majority of ESA (Cesbron-Delauw & Capron 1993).

The abundant 30,000-Dalton protein found on the surface of T. gondii tachyzoites (p30, now renamed Surface Antigen 1, or SAG-1) has been the subject of several vaccine studies. Unfortunately, an initial report suggested that injection of SAG-1 might have an adverse effect on T. gondii immunity (Kasper et al. 1985): these results were never satisfactorily explained. Research has focused on the proper presentation of SAG-1 to the host, through the use of various adjuvants, with some improvements in immunogenicity. One of the first of these studies utilized SAG-1 purified from RH tachyzoites (Bülow & Boothroyd 1991). The greatest protective effects were obtained when SAG-1 was combined with liposomes, when only one of 15 study mice died upon intraperitoneal challenge with 10^5 tachyzoites of the low pathogenicity C strain tachyzoites. Only 11 of 15 control mice died from the C strain challenge, which was apparently less than a lethal dose, since control mice died in the second or third week after challenge. Also, the challenge was not titrated.

Khan et al. (1991) combined SAG-1 with the immunostimulant Quil A, and claimed nearly 100% protection against virulent T. gondii challenge. In this study, bradyzoites of the P strain of T. gondii were used in an oral challenge, which killed 100% of 20 CD1 strain control mice. The survival of 17 of 19 vaccinated mice was statistically significant at the $p = 0.0001$ level. An intriguing aspect of this study was that no brain cysts were found in the vaccinated mice after challenge, although the authors searched for cysts only by phase-contrast microscopy in aliquots of homogenized brain. The authors were also able to show protection of the genetically more susceptible C57BL/6 strain with the SAG-1/Quil A preparation. Again, the total numbers of mice in this study were small, and the authors' claim that the vaccine preparation protects mice from forming tissue cysts after challenge appear premature.

Darcy et al. (1992) examined the sequence of SAG-1 and synthesized selected peptides that were immunogenic in mice. By combining several peptide sequences into octamers, they were able to protect 40% of mice from lethal challenge infection, which killed 100% of controls. The protected mice showed a strong T cell response. These studies suggested that linear sequences of the three-dimensional SAG-1 may be capable of inducing an efficient T cell response, if presented to the host in the proper conformation with other linear epitopes. This study is the strongest evidence for the immunoprotective effects of SAG-1.

The immunobiology of SAG-1 has been extensively studied by Khan et al. (1988). They were able to show that SAG-1 is capable of inducing CD8+ T cells in mice. These cells can lyse *T. gondii*-infected mouse peritoneal macrophages. These studies parallel the later work by Hakim et al. (1991) on the immunobiology of *T. gondii* infection, who were able to show that ts-4-vaccinated mice induce CD8+ T cells that can kill either *T. gondii*-infected or antigen-pulsed host cells. These experiments are of great interest, since *T. gondii* bradyzoites are usually found in host cells other than macrophages. Suzuki and Remington (1988) also associated CD8+ T cells with antitoxoplasma activity.

Anti-SAG-1 polyclonal and monoclonal antibodies can be used to inhibit the invasion of host cells *in vitro* (Mineo et al. 1993). These studies suggested that SAG-1 may be important in host cell invasion. However, a mutant that lacks SAG-1 appears to invade host cells normally, implying that SAG is not necessary for invasion (Kasper & Khan 1993). SAGA may somehow assist invasion, or be located close to proteins that enable invasion, so that antibody binding might induce steric hindrance to penetration.

Angus et al. (1996) have reported on a recombinant plasmid produced by cloning the DNA of p30 with the sequence for tissue plasminogen activator into a plasmid. Vaccination of mice with this plasmid produced a strong antibody response to the p30 antigen compared with controls.

Significant interest has surrounded the subsurface proteins of *T. gondii* known as ROP. Rhoptries are thought to secrete substances used in penetration, and these substances were suspected to be part of ESA, but this has turned out not to be the case (Dubremetz & Schwartzman 1993). The ROPs include the antigenically related proteins of 28 and 58 kilodaltons, which had previously been noted as possible protective antigens in a killed vaccine preparation (Sibley & Sharma 1987). Immune animals and humans express antibodies to these proteins, suggesting that they are of importance in the immune response. ROP-1 and ROP-2 have now been cloned (Herion et al. 1993; Saavedra et al. 1991).

Other subsurface proteins close to the rhoptries, known as GRA, may also be part of the so-called ESA (Cesbron-Delauw & Capron 1993). These antigens are presumably secreted upon penetration of the organism into the host cell, and continue to be secreted by the encysted bradyzoites. These antigens cross-react with tachyzoite antigens, and thus provide the basis for premunition immunity, presumably through the processing of their soluble antigens by immune cells (Hakim et al. 1991). There has also been some interest in the 23-kilodalton dense granule protein, known as GRA-1, as a vaccine (Cesbron-Delauw et al. 1989).

Conclusions

For domestic animals and humans, the only vaccine candidate that demonstrates effective immunity is the temperature-sensitive mutant, ts-4. It protects against challenge by 10^6 organisms of the RH strain in mice (Waldeland & Frenkel 1983). No other vaccine candidate so far described (save drug prophylaxis of infection with a wild strain) can demonstrate a similar level of protection. The ts-4 vaccine has been tested in mice, rats, hamsters, monkeys and pigs. No tests on humans have been done.

When current preparations are compared to the level of immunity achieved with wild strains or ts-4, they are seen to be lacking in immunogenicity. This is easily seen in side-by-side trials of inert preparations versus the ts-4 vaccine, such as those done by Bourguin et al. (1993). Studies of ROPs, SAGs and GRAs are especially intriguing, since they may ultimately offer a means of blocking penetration and achieving sterile immunity that protects the host from acquiring infection. One tissue cyst in an immunocompromised patient could be one too many. However, for use in women of child-bearing age, some have argued that a vaccine need not be so perfect, and subunit vaccines may find practical use in this subpopulation of patients (Bülow & Boothroyd 1991).

Several studies have highlighted a decrease in tissue cyst numbers in vaccinated animals after challenge (McLeod et al. 1988; Khan et al. 1991; Bourguin et al. 1993; Lindsay et al. 1993). In all cases this was documented by simple microscopic counts of aliquots of brain tissue. We are suspicious of the accuracy of these counts. It is very easy to miss small cysts, and cysts may not be evenly suspended in homogenates. Aliquots should be pepsin-digested, diluted ten-fold to a million-fold, and injected into mice to detect bradyzoites (McLeod et al. 1988). Perhaps quantitative polymerase chain reaction studies could be used to document the absence of tissue cysts. However, we believe that mouse titration offers the best answer to this question. Polymerase chain reaction requires high technical competency, is subject to contamination problems and results may be difficult to interpret unless extreme care is taken to use proper controls.

Better methods of selecting antigens for vaccine trials should be sought. Dahl et al. (1987) have suggested selecting vaccine epitopes by competitive ELISA using patient immune sera. This may prove to be a useful technique, but should probably be combined with antigen-specific human T cell clones as a means of linear epitope selection, since numerous adoptive transfer studies (Frenkel 1967; Suzuki & Remington 1988; Hakim et al. 1991) all point to the importance of T cell immunity. Several groups have isolated antigen-specific T cells that may be useful in epitope screening (Sklenar et al. 1986; Khan et al. 1991; Saavedra et al. 1991). Antigen-specific T cells that showed proliferation in response to specific antigens have been further examined for the production of gamma interferon and interleukin-2 (Saavedra et al. 1991). Since these two cytokines are seen as pivotal in the immune response to *T. gondii* (Sharma et al. 1985; Suzuki et al. 1988), it may be necessary to select antigens that can induce their synthesis.

Better knowledge about regional transmission trends would be desirable, to assess the potential for intervention with a vaccination programme should intensive public health measures fail. If a politically acceptable nonviable vaccine is eventually formulated for animals and humans, then its efficacy in the field could be more easily assessed if such baseline data were available.

Summary

There is not a vaccine available for humans and it is unlikely that there will be one in the foreseeable future. In the veterinary field a commercial live vaccine (Toxovax™) for sheep using tachyzoites of the S48 'incomplete strain' of *T. gondii* has been marketed. At present, however, the only vaccine candidate for felines is the live vaccine derived from *T. gondii* strain T-263. Evaluation of its usefulness in domestic felines continues. A subunit vaccine to prevent oocyst shedding in cats remains a distant proposition, since little is known about the interaction of the various intraepithelial stages of *T. gondii* with the immune system in the feline gut.

We know much about the immunobiology of *T. gondii*, and have begun to explore its genome. We should resist the temptation to clone a gene, express it and immediately begin vaccine trials. Many antigens will probably have to be combined before a synthetic vaccine can approach the efficacy of current live vaccine candidates. Successful immunogens may eventually be found, but the challenge in future *T. gondii* vaccine research is to satisfy ourselves that a vaccine is really necessary and cost-effective when compared to prevention or surveillance schemes.

REFERENCES

Alexander, J., Jebbari, H., Bluethmann, H., Satoskar, A. & Roberts, C. W. (1996). Immunological control of *Toxoplasma gondii* and appropriate vaccine design. *Current Topics in Microbiology and Immunology*, **219**, 184–95.

Anderson, R. M. & May, R. M. (1982). Directly transmitted infectious diseases: control by vaccination. *Science*, **215**, 1053–60.

Angus, C. W., Klivington, D., Wyman, J. & Kovacs, J. A. (1996). Nucleic acid vaccines against *Toxoplasma gondii* in mice. *Journal of Eukaryotic Microbiology*, **43** [Suppl. 5], S117.

Berkowitz, R. L. (1993). Should every pregnant woman undergo ultrasonography? *New England Journal of Medicine*, **329**, 874–75.

Bourguin, I., Chardes, T. & Bout, D. (1993). Oral immunisation with *T. gondii* antigens in association with cholera toxin induces enhanced protective and cell-mediated immunity in C57BL/6 mice. *Infection and Immunity*, **61**, 2082–8.

Bülow, R. & Boothroyd, J. C. (1991). Protection of mice from fatal *T. gondii* infection by immunisation with p30 antigen in liposomes. *Journal of Immunology*, **147**, 3496–500.

Buxton, D. & Innes, E. A. (1995). A commercial vaccine for ovine toxoplasmosis. *Parasitology*, **110**, S11–S16.

Buxton, D., Uggla, A., Lovgren, K., Thomson, K., Lunden, A., Morein, B. & Biwett, D. A. (1989). Trial of a novel experimental *T. gondii* ISCOM vaccine in pregnant sheep. *British Veterinary Journal*, **145**, 451–7,

Buxton, D., Thomson, K., Maley, S., Wright, S. & Bos, H. J. (1991). Vaccination of sheep with a live incomplete strain (S48) of *T. gondii* and their immunity to challenge when pregnant. *Veterinary Record*, **29**, 89–93.

Capron, A. & Dessaint, J. P. (1988). Vaccination against parasitic diseases: some alternative concepts for the determination of protective antigens. *Annals of the Institute Pasteurunologie*, **139**, 109–17.

Cesbron-Delauw, M. F. & Capron, A. (1993). Appendix: tentative list of *T. gondii* genes cloned and characterised thus far. *Research in Immunology*, **144**, 77–9.

Cesbron-Delauw, M. F., Guy, B., Torpier, G. et al. (1989). Molecular characterisation of a 23 kilodalton major antigen secreted by *T. gondi*. *Proceedings of the National Academy of Sciences USA*, **86**, 7537.

Choromanski, L., Freyre, A., Brown, K., Popiel, I. & Shibley, G. (1994). Safety aspects of a vaccine for cats containing a Toxoplasma mutant strain. *Journal of Eukaryotic Microbiology*, **41**, 8S.

Daffos, F., Forestier, F., Capella-Pavlovsky, M., Thulliez, P., Aufrant, C., Valenti, D. & Cox, W. (1987). Prenatal management of 746 pregnancies at risk for congenital toxoplasmosis. *New England Journal of Medicine*, **318**, 271–5.

Dahl, R. J., Woods, W. H. & Johnson, A. M. (1987). Recognition by the human immune system of candidate vaccine epitopes of *T. gondii* measured by a competitive ELISA. *Vaccine*, **5**, 187–91.

Darcy, F., Maes, P., Gras-Masse, H. et al. (1992). Protection of mice and nude rats against toxoplasmosis by a multiple antigenic peptide construction derived from *T. gondii* P30 antigen. *Journal of Immunology*, **149**, 3636–41.

Dubey, J. P. & Frenkel, J. K. (1974). Immunity to feline toxoplasmosis: modification by administration of corticosteroids. *Veterinary Pathology*, 11, 350–79.

Dubey, J. P., Baker, D. G., Davis, S. W. et al. (1994). Persistence of immunity to toxoplasmosis in pigs vaccinated with a nonpersistent strain of *Toxoplasma gondii*. *American Journal of Veterinary Research*, 55, 982–7.

Dubey, J. P. & Frenkel, J. K. (1976). Feline toxoplasmosis from acutely infected mice and the development of Toxoplasma cysts. *Journal of Protozoology*, 23, 537–46.

Dubey, J. P., Urban, J. F. & Davis, S. W. (1991). Protective immunity to toxoplasmosis in pigs vaccinated with a non-persistent strain of *T. gondi*. *American Journal of Veterinary Research*, 52, 1316–19.

Dubremetz, J. F. & Schwartzman, J. D. (1993). Subcellular organelles of *T. gondi* and host cell invasion. *Research in Immunology*, 144, 31.

Elwell, M. R. & Frenkel, J. K. (1984). Immunity to toxoplasmosis in hamsters. *American Journal of Veterinary Research*, 45, 2668.

Foulon, W. (1992). Congenital toxoplasmosis: is screening desirable? *Scandinavian Journal of Infectious Disease, Supplement*, 84, 11–17.

Frenkel, J. K. (1967). Adoptive immunity to intracellular infection. *The Journal of Immunology*, 98, 1309–19.

Frenkel, J. K. (1981). Toxoplasmosis, prevention or palliation? *American Journal of Obstetrics and Gynecology*, 141, 359–61.

Frenkel, J. K. (1989). Tissue-dwelling intracellular parasites: infection and immune responses in the mammalian host to *T. gondii*, *Sarcocystis*, and *Trichinella*. *American Zoologist*, 29, 455–67.

Frenkel, J. K. & Escajadillo, A. (1987). Cyst rupture as a pathogenic mechanism of *T. gondii* encephalitis. *American Journal of Tropical Medicine and Hygiene*, 36, 512–22.

Frenkel, J. K. & Smith, D. D. (1982a). Immunisation of cats against shedding of *T. gondii* oocysts. *Journal of Parasitology*, 68, 744–8.

Frenkel, J. K. & Smith, D. D. (1982b). Inhibitory effects of monensin on shedding of *T. gondii* oocysts by cats. *Journal of Parasitology*, 68, 851–5.

Frenkel, J. K., Dubey, J. P. & Hoff, R. (1976). Loss of stages after continuous passage of *T. gondii* and *Besnoitia jellisoni*. *Journal of Protozoology*, 23, 421–4.

Frenkel, J. K., Pfefferkorn, E. R., Smith, D. D. & Fishback, J. L. (1991). A *T. gondii* vaccine for cats using a new mutant. *American Journal of Veterinary Research*, 52, 759–63.

Freyre, A., Choromanski, L., Fishback, J. L. & Popiel, I. (1993). Immunisation of cats with tissue cysts, bradyzoites, and tachyzoites of the T-263 strain of *T. gondii*. *Journal of Parasitology*, 79, 716–19.

Hakim, F. T., Gazzinelli, R. T., Denkers, E., Hieny, S., Shearer, G. M. & Sher, A. (1991). CD8+ T cells from mice vaccinated against *T. gondii* are cytotoxic for parasite-infected or antigen-pulsed host cells. *Journal of Immunology*, 147, 2310–16

Herion, P., Hernandez-Pando, R., Dubremetz, J. F. & Saavedra, R. (1993). Subcellular localization of the 54 kDa antigen of *T. gondii*. *Journal of Parasitology*, 79, 216–22.

Kasper, L. H. & Khan, I. A. (1993). Role of p30 in host immunity and pathogenesis. *Research in Immunology*, 144, 45–8.

Kasper, L. H., Currie, K. M. & Bradley, M. S. (1985). An unexpected response to vaccination with a purified major membrane tachyzoite antigen (P30) of *T. gondii. Journal of Immunology*, **134**, 3426–31.

Khan, I. A., Smith, K. A. & Kasper, L. H. (1998). Induction of antigen-specific parasiticidal cytotoxic T cell splenocytes by a major membrane protein (P30) of *Toxoplasma gondii. Journal of Immunology*, **141**, 3600–5.

Khan, I. A., Ely, K. H. & Kasper, L. H. (1991). A purified parasite antigen (p30) mediates CD8 + T-cell immunity against fatal *T. gondii* infection in mice. *Journal of Immunology*, **147**, 3501–6.

Krahenbuhl, J. L., Ruskin, J. & Remington, J. S. (1972). The use of killed vaccines in immunisation against an intracellular parasite: *T. gondi. Journal of Immunology*, **108**, 425–31.

Leighty, J. C. (1990). Strategies for control of toxoplasmosis. *Journal of the American Veterinary Association*, **196**, 281–6.

Lindsay, D. S., Blagburn, B. L., Dubey, J. P. & Mason, W. H. (1991). Prevalence and isolation of *T. gondii* from white-tailed deer in Alabama. *Journal of Parasitology*, **77**, 62–4.

Lindsay, D. S., Blagburn, B. & Dubey, J. P. (1993). Safety and results of challenge of weaned pigs given a temperature-sensitive mutant of *T. gondii. Journal of Parasitology*, **79**, 71–6.

Mateus-Pinella, N. E., Dubey, J. P., Choromanski, L. & Weigel, R. (1999). A field trial of the effectiveness of a feline *Toxoplasma gondii* vaccine in reducing *T. gondii* exposure for swine. *Journal of Parasitology*, **85**, 855–60.

McCabe, R. & Remington, J. S. (1987). Toxoplasmosis: the time has come. *New England Journal of Medicine*, **318**, 313–15.

McLeod, R., Frenkel, J. K., Estes, R. G., Mack, D. G., Eisenhauer, P. B. & Giboria, G. (1988). Subcutaneous and intestinal vaccination with tachyzoites of *T. gondii* and acquisition of immunity to per oral and congenital *T. gondii* challenge. *Journal of Immunology*, **140**, 1632–7.

McLeod, R., Skamene, E., Brown, C. R., Eisenhauer, P. B. & Mack, D. G. (1989*b*). Genetic regulation of early survival and cyst number after peroral *T. gondii* infection of AxBIBxA recombinant inbred and B 10 congenic mice. *Journal of Immunology*, **143**, 3031–4.

Mineo, J. R., McLeod, R., Mack, D., Smith, J., Khan, I. A., Ely, K. H. & Kasper, L. H. (1993). Antibodies to *T. gondii* major surface protein (SAG-1, P30) inhibit infection of host cells and are produced in murine intestine after peroral infection. *Journal of Immunology*, **150**, 3951–64.

Overnes, G., Nesse, L. L., Waldeland, H., Lovgren, K. & Gudding, R. (1991). Immune response after immunisation with an experimental *T. gondii* ISCOM vaccine. *Vaccine*, **9**, 25–8.

Pfefferkorn, E. R. & Pfefferkorn, L. C. (1976). Arabinosyl nucleosides inhibit *Toxoplasma gondii* and allow selection of resistant mutants. *Journal of Parasitology*, **62**, 993–99.

Pfefferkorn, E. R. & Pfefferkorn, L. C. (1979). Quantitative studies of the mutagenesis of *T. gondii. Journal of Parasitology*, **65**, 364–70.

Saavedra, R., Meuter, F., de Decourt, J. L. & Herion, P. (1991). Human T-cell clone identifies a potentially protective 54-da protein antigen of *Toxoplasma gondii* cloned and expressed in *Escherichia coli. Journal of Immunology*, **147**, 1975–82.

Sharma, S. D., Hofflim, J. M. & Remington, J. S. (1985). *In vivo* recombinant interleukin 2 administration enhances survival against a lethal challenge with *T. gondi. Journal of Immunology*, **135**, 4160–3.

Sibley, L. D. & Sharma, S. D. (1987). Ultrastructural localization of an intracellular *T. gondii* protein that induces protection in mice. *Infection and Immunity*, **55**, 2137–41.

Sibley, L. D., Pfefferkorn, E. R. & Boothroyd, J. C. (1991). Proposal for a uniform genetic nomenclature in *T. gondii*. *Parasitology Today*, **7**, 327–8.

Sklenar, I., Jones, T. C., Alkan, S. & Erb, P. (1986). Association of symptomatic human infection with *T. gondii* with imbalance of monocytes and antigen-specific T cell subsets. *Journal of Infectious Diseases*, **153**, 315–24.

Stray-Pederson, B. & Jenum, P. (1992) Current status of toxoplasmosis in pregnancy in Norway. *Scandinavian Journal of Infectious Disease, Supplement*, **84**, 80–3.

Suzuki, Y. & Remington, J. S. (1988). Dual regulation of resistance against *T. gondii* infection by Lyt-2+ and Lyt-1+, L3T4+ T cells in mice. *Journal of Immunology*, **140**, 3943–6.

Suzuki, Y., Orellana, M. A., Schreiber, R. D. & Remington, J. S. (1988). Interferon gamma: the major mediator of resistance against *T. gondii*. *Science*, **240**, 516–18.

Thorpe, J. M. Jr., Seeds, J. W., Herbert, W. N. P., Bowes, W. A., Maslow, A. S., Cefalo, R. C., Cheschein, N. & Katz, V. L. (1988). Prenatal management and congenital toxoplasmosis (letter). *New England Journal of Medicine*, **319**, 372–3.

Uggla, A., Araujo, F. G., Lunden, A., Lovgren, K., Remington, J. S. & Morein, B. (1988). Immunizing effects in mice of two *Toxoplasma gondii* iscom preparations. *Zentralblatt Fuer Veterinaermedizin Reihe B*, **35**, 311–14.

Waldeland, H. & Frenkel, J. K. (1983). Live and killed vaccines against toxoplasmosis in mice. *Journal of Parasitology*, **69**, 60–5.

Waldeland, H., Pfefferkorn, E. R. & Frenkel, J. K. (1983). Temperature-sensitive mutants of *T. gondii*: pathogenicity and persistence in mice. *Journal of Parasitology*, **69**, 171–5.

Wilkins, M. F., O'Connell, E. & Te Punga, W. A. (1987). Toxoplasmosis in sheep I: effect of a killed vaccine on lambing losses caused by experimental challenge with *T. gondii*. *New Zealand Veterinary Journal*, **35**, 31–4.

Wilkins, M. F., O'Connell, E. & Te Punga, W. A. (1988a). Toxoplasmosis in sheep II: the ability of a live vaccine to prevent lamb losses after an intravenous challenge with *T. gondii*. *New Zealand Veterinary Journal*, **36**, 14.

Wilkins, M. F., O'Connell, E. & Te Punga, W. A. (1988b). Toxoplasmosis in sheep III: further evaluation of the ability of a live *T. gondii* vaccine to prevent lamb losses and reduce congenital infection following experimental oral challenge. *New Zealand Veterinary Journal*, **36**, 86–9.

Appendices: Protocols for treatment and management

Contents

1. Suggested treatment protocols

1.1. IMMUNOCOMPETENT PATIENTS – ACUTE INFECTION

Treatment is *NOT* usually indicated but if required

Adults	Pyrimethamine	100 mg orally twice daily for 1 day then 25–50 mg orally daily for 2–4 weeks
	plus	
	Sulphadiazine	50–100 mg/kg (up to 8 g) orally daily for 2–4 weeks (divided doses)
	plus	
	Folinic acid (leucovorin)	5–10 mg orally daily for 2–4 weeks
Children	Pyrimethamine	2 mg/kg orally daily for 3–4 days then 1 mg/kg orally daily for 2–4 weeks (divided doses)
	plus	
	Sulphadiazine	100 mg/kg orally daily for 2–4 weeks (divided doses)
	plus	
	Folinic acid (leucovorin)	5–10 mg orally daily for 2–4 weeks

NB. Due to the risk of bone marrow suppression, patients on pyrimethamine should be monitored twice a week if possible for haemoglobin concentration, white blood cell count and platelet count.
See also Chapters 4 and 13.

1.2. IMMUNOCOMPETENT PATIENTS – CHRONIC ACTIVE TOXOPLASMOSIS

As for acute acquired toxoplasmosis in immunocompetent patients.
Suggested alternative treatment:

Adults	Azithromycin	500 mg orally daily for 2–4 weeks

See also Chapters 4 and 13.

1.3. OCULAR TOXOPLASMOSIS

Adults	Clindamycin	300 mg orally three times daily for 3–4 weeks
	? Corticosteroids when macula threatened	
	or	
	Pyrimethamine	100 mg orally twice daily for 1 day then 25–50 mg orally daily for 3–4 weeks
	plus	
	Sulphadiazine	50–100 mg/kg (up to 8 g) orally daily (divided doses) for 3–4 weeks
	plus	
	Folinic acid (leucovorin)	5–10 mg orally daily for 3–4 weeks
	? Corticosteroids when macula threatened	
Children	Pyrimethamine	2 mg/kg orally daily for 3–4 days then 1 mg/kg orally daily for 3–4 weeks
	plus	
	Sulphadiazine	100 mg/kg orally daily for 3–4 weeks (divided doses)
	plus	
	Folinic acid (leucovorin)	5–10 mg orally daily for 3–4 weeks
	? Corticosteroids when macula threatened	
Suggested alternative treatments		
Adult	Azithromycin	500 mg orally daily for 3–4 weeks
	or	
	Atovaquone	750 mg orally four times daily for up to 3 months
	? Corticosteroids when macular threatened	

See also Chapters 11 and 13.

1.4. PREGNANT WOMEN

Spiramycin	1 g orally three times daily when maternal infection is suspected or confirmed and continued for remainder of pregnancy.
	If confirmed foetal infection stop spiramycin and substitute:
Pyrimethamine plus	50 mg orally daily until delivery

Sulphadiazine	1 g orally three times a day until delivery
plus	
Folinic acid (leucovorin)	50 mg orally once weekly until delivery

See also Chapters 7 and 13.

1.5. CONGENITAL INFECTION IN NEONATES/INFANTS

Pyrimethamine	2 mg/kg per day for 2 days then 1 mg/kg orally daily for 6 months then 1 mg/kg orally three times/week for 6 months
Sulphadiazine	100 mg/kg orally daily (divided into two daily doses) for 12 months
Folinic acid (leucovorin)	5 mg orally three times/week (increased to 5–20 mg if neutropaenic) then 10 mg orally at 1 month of age or ≥4.5 kg until 12 months of age
Continue treatment from birth to end of first year of age	
If high CSF protein level or retinitis	Prednisolone 1 mg/kg orally daily until inflammation subsides.

See also Chapters 10 and 13.

1.6. TRANSPLANT PATIENTS

1.6.1. Heart, liver and kidney transplant recipient

Adults	Pyrimethamine	100 mg orally twice daily for 1 day then 25–50 mg daily for 4–6 weeks after resolution of infection
	plus	
	Sulphadiazine	50–100 mg/kg (up to 8 g) orally daily (divided doses) – duration as for pyrimethamine
	plus	
	Folinic acid (leucovorin)	5–10 mg orally – duration as for pyrimethamine
Children	Pyrimethamine	2 mg/kg orally daily for 3–4 days then1 mg/kg orally daily for 4–6 weeks after resolution of infection
	plus	
	Sulphadiazine	100 mg/kg orally daily (divided doses) – duration as for pyrimethamine
	plus	
	Folinic acid (leucovorin)	5–10 mg orally daily – duration as for pyrimethamine

1.6.2. Bone marrow transplant recipient

Possible alternative treatments to be considered

Atovaquone	750 mg (liquid form) orally three times daily
or	
Azithromycin	500 mg orally daily

1.6.3. Prophylaxis in heart and liver transplant patients (adult)

Trimethoprim/Sulphamethoxazole (co-trimoxazole)	480 mg orally twice daily for 6 weeks post transplant
Alternative treatment	
Pyrimethamine	5–10 mg orally daily for 6 weeks post transplant
plus	
Folinic acid (leucovorin)	5–10 mg orally daily – duration as for pyrimethamine

See also Chapters 6 and 13.

1.7. PATIENTS WITH MALIGNANCIES

Pyrimethamine	100 mg orally twice daily for 1 day then 25–50 mg orally daily for 3–4 weeks or until symptoms resolve
plus	
Sulphadiazine	50–100 mg/kg (up to 8 g) orally daily (divided doses) for 3–4 weeks or until symptoms resolve
plus	
Folinic acid (leucovorin)	5–10 mg orally daily for 3–4 weeks or until symptoms resolve

NB. Haematological monitoring should be considered due to the risk of bone marrow suppression.

See also Chapters 6 and 13.

1.8. PATIENTS WITH HIV/AIDS

1.8.1. Acute toxoplasma infection and/or toxoplasmic encephalitis in AIDS patients

Pyrimethamine	100 mg orally twice daily for 1 day then 50–75 mg once daily for 3–6 weeks
plus	
Sulphadiazine*	100 mg/kg (up to 8 g) orally daily (divided doses) for 3–6 weeks
plus	
Folinic acid (leucovorin)	10–20 mg orally once daily for 3–6 weeks
*Substitute clindamycin	600 mg (orally/i.v.) four times daily for 3–6 weeks

1.8.2. Alternative/experimental regimens for toxoplasmic encephalitis

Pyrimethamine plus	as above
Azithromycin or	1250–1500 mg orally once daily for 3–6 weeks
Pyrimethamine plus	as above
Clarithromycin or	1000 mg orally twice daily for 3–6 weeks
Pyrimethamine plus	as above
Atovaquone or	1500 mg orally twice daily for 3–6 weeks
Trimethoprim–sulphamethoxazole	(co-trimoxazole) Trimethoprim 5–10 mg/kg, sulphamethoxazole 25–50 mg/kg orally/i.v. four times daily for 3–6 weeks
plus	
Folinic acid (leucovorin)	10–20 mg orally once daily for 3–6 weeks

See also Chapters 5 and 13.

1.8.3. Maintenance/suppressive therapy for toxoplasmic encephalitis

Pyrimethamine plus	25–50 mg orally once daily
Sulphadiazine* plus	500–1000 mg orally four times daily
Folinic acid (leucovorin)	10–20 mg orally once daily
* Substitute clindamycin	300 mg orally four times daily

See also Chapters 5 and 13.

1.8.4. Primary prophylaxis for toxoplasmic encephalitis

Trimethoprim–suphamethoxazole (co-trimoxazole)	One double-strength* tablet orally daily or two double-strength tablets orally twice weekly *double-strength tablet contains trimethoprim 160 mg and sulphamethoxazole 800 mg
Alternative suggested treatments	
Pyrimethamine plus	50 mg orally once weekly
Dapsone plus	50 mg orally once daily

Folinic acid (leucovorin) or	10–15 mg orally given with pyrimethamine
Pyrimethamine plus	25 mg orally twice weekly
Dapsone plus	100 mg orally twice weekly
Folinic acid (leucovorin) or	10–15 mg orally given twice weekly with pyrimethamine
Pyrimethamine plus	50 mg orally once daily
Folinic acid (leucovorin) or	50 mg orally twice weekly
Pyrimethamine plus	100 mg loading dose orally, then 50 mg orally three times weekly
Folinic acid (leucovorin)	15 mg orally three times weekly

See also Chapters 5 and 13.

2. Management of toxoplasma infection in pregnancy

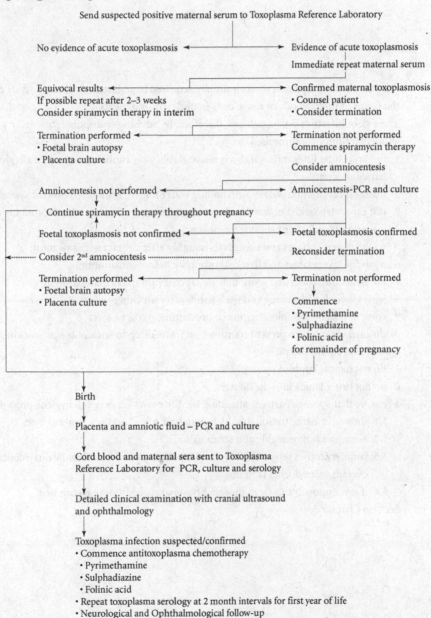

Send suspected positive maternal serum to Toxoplasma Reference Laboratory

No evidence of acute toxoplasmosis ←——→ Evidence of acute toxoplasmosis

Immediate repeat maternal serum

Equivocal results ←——→ Confirmed maternal toxoplasmosis
If possible repeat after 2–3 weeks · Counsel patient
Consider spiramycin therapy in interim · Consider termination

Termination performed ←——→ Termination not performed
· Foetal brain autopsy Commence spiramycin therapy
· Placenta culture
Consider amniocentesis

Amniocentesis not performed ←——→ Amniocentesis-PCR and culture

Continue spiramycin therapy throughout pregnancy

Foetal toxoplasmosis not confirmed ←——→ Foetal toxoplasmosis confirmed

Reconsider termination

Consider 2ⁿᵈ amniocentesis

Termination performed ←——→ Termination not performed
· Foetal brain autopsy
· Placenta culture Commence
· Pyrimethamine
· Sulphadiazine
· Folinic acid
for remainder of pregnancy

Birth

Placenta and amniotic fluid – PCR and culture

Cord blood and maternal sera sent to Toxoplasma
Reference Laboratory for PCR, culture and serology

Detailed clinical examination with cranial ultrasound
and ophthalmology

Toxoplasma infection suspected/confirmed
· Commence antitoxoplasma chemotherapy
 · Pyrimethamine
 · Sulphadiazine
 · Folinic acid
· Repeat toxoplasma serology at 2 month intervals for first year of life
· Neurological and Ophthalmological follow-up

See also Chapter 7.

3. Hygiene measures to prevent infection

Infection with *Toxoplasma gondii* is usually acquired by ingestion of either oocysts excreted in the faeces of infected cats or tissue cysts in undercooked meats.

The risk of infection can be reduced, therefore, by advising susceptible patients (e.g. pregnant women, immunocompromised) to:

1 not empty cat litter trays – if this is unavoidable wear rubber gloves and wash gloves and hands afterwards;
2 disinfect cat litter trays daily with boiling water for five minutes to prevent sporulation;
3 not eat undercooked or raw cured meat, only eat meat that has been thoroughly cooked;
4 wash hands well after handling raw meat;
5 wash kitchen surfaces and utensils thoroughly after contact with raw meat;
6 wash fruit, vegetables and lettuce thoroughly before consumption;
7 not drink unpasteurized goats' milk or eat dairy products made from it;
8 wear gloves for gardening and wash hands after touching soil;
9 cover children's sandpits after use so preventing access to cats.

Additional measures to prevent transmission from sheep to susceptible patients in an agricultural environment:

1 do not handle lambing ewes;
2 do not bring lambs into the house;
3 ensure that spouses/partners attending lambing ewes observe full hygiene procedures:
    3.1 shower or bathe thoroughly, including hair, after handling lambing ewes;
    3.2 wash hands thoroughly and scrub nails;
    3.3 launder clothes separately. Susceptible patients should not handle dirty/contaminated overalls worn during lambing;
    3.4 if it is impossible to clean thoroughly, separate bedrooms are advised.

See also Chapter 3.

4. Classification system and case definitions of *Toxoplasma gondii* infection in immunocompetent pregnant women and their congenitally infected offspring

Patient group	Category of infection	Case definition
1. Primary maternal infection during pregnancy	1.1. Definite	1.1.1. Seroconversion – both samples taken after conception[a]
		1.1.2. Positive culture from maternal blood[b]
	1.2. Probable	1.2.1. Seroconversion – first sample taken within 2 months of conception
		1.2.2. Significant rise of IgG titres, and presence of IgM and/or IgA[c]
		1.2.3. High IgG titres, presence of IgM and/or IgA and onset of lymphadenopathy during pregnancy[c]
		1.2.4. High IgG titres and presence of IgM and/or IgA in second half of pregnancy[c]
	1.3. Possible	1.3.1. Stable high IgG, without IgM, in second half of pregnancy[c]
		1.3.2. High IgG and presence of IgM and/or IgA in first half of pregnancy[c]
	1.4. Unlikely	1.4.1. Stable low IgG, with or without IgM[c]
		1.4.2. Stable high IgG, without IgM, in early pregnancy[c]
	1.5. Not infected	1.5.1. Seronegative (during pregnancy)
		1.5.2. Maternal preconception seropositive sample
		1.5.3. Positive IgM and/or IgA without appearance of IgG[c]
2. Foetal infection	2.1 Definite	2.1.1. Positive culture from foetal tissue, foetal blood, or amniotic fluid[d]
		2.1.2. Histopathological demonstration of parasites in foetal tissue

Patient group	Category of infection	Case definition
		2.1.3. Demonstration of toxoplasma DNA in amniotic fluid or in foetal blood or foetal tissue
	2.2. Probable	2.2.1. Positive IgM and/or IgA in foetal blood
		2.2.2. Persistent ultrasound findings and definite or probable primary maternal infection during pregnancy[e,f]
	2.3. Possible	2.3.1. Persistent ultrasound findings and possible primary maternal infection during pregnancy[e,f]
		2.3.2. No positive foetal findings, but definite primary maternal infection during pregnancy[f]
	2.4. Unlikely	2.4.1. No positive foetal findings, but possible primary maternal infection during pregnancy[f]
	2.5. Not infected	2.5.1. Seronegative mother
		2.5.2. Positive IgM and/or IgA in mother without appearance of IgG[c]
		2.5.3. Maternal preconception seropositive sample
3. Congenital infection in infants	3.1. Definite	3.1.1. Positive culture from cord blood or body tissues obtained within the first 6 months of life[g]
		3.1.2. Confirmed histopathological demonstration of parasites in body tissues obtained within the first 6 months of life[g]
		3.1.3. Rise in IgG titres within the first 12 months of life, with or without clinical signs of the classic triad
		3.1.4. Persistently positive IgG beyond the first 12 months of life, with or without clinical signs of the classic triad[h,i]
		3.1.5. Positive IgM within the first 6 months of life[i,j]
		3.1.6. Positive IgA within the first 6 months of life [k]
	3.2. Probable	3.2.1. Positive culture from placental tissue
		3.2.2. IgM positive between 6 and 12 months, but no previous serological test results for comparison

Patient group	Category of infection	Case definition
		3.2.3. Retinochorioditis and/or hydrocephalus/cerebral calcification and definite primary maternal infection during pregnancy, no other results available[l]
	3.3. Possible	3.3.1. Retinochoroiditis and/or hydrocephalus/cerebral calcification, but no infant serological tests or knowledge of maternal infection[l]
		3.3.2. One of the clinical signs of the triad present, positive IgG, but no knowledge of maternal infection
	3.4. Unlikely	3.4.1. Continuous decline in IgG titre without IgM and/or IgA, with or without clinical signs up to the first 6 months of life, without treatment
	3.5. Not infected	3.5.1. Seronegative within the first 12 months of life, without treatment[m]
		3.5.2. Seronegative 6 months after finishing treatment
4. Individuals over 1 year of age (for whom no information is available for the first year of life	4.1. Definite	4.1.1. Not applicable
	4.2. Probable	4.2.1. Typical retinochoroiditis and IgG-positive patient, definite primary maternal infection during pregnancy
		4.2.2. Typical retinochorioditis with hydrocephalus and/or cerebral calcification[l]
	4.3. Possible	4.3.1. Typical retinochorioditis and IgG-positive patient, maternal IgG positive or unknown[l]
	4.4. Unlikely	4.4.1. Not applicable
	4.5. Not infected	4.5.1. Seronegative offspring
		4.5.2. Seronegative mother
		4.5.3. Maternal seropositive sample preconception

[a]Should be confirmed by third sample.
[b]Culture includes both tissue culture and mouse inoculation.
[c]At least two samples taken 3 weeks apart during pregnancy.
[d]Risk of contamination by maternal blood reduces diagnostic value.
[e]Ventricular dilation and/or echogenic intracerebral lesions.
[f]If ultrasound alone is performed, classification is not possible.

[g]Primary infection of infants up to 6 months of age considered very unlikely.

[h]IgG titres may be modified by treatment.

[i]Ideally, infants should be tested monthly.

[j]Excluding samples within the first 2 days of life.

[k]Excluding samples in the first 10 days of life.

[l]Retinochoroiditis should be confirmed by an ophthalmologist.

[m]Very rarely, trace levels of IgG may be found for a few more months.

General note: ideally tests should be confirmed by another method or by another laboratory. It is the responsibility of the laboratory performing the test to define high and low IgG titres, but a titre equal to or greater than 200 IU is generally considered high. Specific antitoxoplasma chemotherapy may modify a rise in IgG titres.

(with permission) Lebech, M., Joynson, D. H. M., Seitz, H. M., Thulliez, P. et al (1996). *European Journal of Clinical Microbiology and Infectious Diseases*, **15**, 799–805.

Index